Analysing Interactions in Childhood

Analysing Interactions in Childhood

Insights from Conversation Analysis

Hilary Gardner PhD
Lecturer and Speech and Language Therapist
Department of Human Communication Sciences, Sheffield University

Michael Forrester PhD
Senior Lecturer
School of Psychology, University of Kent

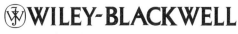

A John Wiley & Sons, Ltd., Publication

Library of Congress Cataloging-in-Publication Data

Analysing interactions in childhood: insights from conversation analysis / [edited by] Hilary Gardner, Michael Forrester.
    p. cm.
  Includes bibliographical references and index.
  ISBN 978-0-470-76034-5 (pbk.)
  1. Conversation analysis.   2. Childhood.   I. Gardner, Hilary.   II. Forrester, Michael A.
  P95.45.A48 2010
  302.3'46–dc22

                                                                      2009028755

A catalogue record for this book is available from the British Library.

Set in 10/12.5pt Sabon by Graphicraft Limited, Hong Kong
Printed and bound in Singapore by Fabulous Printers Pte Ltd

1 2010

Contents

Foreword

Conversation analysis (CA), as amply demonstrated in the chapters of this book, has much to contribute to the study of children and their interactions. Children are in the process of emerging membership in society as well as of developmental change. They can be, from early on, full partners in communicative interchanges but with developing possibilities of how such participation can be carried out. Thus there is an interesting explanatory tension between the more totalising concepts of 'traditional' developmental psychology – 'child', 'adult', 'competence' and 'context', for instance – and the detailed analyses of CA, with its emphasis on the moment-to-moment search for intersubjective understanding. Reading the chapters of this book led me to a number of insights about the possibilities for a fruitful interchange.

First, conversation analyses can provide a corrective to a mundane developmental account that concentrates on just saying what a child cannot do at one particular age and can do at a later stage. Many of the analyses presented here suggest that when talk between children and their interactants is examined in detail, very young children can and do show an ability to identify misunderstandings on the part of the other, and to correct them in speech. Since it is increasingly apparent that preverbal infants show a range of intersubjective skills, CA may well help us to work out how these are mapped into language and used in talk. Undoubtedly 'mapping' is the wrong analogy because whatever it is that children know about other minds before starting to speak, they have to learn how language works in usage. As is shown by the analyses on misunderstanding and on the work done by both the child and others on repair, this is not a straightforward matter. These analyses could contribute a great deal to our understanding of the child's developing control of language 'in use' and, therefore, to a much more complete account of language development.

Second, many of these chapters are relevant to the question of children's 'membership' of societal contexts and their 'membership rights', defined both externally and in the moment-to-moment exchanges of conversation. These analyses show the affordances that can be provided to children by their interactants and how this can vary from moment to moment. They also show how children can accept, reject or resist conversational moves by others to constitute them in a particular membership category. This is particularly important for those working with children in professional contexts and the chapters in the latter part of the book analyse these types of interactions and are extremely revealing on this score. I think professionals working in these contexts will find them interesting and useful when reflecting on their own practices and how they might want to adjust or change them.

My hope is that we will be able to find a way (1) to put together the types of analyses laid out in the chapters of the book with the more traditional concerns of developmental psychology and linguistics, and (2) to take the insights of CA and use them to inform the theoretical question of the factors influencing children's development generally and their increasingly sophisticated grasp of language and its uses in particular. To do this will require those involved in CA to be prepared to compare across situations and individuals – almost inevitably involving some quantitative analysis – and for the insights that arise from CA to be seriously integrated with other theoretical frameworks. This book provides an excellent basis for the latter aim.

Elena Lieven

Max Planck Institute for Evolutionary Anthropology, Leipzig and University of Manchester

Introduction

HILARY GARDNER and MICHAEL FORRESTER

The aim of this volume is to bring together contributors who are not only leading researchers in the rapidly developing field of conversation analysis (CA) but who also focus on aspects of childhood interactions. Traditionally, CA has been mainly concerned with everyday adult talk in order to establish the rules and regularities that ease the path of such mundane interactions. In all CA work, there is a preoccupation with turn-by-turn sequential properties of talk that goes beyond taxonomic categorisation of individual utterances. No detail of form, magnitude or timing, in gesture, talk, gaze or sequential placement, is seen as irrelevant to the interaction. Conversation analysts view talk as situated action: acknowledging, describing and examining conversational structures and conventions, in the same way that, more traditionally, linguists structure phonology, morphology and syntax. Schegloff (1987) used the phrase 'talk in interaction' and details 'syntax for conversation' (see Schegloff 2007) showing that idealised linguistic rules and grammatical 'correctness' are less necessary to meaningful interactions than might be supposed. For a full exposition of the theory of CA there are several publications that can be recommended such as Schegloff (2007) or Hutchby and Wooffit (2008).

The focus in this collection on children's interactions is partly motivated by a key issue for conversation analysis, that of intersubjectivity, which is taken here to be the constant production, recognition and display of mutual 'understandings' between speakers during conversation. This is not dissimilar to those in child development who have emphasised the significance of interactional synchrony for intersubjective relations in early childhood. Some writers in child CA have also emphasised the importance of intersubjectivity for early development (Hutchby and Moran-Ellis 1998) yet with a particular focus on the sequential detail of interaction on a turn-by-turn basis. Needless to say, understanding the emergence of children's communicative skills and abilities will be closely linked to whatever we take to be the essential attributes of engaging in intersubjective relations. In conversation analysis the primary mechanism for the maintenance of intersubjectivity is the organisation of repair – a view shared by various contributors to this volume.

In interaction, participants seek to establish intersubjectivity and make explicit displays of their understanding of cultural and language phenomenon through talk. In seeking to understand how children gradually learn what is involved in recognising and maintaining intersubjectivity as part and parcel of the infrastructure of interaction, conversation analysts set aside the complex issues surrounding cognitive and emotional dimensions that might bear on a complete developmental explanation and focus instead on highlighting the fine detail of the local discursive context. Wootton (1997), for example, has commented that it is from learning how to utilise mutual understandings and 'interpersonal alignments' that the child's cultural awareness is fashioned.

Given the recognition that the moulding of intersubjectivity is interdependently related to whatever self-righting mechanisms are in play in the localised sequence of interaction, it comes as no surprise that procedures surrounding repair practices in child conversation are of particular interest to the researchers in this volume. Whether initiated by adult or child, the numerous ways in which adjustments, reformulations, clarifications and whatever serve as repair is a theme that permeates many of the chapters. The repair may be self-initiated or initiated by the recipient ('other initiated'); for instance, instigated by the adult in order to make his or her meaning more transparent to the child, or to help the young conversational partner to correct its own misunderstood utterance. These repairs may be overtly marked or embedded in the talk. The child itself may seek clarification from the adult or recognise particular inefficiencies in its own talk and seek to self-repair. The area in which CA can complement other psychological and linguistic research traditions that examine repair practices, is in the central place given to the interdependence between the production and recognition of trouble sources and repair. Where, when and how the utilisation of repair changes over the long and short term (and not necessarily with reference to a developmental focus) is illustrated in several contexts throughout this volume.

Significant, then, for understanding the isues that shape the child's emerging linguistic skills is the orientation that children, and those with whom they interact, have towards the production and recognition of mutual understandings. This social constructivist view of development brings into focus the subtle changes in association produced by the child, which are often shown to be highly sensitive to the communicative sequence in which they occur. Systems of repair, as outlined above, which deal with troubles in talk, contribute to this change; however, how such repair organisation operates is not dependent solely on lexicalisation. Conversation analysis pays equal attention to embodiment of meaning through action, gesture, timing, emphasis and the use of physical context. The finest detail of change in terms of timing, phonetic output, intonational change and the sequential positioning of utterances are all of potential significance, reflected here in the different considerations the contributors highlight in the volume.

As can be seen from some of the discussions already extant in this introduction, CA research on children's interactions is not solely concerned with development in the traditional sense and, indeed, draws attention to problems associated with the assumption that behavioural change is necessarily developmentally significant (see Forrester, this volume). Instead, CA looks at how the child begins to engage with the world through talk and other interactional modalities. Wootton (1997), in his seminal work *Interaction and the Development of Mind*, talks of the acculturation of the child through emerging intersubjective understandings that are locally derived – that is, pertaining to very recent cultural and moral events. Certainly, CA studies with a child focus are unique, as those skills and abilities that might be central to the display of such understandings, and how they could develop, must be mapped out precisely, which necessitates a close examination of the fine detail of children's early interactions – both with adults and with each other.

CA adopts the view that in order to become fully fledged 'members' of a culture, children have to learn how to recognise and produce talk that displays to others around them their understanding of 'talk' as an accountable set of social practices. Displays of asymmetry in knowledge, power and understanding between conversational partners, as children gradually attain membership, is inherent in this view of talk in interaction. This theme is developed, for example, by Forrester (Chapter 3) with a very young child in the home; by Hutchby (Chapter 8) with adult–child counselling data; and by Sidnell (Chapter 6), where the context is that of child–child interaction outside the home. Clarke and Wilkinson in Section 3 also find that issues of acceptance arise in their analysis of interactions between children with cerebral palsy. Membership can be seen to be of clear significance to the participants in talk across the span of childhood experiences.

Many of the broader theoretical and methodological preoccupations of conversation analysts, working with any type of data, are reflected in the contributions to this volume. One such preoccupation is that of the relevance of notions such as a preset context or identity. Conversation analysts are somewhat cautious regarding the relevance, use and value of definitive category formulations such as child, adult, typical or ayptical development, family or gender status. The ethnomethodological background of CA requires the focus to be participant-oriented where possible, and thus CA often seeks to unpick the displayed orientations of the speakers and show how these are constituted within the interactional sequence. In the Foreword to *Applying Conversation Analysis* (Richards and Seedhouse 2005), Paul Drew draws attention to the potential power of the convergence of applied linguistics and CA as research methodologies. He exposes inherent presuppositions by comparing two different bodies of data distinguished by labels such as 'classroom' versus 'ordinary' talk – something that has been common practice in applied linguistics but may be dealt with differently in CA. In CA the detail of the analysis should indicate how the participants are orienting to the terms of those differentials in aspects of turns at talk. This ethos is developed within the research writings in this book and certain contrastive phenomena in child–adult talk may become obvious across bodies of data, regardless of the specific labels they reference. This editorial draws attention to some of those common themes.

One of the subdivisions imposed in creating the three sections of this book concerns the investigation into more stylised forms of talk – for example, those employed in professional and other institutional settings. CA has shown how much an institution's ethos and practice may be enacted through talk and, therefore, has proved to be an appealing methodology in applied research. The point at which institutional talk impinges on children's lives will be an issue for this volume and will encompass aspects of membership, asymmetry in relationships, and displays of the acquisition of cultural (and other) knowledge. To return to the idea of 'context' here is to return to a crucial theme in CA. Context is not simply a physical phenomenon but is continuously created and shaped, renewed or changed by each turn in the talk itself. And so an interaction that constitutes a medical consultation or therapy is recognisable as such whether it occurs within a child's home or within a clinical setting. The child's identity also may change as seen by the participants' orientation, turn by turn, from 'patient' to 'child' to 'expert' on his or her own illness.

We will now consider the thematic aspects of the three sections in this book, not just how they cohere but also with an eye to how issues are carried through various chapters across the subdivisions.

Section 1: Interactions between typically developing children and their main carers

The first and longest section is concerned with typically developing children, that is, those not labelled as having any form of developmental disability and engaged in everyday talk with their primary caregivers within the home. The subject matter in these chapters is certainly that of the development of conversational skills and the role of the adult in inculcating the child into appropriate social and linguistic practices. Local sequential issues are always inextricably linked to wider issues of the child's emerging membership within society, as outlined above. Focus is on the complex and meaningful layering of talk with gaze, gesture and other resources, not just because of the child's rudimentary and emerging linguistic skills but because these skills are very much part of the communicative framework at any age. The section starts with the inclusion of a hitherto unpublished article that must be viewed as a substantial piece of early childhood CA – a tribute to the late Dr Clare Tarplee, who died suddenly in 1999 just as she was establishing her postdoctoral research career. It addresses the inherent difficulties of using global categories to describe mechanisms of language development in mother–child talk such as 'feedback', imported from the field of learnability and the theoretical modelling of mental processes. Instead, by looking in fine detail at displays of intersubjective understandings, on a turn by turn basis, it shows the child's sensitivity to sequential implicature. The attention to phonetic detail is a marked feature of this chapter and raises interesting questions about the notion of a recognised word or words in child utterances and what constitutes repair.

The work of Corrin (Chapter 2), looking at children of a similar stage of linguistic development to Tarplee, also displays clearly how CA can inform important questions in child language research through microanalysis. Seemingly insignificant and over-looked types of repair are identified as key opportunities to learn about the crucial placement of talk in the context of other moves and, on a broader basis, display the mother as affording apprenticeships in the organisation of social practices central to pragmatic development. The works of Corrin (Chapter 2) and Laakso (Chapter 5) both question the rubric that children's self-initiated self repair might emerge out of earlier social practices where adults routinely draw the child's attention to an error. It would seem that this is not inherently the case, but that self-initiated repair comes very early in communicative, protoverbal development, on a par with the former. Both authors focus on instances where there are different orientations during play activity on the part of adult and child and repair may seek to establish a joint focus. In Laakso's Finnish data the issue of cross-cultural relevance is raised. It would appear that Finnish parents may have a propensity to other-correct very young children, rather than other-initiate a repair by the child, as has been found in similar data from the UK. Repair is revealed as a dynamic system as the child progresses linguistically and in age.

Tony Wootton's work on a young child's use of 'actually' (Chapter 4) is a very subtle analysis of what might be considered to be a relatively rare and somewhat dispensible word in a child's vocabulary. Through highlighting the general features of use, and the enactments of departures from such use, we are shown precisely the insights that a developmental focused conversation analysis can bring. The child's use of 'actually', when looked at very carefully, suggests a line of developmental enquiry well beyond the use of the particular word. The fact that this word is used heavily over a short period of time and then falls away is an interesting exemplar of a child's active engagement with the processes of word learning and developing usage.

Forrester (Chapter 3) overtly addresses theoretical issues in ethnomethodologically informed CA and its relationship to child developmental research. This major debate is exemplified by a child's display of orientation to her own 'half–membership' in society through her interactions with an adult family member, and raises questions about the implicit or explicit benchmarks of cultural competence. The theme of membership is revisited in several chapters later in the book.

Section 2: Childhood interactions in a wider social world

As children grow they are likely to enter into, or be party to, interactions in a wider range of contexts outside the home, including those that are institutional in nature. Here their entry into society and their place within it is marked by a power ratio of the expert and the less expert (which also occurs between adults but the power relation may be exacerbated by the very status of being a child). Children may need to acquire adaptive interactional skills to accommodate the particular rules and practices of types of institutional talk. Alternatively, as in some instances in this volume, they may resist full cooperation with the institutional morés advanced by the adult (see Hutchby, Chapter 8). One can contrast the relaxed and embedded nature of learning at home as compared to the more direct didacticism of the school setting. There may be some commonalities despite the contextual differences, especially in the construction of repair, which has at its heart the notion of instruction. In Pike's work (Chapter 9), involving a child and teacher engaged in a mathematical problem, the development of teacher scaffolding of child learning is analysed in fine detail. In repair the adult's dispreference for other-repair/correction is extant, yet it is shown through the analysis that this dispreference can be self-defeating – and even outside the conscious awareness of both participants involved. Demonstrating an orientation to intersubjective understanding in context is shown to be more complex than often suspected. The theme of teacher–child talk is explored further in Section 3 of this book. The analysis details the tensions inherent in the finely honed interplay between learning aimed at a greater goal, such as maths or language structure, and learning how to interact successfully in the local context. The theme of learning at home and in a more controlled setting is taken up again in the final section of the book where Tykkyläinen (Chapter 12) compares clinical data to that of mother–child interaction.

How far children are involved in, or have control of, discussion of their own lives and needs is illustrated by both Cahill's analysis of triadic GP consultations regarding a child's health (Chapter 7) and Hutchby's work on counselling data (Chapter 8). Despite the move in health psychology towards more open and informed doctor–patient interaction, Cahill's work highlights the very rare and constrained nature of doctor–child interaction, even when potentially supportive adults (parents) are in attendance. This chapter arises from research directed towards enhancing communication in professional settings and indicates how doctors could facilitate child participation through the use of address terms and other interactional resources.

Hutchby (Chapter 8) engages with child counselling data and contributes to a theme taken up by both Forrester (Chapter 3) in mundane talk and Sidnell (see below): that is, the significance of 'half-membership' rights and how children produce talk such that it displays an orientation to conventions of adult–child membership categories. The difficulties and challenges that children face when interacting in contexts/circumstances in which other social conventions predominate are highlighted. Also discussed are the subtleties involved in inviting a child's participation in such contexts, and the extent to which 'feelings talk/therapeutic vision' is something that children may have no recognition of, or indeed have resistance towards.

The theme of children's displays of membership categories is discussed further in the work of Sidnell in Section 2 of this volume (Chapter 6). The data arises from a preschool setting and stands out from the other chapters in this section as it concerns children talking together with no adult involvement. He shows that children of different ages may have different interactional concerns and, like Forrester in Chapter 3, urges caution with regard to the explanatory value of developmental stages. Sidnell reminds us of the dangers of developmental 'hegemony', in the sense of explaining away change over time, which may simply be appealing to a general or grander-scale developmental theory. Other concurrent concerns need to be unpicked – in particular how children's skills can be constrained by their own overemphasis on assumed shared knowledge with their conversational partners.

Section 3: Interactions with children who are atypical

The final section of the book comprises a set of chapters looking at interaction with children who are regarded as being 'atypical' in that they face challenges to the enactment of what are considered typical communicative processes. The children are variously those with cerebral palsy, autistic spectrum disorder, the deaf and those with specific speech and language difficulties. It cannot be presumed that a developmental 'lag' in communication is present and the authors explore issues of different and adaptive practices, rather than those concerning delay. There is evidence that interactional participants may not orient to disability or difference at all, at least in the terms set out in the wider society. The same issues, such as those of intersubjectivity and membership in their societal context, are seen to be have a form of orientation. Certainly a deficit model is routinely eschewed in favour of revealing interactional competencies hitherto overlooked. The role of professional adults, such as teachers and therapists, in supporting language and other learning is presented alongside work on more mundane interactions with peers and parents. How much CA should be used to describe professional interactions with a view to evaluating and subsequently enhancing practice and intervention is a current issue for researchers of institutional talk. Certainly the samples given here are exemplars of the value in teasing out skills and strategies that might otherwise remain implicit and embedded in talk that is obviously aimed at more global targets.

The last chapter in this section (Chapter 13 by Clarke and Wilkinson), is a good example of the problematic contrast of difference with disability, where children with cerebral palsy are using electronic communication aids. This chapter stands out as an example of children just being themselves rather than being engaged in an overt learning process. The subtle nature of the communication that takes place between children with speech and those using an alternative means of communication, demonstrates how CA studies of children in different contexts can highlight the 'doing being ordinary' of every-day interaction for them. In many ways the concerns of these children talking together are very much the same as those in Sidnell's chapter (Chapter 6), that is, concerns about belonging and acceptance with peers. For CA itself, the use of 'alternative', electronic communication challenges contemporary CA conventions such as those regarding the 'transition relevant pause' or 'turn constructional unit'. This chapter also reminds us (as does the chapter by Radford and Mahon) of the care we need to exercise when defining a 'turn at talk'.

Radford and Mahon (Chapter 11) examine gaze and gesture in classroom interactions between children with language learning needs (deaf children and children with specific language difficulties) and their teachers. The authors' detailed analysis raises questions about the exact nature of a 'turn' in adult–child interactions (particularly in this context) and introduces the notion of a 'shared' turn. What constitutes an overlap is subtle and not immediately recognisable as such, when the adult may orient to gesture in overlap as a non-competitive turn-getting move. While the emphasis of the learning experience might be directed to symbolic language, there is clear attention to the relevance of multimodal communicative practices and their contribution to turn construction. The analysis addresses the multilayered nature of adult–child interaction and thus questions such notions as 'joint attention' and similar assumptions underpinning more typical adult–child interaction, picking up on issues discussed in earlier chapters.

The deliberate exploitation of multimodal resources by professionals in didactic contexts is revisited in the two remaining chapters: Tykkyläinen (Chapter 12), looking at speech and language therapy; and Stribling and Rae (Chapter 10), looking at complex teaching interactions.

Stribling and Rae look at social practices inherent in establishing intersubjectivity and scaffolding of (learning) with a child who has severe disabilities in a classroom context. The role of the support participant and the sequential consequences of 'triadic' autistic child/support person and teacher interaction are explored in fine detail and reveal the organisational subtlety and crucial timing of recipient sensitive management of learning support. The authors point out that, however much the child might be learning about elementary principles of mathematical subtraction, she is equally learning about participation frameworks that can contribute to her learning.

Tykkylainen, like Cahill, suggests that findings from CA can be used to enhance professional practice: a direct comparison of repair between typical children playing with their mothers and children with SLI (Specific Language Impairment) undertaking tasks in speech and language therapy. The author looks at possible institutional differences in the setting up of learning situations and the differences that are inherent due to the nature of the child's difficulties. While both sets of children, typical and atypical, made repair initiations only rarely, there were qualitative differences in the ways the language-impaired children sought repair in this institutional setting. The work focuses on the adult use of multimodal resources in support of the child achieving success with linguistic targets. The child with SLI is additionally shown to be sensitive to multimodal cues and to work hard at maintaining intersubjectivity in extended repair sequences.

It is hoped that this volume will further the appreciation of fine detailed analysis as a mechanism for understanding the nature of human communication and its development. The impact of CA as a discipline can only be enhanced by methodological expansion into the developmental and applied areas. To a great extent children can be viewed simply as people interacting, in search of the same or similar outcomes to adults. It is interesting therefore, as analysts, to consider what rules of talk, established through analysis of adult mundane talk, are relevant to children or how, why and within what particular contexts do children learn the skills necessary to engage fully in conversational contexts. By questioning assumptions inherent in macrolevel quantitative and qualitative research, CA has already opened the way to new interdisciplinary collaborations. Certainly we take the view that CA–child research can supplement and enlarge our understanding of children's behaviour. Hopefully, future developments and collaborations can continue to flourish in the light of new understandings brought about by CA.

Acknowledgements

With grateful thanks to ESRC Grant RES-451-26-0138, which funded the seminar series from which the impetus for this volume arose. Thank you, also, to all the attendees whose stimulating discussion helped us to further the project.

References

Drew, P. (2005) Foreword. In K. Richards and P. Seedhouse (eds), *Applying conversation analysis*. Hampshire: Palgrave Macmillan.

Hutchby, I. and Moran-Ellis, J. (1998) *Children and social competence*. London: Falmer.

Hutchby, I. and Wooffitt, R. (2008) *Conversation analysis* (2nd edition). Cambridge: Polity.

Schegloff, E.A. (1979) The relevance of repair to syntax-for-conversation. In T. Givon (ed.), *Syntax and semantics, Vol. XII: Discourse and syntax* (pp. 75–119). New York: Free Press.

Schegloff, E.A. (1987) Between macro and micro: Contexts and other connections. In J. Alexander, B. Giesen, R. Munch and N. Smelser (eds), *The micro-macro link* (pp. 207–234). Berkeley and Los Angeles: University of California Press.

Schegloff, E.A. (2007) *Sequence organisation in interaction: A primer in conversation analysis I*. Cambridge: Cambridge University Press.

Wootton, A.J.W. (1997) *Interaction and development of mind*. Cambridge: Cambridge University Press.

Contributors

Patricia Cahill, MRCGP
General Practitioner Researcher
University of East Anglia
Ipswich, Suffolk
UK

Michael Clarke, PhD
Lecturer
Psychology and Language Sciences
University College London (UCL)
Chandler House
London
UK

Juliette Corrin, PhD
Hon Research Fellow and Speech
    and Language Therapist
Psychology and Language Sciences
University College London (UCL)
Chandler House
London
UK

Michael Forrester, PhD
Senior Lecturer
School of Psychology
Keynes College
University of Kent
Canterbury, Kent
UK

Hilary Gardner, PhD
Lecturer and Speech and
    Language Therapist
Department of Human
    Communication Sciences
Sheffield University
Sheffield
UK

Ian Hutchby, PhD
Professor of Sociology
Department of Sociology
University of Leicester
Leicester
UK

Minna Laakso, PhD
Senior Lecturer and Docent
Department of Speech Sciences
University of Helsinki
Helsinki
Finland

Merle Mahon, PhD
Senior Lecturer
Deafness, Cognition and
    Language Research Centre
University College London
London
UK

Chris Pike, PhD
Principal Lecturer
Applied Social Sciences
Canterbury Christ Church University
Canterbury, Kent
UK

Julie Radford, PhD
Senior Lecturer in Special and
    Inclusive Education
Department of Psychology and
    Human Development
Institute of Education
University of London
London
UK

John Rae, PhD
Reader in Psychology
School of Human and Life Sciences
Roehampton University
Whitelands College
London
UK

Jack Sidnell, PhD
Associate Professor
Department of Anthropology
University of Toronto at Mississauga
Missisauga
Canada

Penny Stribling, PhD
Lecturer
School of Human and Life Sciences
Roehampton University
Whitelands College
London
UK

Tuula Tykkyläinen, PhD
Researcher, Speech and
    Language Therapist
Department of Speech Sciences
University of Helsinki
Helsinki
Finland

Ray Wilkinson, PhD
Clinical Reader in Language and
    Communication Science
Neuroscience and Aphasia
    Research Unit (NARU)
School of Psychological Sciences
University of Manchester
Manchester
UK

Anthony Wootton, PhD
(Retd Senior Lecturer in Sociology)
University of York
York
UK

Section 1

Interactions between typically developing children and their main carers

Chapter 1

Next turn and intersubjectivity in children's language acquisition

CLARE TARPLEE (1962–1999)

Edited by
Michael Forrester and Anthony Wootton

Introduction

There is now a substantial research tradition within child language study which takes as its focus the language addressed to young children (e.g. Gallaway and Richards 1994). This research tradition has consolidated, developed and broadened in outlook since gathering momentum in response to nativist claims in the 1970s. Over the intervening period, one can chart a shift in emphasis from early concerns with the description of a child-directed register, to a more recent drive to understand the nature of the interactions between child and adult. Such a shift is documented by two review articles within that collection. Snow, charting changes between the late 1970s and early 1990s, writes, 'the analysis of input moved from being located in the study of registers to being located in the study of discourse analysis' (1994: 6); while Pine reports recognition of 'the need to consider the interactive context in which CDS [child-directed speech] occurs if we are to understand exactly how it operates' (1994: 18). Commentaries on the field, then, suggest that work in this research tradition can now lay claim to a sensitivity to the workings of the conversational interactions between adult and child which are the site of children's language development.

A particular impetus for research into the language addressed to children has come from learnability theory and the 'no negative evidence' debate (e.g. Brown and Hanlon 1970; Morgan *et al.* 1995), which concerns the sufficiency with which children learning language are supplied with indications that their ungrammatical productions are indeed ungrammatical. In itself, the point at issue here is quite specific, and applicable to a particular research enterprise. It amounts to a logical problem pertaining to the child's ability to recover from the overgeneralisation of grammatical rules in the deduction of an adult-like grammar – a debate that informs the extent to which innate capacities are built into theoretical models of language acquisition. These concerns have provided fuel for a long-running debate which has become much wider in scope. Following a catalyst article by Brown and Hanlon (1970), some have endorsed their finding that children do not receive negative feedback following their ungrammatical productions (e.g. Morgan and Travis 1989; Marcus 1993; Morgan *et al.* 1995), while others have argued that they do (e.g. Bohannon and Stanowicz 1988; Moerk 1991; Farrar 1992; Furrow *et al.* 1993; Penner 1997). Following Hirsh-Pasek *et al.* (1984), some have widened the scope of what might constitute negative evidence and looked at more implicit forms of feedback (e.g. Demetras *et al.* 1986; Morgan and Travis 1989; Saxton 1993, 1997). Some studies have considered the role of feedback in relation to phonological and lexical development (Bohannon and Stanowicz 1988; Huttenlocher *et al.* 1991; Harris 1992), while others have considered similar issues in relation to atypical populations of learners, such as children with specific language impairment (Nelson *et al.* 1996) and deaf children (Harris 1992). It is striking, however, that in this broader arena the terms of the debate remain those pertaining to theoretical modelling. These studies make abundant use of terms like stimulus, input and feedback – terms which implicitly present language development as a computational mental process of grammar deduction.

What one finds, then, in the literature, is a debate which on the one hand claims to value an understanding of the nature of adult–child discourse and to locate language development within social interaction – while on the other claims to be steeped in terms and concepts which locate language development firmly within the individual child's head. What I want to do in this chapter is to take one of those terms – feedback – and consider some of the limitations of this concept for understanding both how adult–child interaction works and how the nature of that interaction may have a part to play in facilitating children's language development. By presenting an interactional analysis of some data, I hope to indicate how a greater understanding of the working of conversational interaction, as uncovered by those working in the tradition of ethnomethodological conversation analysis (see, for example, Levinson 1983; Heritage 1984a; Wootton 1989) might illuminate and advance this important area of child language research.

Feedback

Feedback is a term which has been imported into studies of adult–child discourse from theoretical models of learning and deduction. In terms of sensitivity to the dynamics of social interaction, it takes us a step further than input (still heavily used in these studies), which implies that an adult's contributions to an interactional adult–child exchange can be stripped away and summed as an entity, each contribution divorced from the local interactional context in which it was embedded. Input, in other words, represents a one-way phenomenon. Feedback, on the other hand, incorporates a recognition of the two-way nature of dyadic talk, since it describes a relationship between two (generally consecutive) turns – the relationship of an adult's response to a prior child production. But it is severely limited as an analytic concept applied to interactive talk, since its bounds are set at those two turns. The concept allows no consideration of the part played by later turns in the emergent relationships between earlier, adjacent ones.

Let me illustrate some of the problems caused by this limitation inherent in the concept of feedback by considering how the concept is employed in the work of Moerk (1991), whose work is more sequentially sensitive than that of many in the field. Moerk sets out to refute the claim, often made in the literature, that 'negative evidence' is not a feature of adult–child talk. He does this by presenting numerous transcript examples of sequences in which adults correct children's linguistic errors. The wealth of examples presented is effective both in demonstrating the prevalence of these kinds of sequences, and in broadening out the rather constricted view of these issues as presented by learnability theorists. The analysis is nonetheless limited, however, by the fact that the 'feedback cycles' which Moerk illustrates consist principally of just two turns – an ungrammatical utterance of some kind from the child and a correction of some kind from the carer. There is (in most cases) no consideration of the child's response to this 'feedback' turn, and thus no attention is paid to how different kinds of 'corrective' carer responses are treated by the child. This limitation has at least two consequences. Firstly, it prevents us from gaining any understanding of how different carer responses may carry different implications for what the child does next. Consideration of such matters could in turn help us to understand just how certain adult utterances present usable information to the child. Secondly, omission from the analysis of the child's response to these adult turns also leaves Moerk with no warrant for categorising the adult utterances as corrections – since we cannot tell whether the child treated them as such. This categorisation, then, can be done only on an intuitive basis. Since a concern of this work is with establishing the extent of corrective information available to the child, this omission is a significant one.

A further problem with the concept of feedback is one which has beset studies in this area. Adult response types have typically been categorised according to their structural relationship to preceding child turns. Categories such as 'recasts' – some instances of which function as corrections and others of which do not – are typically used. Some work (Marcus 1993; Morgan *et al.* 1995) has identified a problem with this – but the way in which the problem has been formulated fails, in my view, to address what is really the issue. In essence, the problem is conceived by these researchers as being a problem for the child, rather than a problem of approach. Morgan *et al.* (1995), for instance, argue that, since recasts are not easily discriminable as a class by children, who will also be unable to identify recasts as corrections (since some are not), recasts are unlikely to supply the child with any 'evidence' to make use of. The implication here is that, in looking for ways in which adult responses may provide useful information to the language learning child, we are simply looking for identifiable classes of response types which act as a signal for the child by routinely marking ungrammatical utterances. We are looking, in other words, for a signalling code which the child can crack.

What I hope to illustrate in this chapter is that we cannot afford to ignore the nature of adult utterances in the way that this line of research appears to do. It might very well matter whether an adult produces a clarification question or a correction, for instance, since these actions implicate different next actions on the part of the child, and in particular offer different kinds of opportunities for the child's rehearsal of target items. The problem is that the categories typically employed in feedback studies are formulated in terms of the kinds of grammatical information they contain. Instead of formulating categories in terms of the kind of grammatical information they contain I hope to illustrate the benefits of looking at adult turns as interactional objects, objects which are, on that basis, identifiable to the child.

Method

The analysis which follows makes use of the procedures of conversation analysis, and draws on some important insights uncovered by that tradition, pertaining to the relationship between a turn at talk and its prior. My intention is to illustrate how we might arrive at a clearer understanding of the relationship between adult turns and child turns in child–adult talk – and to suggest how we might bring such an understanding to bear on what is a fundamental debate in child language – the role of 'negative evidence'.

The data presented is taken from a study of naturally occurring dyadic interactions taking place between normally developing children aged between 1;7 and 2;3 and their carers (see Tarplee 1993). The recordings were made by the carers themselves in their own homes, and at the time of recording, the carers were unaware that their own part in the talk was to be an object of study. The data extracts presented have been transcribed according to the notation conventions generally adopted in conversation analytic work (see Atkinson and Heritage 1984; ix–xvi), with the additional use of symbols of the IPA enclosed within square brackets.

The analysis begins with data drawn from a particular setting – that of picture labelling from books. Since the interest here is to identify features of the social interactions in which a young child engages which might facilitate for the child the language-learning task, then an appropriate place to start looking is at an instructional activity. Picture labelling from books is clearly an activity which is often engaged in by carers and young children, and featured in all the recordings that were gathered for the study. Picture labelling is an activity where linguistic testing, instruction and rehearsal take place naturally.

Analysis

Picture labelling as an instructional routine

Picture labelling is clearly an activity in which a young child's linguistic skills can be directly addressed and worked on, and it is worth considering just how this 'instructional' work is achieved. Extracts 1.1 and 1.2 display picture-labelling talk.

Extract 1.1

```
1    Adult:   wha:t:'s: that
                  (1.8)

2    Child:   e:lephant =

3    Adult:   = (hh)'a:t's ri:ght
```

Extract 1.2

```
1    Adult:   a::nd what's that
                  (3.3)

2    Child:   [ba·ɪdənə·ˀtʃɐʊəsʲ]
                  (.)
```

3+1   Adult: n:o tha̲t's the rhi:no̲ceros tha̲t's the-
                  (1.7)

2   Child: [ɪdɛpʰɔdːʊˑmː] [ə( )]

3   Adult: [(hh) hippopo̲ta(h)mus

3   °yes°=
       Child: =what's this

In both cases we can see a basic three-part structure to the labelling sequence, which has been indicated by numbering in the left-hand margin: there is an elicitation from the carer, a label from the child, and in third position a receipt from the adult of the child's label. In Extract 1.2, the adult's *no that's the rhinoceros that's the-* is a turn which contains both a third part to one labelling sequence and a first part to a next. *No that's the rhinoceros* (with contrastive stress – by means of on-syllable pitch movement – on *that's*) receipts the child's erroneous first label, while in the same turn *that's the-* (on level pitch in mid-range) serves as a 'fill-the-blank' type elicitation, inviting the child to produce a repaired attempt at the label. We can see in these two examples that the third-position receipt can either affirm the child's label (*that's right* in Extract 1.1, *hippopotamus yes* in Extract 1.2), or it can reject it (*no that's the rhinoceros* in Extract 1.2). We can also see that a third-position receipt which affirms that a child's label can be designed in different ways. *That's right* in Extract 1.1 affirms without reproducing a version of the label, while *hippopotamus yes* in Extract 1.2 combines a version of the label with a confirmation marker. Extract 1.3 illustrates a third design for affirming receipts found in the corpus:

Extract 1.3

1   Adult: o [oh]   who's tha̲t
    Child: [ë̆h]
                    (1.0)

2   Child: li̲:on

3   Adult: l̲:i̲::on
                    (5.0)
    Child: °norah°

Here affirmation is done without any confirmation marker of any kind, but simply with a version of the label.

The carer's receipting turn in third position in a labelling sequence

When considering how 'instructional' work is accomplished in these labelling sequences, it is clear that the turn which regularly occupies third position in these three-part structures – the adult's evaluative receipt of a child's labelling turn – is of central importance. This kind of turn within a three-part sequence has often been identified in the literature as characteristic of classroom and other styles of pedagogic interaction.

This is because one accomplishment of an evaluative receipt in third turn position after a question is to specify that question as having held a particular status. Searle (1969:66) makes the distinction between what he terms 'real' and 'exam' questions in talk:

> In real questions the speaker wants to know (find out) the answer; in exam questions, the speaker wants to know if the hearer knows.

Heritage (1984a) nicely demonstrates the options available to a questioner to constitute a question as one or other of these alternative actions, by virtue of the action that the questioner takes directly after a co-participant's answer. Since, as Heritage (1984a: 286) points out,

> In a 'real' question, the questioner proposes to be ignorant about the substance of the question and . . . projects the intended answerer to be knowledgeable about the matter.

Then questioners of 'real' questions typically receipt their answers with the use of a particle like *oh* which, as Heritage elsewhere explicates (Heritage 1984b), marks its speaker as having undergone some change of state in knowledge or orientation. In mundane conversation one therefore finds three-part *question–answer–receipt* sequences of the following form:

```
(Frankel: TC:1:1:13–14:ST) (Heritage 1984b: 308)
    S :   .hh When d'ju get out. Christmas week or the week before Christmas
    G :   Uh::m two or three days before [Ch  ] ristmas,
    S :                                  [Oh :,]
```

In such a sequential position, the use of *oh* marks its speaker as having undergone a change of state from ignorance to knowledge, through receipt of a co-participant's answer, and therefore as NOT having been in possession of this knowledge when the question was asked.

By contrast, a third-position receipt which evaluates an answer to a question, proposes instead that the questioner has undergone no such change of state of knowledge, but has been already in possession of the information elicited by the question. An evaluative receipt, then, types a question as having been of the 'exam' type – a question produced in order to test its recipient's knowledge.

There is nothing new in the association of this structure of talk with instructional activity: the recurrence of this kind of questioning sequence in classically pedagogic settings such as in the interaction between teacher and pupils in classroom lessons has often been noted by researchers working in different research traditions. This three-part structure has been described and associated with instructional modes of interaction (e.g. Sinclair and Coulthard 1975; McHoul 1978; Mehan 1979; Lerner 1995), however, few researchers have been concerned with a systematic explication of just how this kind of sequence accomplishes instructional work.

A third-position evaluative receipt after a question characterises the questioner not only as being already in possession of the information being solicited, but also, by virtue of having access to that information, as being in a position to measure the correctness of the elicited answer. This means that the child is being provided with a particularly important kind of 'feedback' here, over and above the message that *elephant* and *hippopotamus* are appropriate labels and *rhinoceros* is not. The adult is standing as arbiter over the linguistic appropriacy of the child's productions, and means that the child's answer itself, framed in this way, becomes a particular kind of object. It is not an informing, as many answers to questions are, but a display. The child's turn in a picture book labelling sequence, since it implicates an evaluative response from the adult, takes on the status of a performance, a presentation of certain skills, offered to the adult for acceptance or rejection – offered, that is, to be worked on in some way. In the examples we have so far seen, it is lexical knowledge that is being tested. A child's labelling turns, then, present a display of certain of the child's linguistic abilities, and explicitly offer them to the adult to be worked on in those terms.

It was seen earlier that there are essentially two kinds of work which the adult's evaluative receipt may perform. It may explicitly accept and affirm the child's prior action, or it may indicate non-acceptance and instigate repair on it. By means of the regular occurrence of the adult's third-position evaluative receipt, one or other of these two courses of action is routinely taken. An important consequence of this is that the child is given reduced opportunities for a critical monitoring of her own turns, since responsibility for such monitoring is, by virtue of that third-position turn, conferred upon the adult. In the corpus, the children were very rarely seen to initiate repair on their own labelling utterances. As the adult's evaluative receipt regularly follows very swiftly from the child's labelling attempt, without delay, then actual opportunities for this kind of initiation are minimised – just as the expectation of its occurrence may inhibit the critical monitoring that would motivate it. One kind of 'feedback' available to the child in these sequences, then, is that the charge of monitoring the child's utterances for her linguistic 'correctness' is taken away from the child and laid at the door of the adult – a feature that would seem to be crucial to this talk's pedagogic nature.

There is also another kind of 'feedback' implicit in a carer's evaluative receipt which follows a child's labelling utterance. Consider Extract 1.4.

Extract 1.4

1   Child: [tʳa̬dɪ̬ə̯θ]

2   →   Adult: <u>tee:</u>th

3   →   Child: [t̬iːjəʰ]

Here the carer follows the child's initial attempt at the label *teeth* with a repetition of the label – a turn design we have already seen accomplishing the work of evaluative receipt. However, compare this extract with Extract 1.3, in which, following the carer's repetition of the child's label, there is a five-second silence and the child moves on to label another picture. In other words, the repetition affirms the child's label and ends that particular labelling sequence. In Extract 1.4, on the other hand, the carer's version of the label prompts a second, repaired, attempt at *teeth* by the child. Examples such as Extract 1.4 show us that the picture-labelling activity presents opportunities, not only for working on the child's lexical skills, but for engaging with the child's developing articulatory skills as well. The carer's utterance of *teeth* serves as an affirmative receipt as far as the lexical choice made by the child is concerned, but it invites repair at a phonetic level. This example also shows us that the labelling activity is not just concerned with the testing of a child's linguistic skills: it offers opportunities for rehearsal of development skills on the part of the child. And in terms of 'feedback' made available to the child, a consideration of Extracts 1.3 and 1.4 makes apparent that what looks to be a similar object – a carer's repetition of a child's prior labelling attempt – can do two very different kinds of work, and have very different implications for what follows it. In Extract 1.3, the repetition affirms the child's lexical choice, requires no further work from the child and effectively ends the labelling sequence. In Extract 1.4, by contrast, the repetition invites the child to have another go at articulating the label. As well as the 'feedback' inherent in these responses (that the child's production of *lion* in Extract 1.3 is lexically appropriate and articulatorily adequate, while the child's production of *teeth* in Extract 1.4 is lexically appropriate but articulatorily leaves room for improvement), it is also important to consider how the child is able to distinguish between instances of a carer's repetitions which make one rather than the other of these two courses of action (end of talk on a given picture versus phonetically repaired attempt at the label) relevant. (See Tarplee 1996, for an attempt to tease out some of the subtleties of this distinction in prosodic terms.)

Picture labelling: summary

In picture labelling, both lexical and articulatory skills are worked on, not only by being tested, but also by rehearsal. It can be seen that the carer's third-position receipt in a labelling sequence is crucial to this instructional work, and provides 'feedback' on at least three levels. Firstly, it can explicitly affirm or reject the appropriacy of the child's labelling attempt (both in lexical and articulatory terms). This is a similar kind of 'feedback' to that most often attended to in the literature (although there the concern is usually with syntactic appropriacy). Secondly, there is a level of 'feedback' which the literature usually misses. This is that the carer's response to the child's utterance has implications for what the child does next. Thirdly, the fact that there is this kind of evaluative response at all has implications for the whole tenor of the talk, since it casts carer and child into the roles of instructor and instructee, reducing opportunities for the child to engage in a critical self-monitoring of her own utterances.

The remainder of the analysis considers similar features in ordinary adult–child conversations.

The incidence of labelling sequences outside picture book settings

A first point to note about the conversational data is that labelling sequences taking the same three-part structure as in picture book settings are found prompted by play with jigsaw puzzles, crayons and toy animals. The adults and children in the corpus also regularly engage in similar testing and naming activities, centring on people and objects figuring in the child's recent experience (Extract 1.5).

Extract 1.5

1   Adult: can you remember wh<u>o</u> came y<u>e</u>sterday <u>ian</u>
                     (1.2)
     Child: m:a:mmy

1   Adult: who came t-   who <u>ca:</u>me
             (0.6)

1   Adult: who came round y<u>e</u>sterday
             (0.8)

2   Child: [d'ɔ̰·ẽ]
             ḭ
                      (0.9)

3   Adult: <u>j̊:a:</u>ne
             (1.0)

2   Child: j[ane

3   Adult: [ja-

Labelling elicitations can even be built out of the child's preceding talk. In Extract 1.6, the completed utterance constructed from a fill-the-blank task itself becomes a further labelling elicitation.

Extract 1.6

((*the child has been engaged in sound play around the word dodie – this child's word for dummy*))

1   Adult: wh<u>o</u> h<u>as</u> a:-
             (0.6)

2   Child: d<u>o:</u>die

3   Adult: who has a <u>do:</u>die
             (1.0)

4   Child: l<u>ew</u>is: [( )

5   Adult: [<u>lew</u>is does y<u>e</u>s

The adult picks up on the child's prior sound play around the world *dodie*, and builds a fill-the-blank construction with *dodie* as its target. This construction, completed by the child with *dodie*, is itself an eliciting question, and the child's *dodie* is not evaluatively receipted by the adult. The adult then asks the child *who has a dodie* and it is the child's response to this WH-question (*Lewis*) that receives an affirmation from the adult (*Lewis does yes*). Finally, Extract 1.7 illustrates how the labelling activity performed in this greater range of settings goes beyond simple lexical testing and involves, like picture book labelling, rehearsal on the child's part.

Extract 1.7

1   Adult: know what th<u>at</u> is
             (0.8)

2   Child: u:h
             (1.2)

3   Child: what's <u>this</u>

4   Adult: that's a t:ree
         (1.0)

5   Adult: what is it
         (0.9)

6   Child: tree:

7   Adult: mm shall we put some more leaves on

Here, the child responds to the adult's eliciting question by turning it back on the adult with *what's this*. The adult responds with an informing turn, *that's a tree*, which is not immediately met with a child version. That it invites a child version, however, is made apparent by the adult's following it up, after one second, with a prompting question, *what is it*. The child responds to this with a version of the target, *tree*, which the adult then receipts (*mm*). These sequences, then, are concerned not only with the retrieval of known labels, but also with the articulation and rehearsal of unknown ones. That is, they work on the child's linguistic abilities in just the same ways as picture book labelling sequences.

The pervasiveness of labelling

It is apparent that labelling is an activity that is engaged in by adults and young children in a wide range of situational contexts. The fact that adults and young children label many different sorts of objects around them is important in highlighting the many opportunities that arise for a young child and adult to become involved in working on the child's linguistic skills. This observation alone is sufficient to undermine any characterisation of labelling talk as a specialised, context-specific style of interaction. What is much more important, however, is the fact that labelling does not rely on there being any physical objects or representations present to be labelled. Not only can the child's familiarity with objects, people and experiences from memory be called upon, at any time, for participation in bouts of labelling, but it has been seen that the adult can also pick up on the child's preceding talk to build labelling targets out of it. If a child's own spontaneous utterances can be built, by the adult, into fill-the-blank labelling constructions, then it would seem that any number of things can be characterised as 'labelable'. Labelling, then, becomes an activity which is constituted by the talk taking a particular three-part structural design, involving the display and evaluation of the child's linguistic knowledge. The analysis presented here has shown that talk between child and adult can take this structure in a potentially boundless range of contexts.

Beyond labelling sequences: carers' receipts of children's non-labelling utterances

Consideration of the conversational data suggests that this kind of evaluative receipting turn is widely prevalent in adult–child interaction, and in positions other than in third-turn position in a labelling sequence. If an evaluative receipt types its speaker as having been in possession of the information presented in a prior utterance before that utterance was produced, it may do that work in sequential contexts other than in third turn after a question.

Consider Extracts 1.8–1.10.

Extract 1.8

((This extract opens with the adult making a request for the child to pass her some keys))

1		Adult:	can I <u>have</u> the<u>m</u>
2		Child:	<u>u</u>hh <u>n:o</u>::=
3		Adult:	=o(h)h y(h)ou <u>t:ea:</u>sing m(h)e ·hh y(h)ou
			little mo:ns:<u>ter</u>
			(0.6)
4		Child:	[m<u>ʌ</u>ᵊç·tï]
5	→	Adult:	<u>mo:</u>nster y<u>es</u>

Extract 1.9

1		Adult:	these are a p<u>air</u> of [wʌːïdfʊẽn·sː]
2		Child:	[b⁻ẹːᵊs̩·ẹʰ]
3	→	Adult:	w(h)<u>i</u>(h)de <u>fr(h)o</u>(h)nts y(h)<u>e</u>(h)s: ·hh

Extract 1.10

((child playing with toy cow and fence))

1		Adult:	's <u>cow</u> behind the <u>fe</u>nce isn' it
			(4.2)
2		Adult:	u:h (.) sitting <u>o</u>n the fenc:e (.)
			that's a good place to <u>be</u>
			(.)
3		Child:	[ïˀtsəïfẹ̃ᵊnˀs·]
4		Adult:	m (h)y(h)e(he)s
5		Child:	[nẹs(l)izanẽ̞fᵋˀts]
6	→	Adult:	sitting <u>on</u> the <u>fe</u>nce y<u>es</u>

In each case, the arrowed adult turn carries a version of the child's prior utterance, and a confirmation marker, *yes*. The adult, then, appears to be confirming what the child is saying. But in every case, too, the child's prior utterance which the adult is confirming turns out to be a version of part of the adult's turn which preceded it; that is, it is a partial imitation of that turn. These child turns represent the picking up of part of that turn and an attempt at articulating it. What the adult is doing, then, by producing a confirmation in next turn, is confirming these child utterances AS appropriate imitations – as being an acceptable version of what she herself just said.

In Extract 1.8, the child's imitation, [mʌ̃ˀᵊçˑtï], of the adult's *monster*, is phonetically quite close to the adult target. In Extract 1.9,[1] on the other hand, the child's [bˀʏ̝ːᵊşˑe̝ʰ] looks, on the face of it, very unlike the adult's [wʌːïdfʊ̃n̩ˑsː]. However, there are similarities. Both utterances open with labiality ([bˀ] and [w]) and a vocalic portion with an open, backish and unrounded quality which moves to around mid height. The consonantal portion in both utterances has friction coinciding with voicelessness ([şˑ] and [f]), and also alveolarity ([şˑ] and [d]). In the latter part of both utterances there is a vocalic portion with a mid-high quality. In rhythm, too, the two utterances are closely matched, with a long first vocalic portion in both cases, which also carries an increase in loudness. There are, then, several shared features between the two versions, which seem to be enough for the adult to treat the child's version as a version of her own utterance, and, moreover, to confirm it as such. And in Extract 1.10, the child's first version, [ïˀtşɔ̈ïfɛ̠ˀn̩ˀşˑ], receives a confirmation marker alone (*yes*), while a second, phonetically improved version, [nɐ̠s(l)izanɛfᶜɛˀtş], receives a confirmation comprising, like those in Extracts 1.8 and 1.9, a repeat of the child's turn and *yes*.

In these examples, then, the adult is following a child turn with an explicitly evaluative response, and thereby is putting herself in a particular relationship to what is contained in the child's turn. To highlight the fact that it is the linguistic content of the child's turns which is being evaluated in these cases, compare Extracts 1.8 to 1.10 with Extract 1.11.

Extract 1.11

(('*telephone*' has just been mentioned))

1	Child:	j̠ossy 'n a telepho:ne
		(0.6)
2	Child:	[dᶻɔ̃çiˑnɛtɛtʰ]
3 →	Adult:	i yea j̠ossy was on the telephone wasn't
4 →		she

In this sequence, the child's opening turn is an observation, concerning a friend and a telephone, which he begins to repeat in face of no response from the adult (although his second version, for whatever reason, trails off in the middle of the word *telephone*). And what is being ratified here by the adult's evaluative receipt is the propositional content of that observation – the fact that Jossy was indeed on the telephone. This kind of sequence would appear to be part of the constitution of an adult–child relationship whereby the adult is credited with a greater degree of knowledge than the child, and is granted, moreover, a higher level of authority on the validity of the child's reported observations. A relationship (which is in part constructed by this very kind of talk) holds between the two participants, such that the adult is in a position to ratify the child's statements.

---

[1] It is apparent from the talk surrounding this extract that what is being talked about is a pair of Y-fronts. The adult, however, in both her utterances, can be clearly heard to articulate *wide fronts*.

In Extracts 1.8 to 1.10, too, the adult is casting herself as arbiter – but not, in these cases, as arbiter over the accuracy of the propositional content of the child's turns. Indeed, it would be difficult to identify the propositional content of the child's [mʌ̃²ç·tï], [b⁻ẹ:²s̩·ẹʰ] and [ⁱ²ts̩əⁱfẹ³n²s̩·] in this sequential position. Instead, she appears to be evaluating their status as acceptable imitations of her own speech – that is, to be appraising their merit as linguistic productions. The child, by imitating the adult's utterances, treats those utterances as constituting some kind of target. The adult, by confirming those imitations, treats them as having hit that target. In other words, the child's contributions here are being attended to in their capacity as articulatory objects.

Next turn ratification of linguistic content in other sequential contexts

Occurrences of the child's picking up parts of the adult's talk in the way illustrated in Extracts 1.8 to 1.10 are common in the corpus. So, too, are instances of the adult opting to deal with such imitations by confirming them, as just illustrated. What is notable about those three examples, however, is that, in each case, the adult turn which forms the basis for imitation is relatively unconstrained with regard to the range of possible next utterances which it projects. That is to say that the three adult utterances – *you little monster*; *these are a pair of wide fronts*; and *uh sitting on the fence that's a good place to be* – occupying the sequential positions which they do, place few restrictions on what may follow them as a relevant next turn at talk. None, for example, is a question making an answer a relevant next action for the child to take. Instead, they are contributions to the talk which may be followed, unaccountably, by any of a wide range of next actions. For the child to follow them with an imitation, then, and for the adult to confirm that particular next action as an appropriate one to take – that is, for both participants to take 'time out' to deal with linguistic aspects of the ongoing talk – does not interfere in any significant way with the interactional business of the exchange. Indeed, one could build a case that adult–child talk at this age very readily allows such linguistic matters to become the main interactional business.

This focus on the performative aspects of the child's talk becomes more noticeable, however, in instances where such matters interrupt an ongoing interactional sequence which looks, at its outset, to be taking a more clearly specified direction. Consider Extract 1.12.

Extract 1.12

1		Adult:	(alright) do you want to g<u>e</u>t some <u>du:</u>plo <u>out</u> (0.7)
2		Child:	e ·hh hh <u>slippers</u>
3	→	Adult:	°y(h)e(he)s slippers° ·hh do you
4	→		w<u>a</u>nt to g<u>e</u>t some <u>du:</u>plo out=
5		Child:	=<u>no:</u>
6		Adult:	<u>no</u> <u>wha</u>t do you <u>wa</u>nt then

```
7        Child:    I: (got) a slippers    o : [n
                      (want)

8        Adult:                            _(h)[you w(h)an-_ you
                      wa(h)nt to pl(h)ay w(h)ith your slippers
```

The adult's first turn presents the child with a question, *do you want to get some duplo out?*, and is therefore a turn which carries quite specific implications for what is to follow: on its completion, an answer to that question is what is made relevant. However, the child's following turn, *slippers*, appears not to be, in any intelligible sense, an answer to the adult's question – nor, indeed, any kind of contingent response to it (as, for example, a response such as *I don't know*). Nor is it, unlike those child turns considered in the previous extracts, any kind of version of part of the adult's prior turn. But it, too, like the child turns in those extracts, receives an affirmative response from the adult – this time with a turn in which the ordering of the two elements, confirmation marker (*yes* produced with laughter) and a version of the child's utterance (*slippers*), are reversed (*yes slippers*).

Directly after her affirmative *yes slippers*, the adult draws breath and, within the same turn, presents again her opening question, *do you want to get some duplo out?*. This is an exact redoing of her question in the first line of the extract – not only in its syntactic construction, but also in its pitch configuration, rhythm and loudness. The earlier part of her turn, *yes slippers*, is marked out from this redoing by being quieter, and by a speeding up of tempo over *slippers*. This second version of the question is thus marked as a 'restart' (see Local 1992), a redoing of her opening question – but not as one which makes explicit an orientation to the question's not having been addressed the first time round. One way of displaying such an orientation would have been to reformulate the question in some way, and thereby to address the child's disattendance to it. An example is supplied in Extract 1.13 (an extract from a picture book labelling sequence).

Extract 1.13

```
1        Adult:    ooh ((points)) what's that
                      (2.8)             ((child moves about in chair))

2   →    Adult:    what is it
```

The adult's second question in this extract is presented, not as a redoing of his first one, but as a follow up to it. It credits the child with having registered the question, but not, for some reason, being disposed to address it. This is quite different from what happens in Extract 1.12. Nor, in Extract 1.12, is the redoing produced louder or on higher pitch than the original question, like the restarts (in adult–adult conversation) which Local (1992: 285ff) describes, which thereby seem to be presented as entirely new contributions to the exchange. In this case, both pitch and loudness between the two versions are closely matched, so that the second version comes off as a straightforward rerun of the first. The intervening talk – the child's *slippers* and the adult's response *yes slippers* – is thus framed as an 'insertion sequence', which takes a kind of side step out of the ongoing business of the talk.

Such insertion sequences are not uncommon in question–answer structures in talk. Recurrently, however, these insertion sequences turn out to be contingent on the original question. The following example has been taken from Schegloff (1972: 78):

    A: Are you coming tonight?
    B: Can I bring a guest?
    A: Sure.
    B: I'll be there.

In this case, the insertion sequence (*Can I bring a guest? – Sure*) itself takes the form of a question–answer sequence, and can be seen to be contingent on A's original question – to be a step taken on the way to arriving at the answer to that question, which is produced in the fourth turn.

    Now, in Extract 1.12, the child's turn *slippers* may indeed be, as far as he is concerned, a contingent response to the adult's opening question, *do you want to get some duplo out?*. As the sequence turns out, we may be able to suggest that what the child meant by uttering *slippers* here was something to the effect of 'No, I don't want to get some duplo out: I want to play with my slippers'. However, it is not treated in this way by the adult. In the extract cited above, A treats B's *Can I bring a guest?* as contingent on the original question, by providing a response (*Sure*), but in Extract 1.12 the adult, by running off her original question again, instead treats the insertion sequence which opens with the child's *slippers* as a non-contingent, parenthetical sequence of talk.

    In Extract 1.12, then, the adult and child take time out from a question–answer sequence for the child to produce an utterance, *slippers*, and for the adult to produce an affirmative response to it. At least, this is what the adult's replay of her question constructs the participants to be doing. What remains to be considered is the order of work which is accomplished by this insertion sequence.

    A first observation is that the adult could have replayed her question directly after the child's *slippers* – could, that is, have treated the child's *slippers* not only as non-contingent on her question but also as not inviting an adult response. Instead, she opts to respond affirmatively to the child's turn. Given that the child's turn is treated as one which invites acknowledgement of some kind, one possibility which could be argued for is that the adult is treating the child's *slippers* as a noticing on the child's part, which happens to have broken into an ongoing sequence of talk, and that she is affirming it on that basis. This possibility cannot be entirely refuted. However, it is notable that the adult, in selecting from a number of turn-type options which might have done this work, such as *yes*, or *yes there are your slippers*, or *yes aren't they nice*, for example, selects a turn-type which combines a confirmation marker with a repeat of the child's utterance – a turn-type which has been seen, throughout the analysis so far presented, to do the work of confirming a child's utterance on linguistic grounds. It is plausible, then, that what the adult's *yes slippers* in this sequence is doing, like the corresponding adult turns in Extracts 1.8 to 1.10, is ratifying the child's prior turn with reference to articulation rather than with regard to interactional significance.

The pervasiveness of affirmation as a locally relevant next action

It has been seen here that an adult's affirming receipts, in next turn position after a child's utterances, are not restricted to being a feature of a particular species of interactional activity which we might call 'labelling', but are a much more pervasive feature of adult–child talk. By an adjacently placed affirming receipt, the adult can ratify both the propositional content of a child's turn, and also its adequacy as a linguistic production. The young child often picks up parts of an adult's utterances for articulation – that is, seems to treat the adult's talk as a resource from which to select bits of language to experiment with – and the adult, by the use of an affirming receipt, can approve these rehearsals and displays. In doing this, the adult is treating the child's utterances, not as sequentially located contributions to the interactional business of the talk, but as articulatory performances. Where such reference takes place in the midst of an ongoing sequence of talk and subsequently alters the ongoing sequence of the interaction, it becomes particularly apparent that the child's talk is being marked out from the interactional context in which it occurs, in order to draw attention to its linguistic merits.

A consideration raised by the analysis presented here is that, since the adult can take 'time out' from certain kinds of interactional sequence (like a question–answer structure) to affirm a child's utterance on linguistic grounds, it may be that there are few, or even no, restrictions on where, in sequential terms, this kind of affirmation may be produced. This raises the question of whether this kind of affirmation may occur in child–adult interaction in a rather similar way to the occurrence of its converse – repair – in talk generally. Repair is a phenomenon that is locally relevant throughout talk. While there are organisational principles governing the precise details of how and when repair is managed in various ways (see Schegloff *et al.* 1977), it is nonetheless a general principle of talk-in-interaction that participants may, at any point in the talk's progression, divert from the course of its immediate interactional business to deal in some way with problems which arise concerning the transmission or interpretation of that talk. In ordinary mundane conversation between adults, participants may, on occasion, be impelled to correct a co-participant's errors in the realm of pronunciation or word choice. They will rarely be moved to affirm such things, since, generally speaking, they are not attuned to the kind of linguistic monitoring of their co-participant's talk which would motivate such affirmation. Utterances which are linguistically unproblematic will simply be 'not repaired', and allowed to pass unhindered, affirmed, that is, by default. But in adult–child interaction – at least in interactions involving children of the age group under consideration here – it may be that adults are engaged in just this kind of linguistic monitoring of the child's talk, such that affirmation of a child's productions becomes, like repair, a locally relevant next action for the adult to take, throughout the progress of the talk.

Discussion

The analysis presented here represents an alternative approach to investigating ways in which the young child's linguistic environment may facilitate language development. It suggests that current conceptual frameworks within which these matters are typically studied are severely limited. Notions such as input and feedback underestimate the intricacy of the mechanics of social interaction, and thus present an oversimplified picture of the adult–child interactions which must form the site of such investigations. In attempting to overcome some of these limitations, the analysis presented above has kept sight of two fundamental characteristics of social interaction which have long been established tenets within the tradition of conversation analysis. These are sequential implicature and the analytic importance of next turn. It is worth giving some further consideration here to the significance of these two notions, and to some of the ways in which they might usefully inform work in this area.

Sequential implicature

Sequential implicature or sequential implicativeness (Sacks 1995, winter 1970, Lecture 4; Schegloff and Sacks 1973) essentially amounts to the insight that contributions to an interaction are not randomly ordered with respect to one another, but certain actions in talk make relevant certain other actions that follow them. Within the conceptual framework of 'feedback', an adult feedback turn is regarded only with respect to its retrospective stance – its relationship with the prior turn. What is missed is the fact that this adult turn is itself a prior to a next action of some sort – and that it carries its own sequential implications, or set of expectations concerning what might properly occur next. By looking at a child response to such a turn, one can begin to uncover the sequential implications of particular utterance types (such as, say, clarification questions or corrections) – and start to build a picture of just what kinds of information (grammatical and otherwise) they are making available to the child. This notion of sequential implicature has informed the analysis presented above.

Analytic importance of next turn

A second important insight, uncovered by conversation analysis and lost in the restricted concept of feedback, is related to sequential implicature. Turns at talk are built to be understood as contingent upon one another, so that each next turn displays to its recipient how a prior turn has been received and understood. Hence, next position or next turn has a special status in the analysis and interpretation of talk (for both analysts and participants) as 'a basic structural position in conversation' (Drew 1990: 5) and 'an analytic object' (Sacks 1995, spring 1972, Lecture 4). This is because, as Heritage (1984a: 244) notes, considering pairs of utterances, 'however the recipient analyses the first utterance and whatever the conclusion of such an analysis, some analysis, understanding or appreciation of the prior turn will be displayed in the recipient's next turn at talk'. The way in which the concept of feedback misses this important insight is apparent in a question posed in a feedback study by Demetras *et al.* (1986: 277). They ask, 'If one considers both implicit and explicit feedback, and non-adjacent as well as adjacent feedback, how much feedback is available in speech to young children?' The answer must be that young children receive feedback on all of their utterances, just as adults in turn receive feedback on all of their utterances, which may indicate to the adult how that initial feedback has been received by the child, and so on, recursively. That is, talk is collaboratively constructed in such a way that participants display for one another, most fundamentally in next turn position, an understanding of how a prior turn has been received and what its import has been taken to be, and that by this continual process throughout the progress of talk, intersubjective understandings are reached. Analytically, this conceptualisation of next turn as a crucial site for the display of intersubjective understandings takes us a considerable way further than the notion of feedback in our understanding of the relationship between adjacent utterances in interactive talk.

Conclusion

The analysis presented in this chapter indicates that, in considering the relationships which pertain between an adult's response and a preceding child turn, a number of levels of 'feedback' can be taken into account. Beyond the explicit linguistic feedback inherent in adult turns which present as affirmations or corrections, we must consider the ways in which such evaluations target different aspects of a child's turn (phonetic as opposed to lexical, for instance). Crucially, we need to attend to the various ways in which an adult's response can implicate particular next actions from the child. And finally, we need to consider the kind of 'feedback' conveyed to the child by the very occurrence of an adult's evaluative responses. The latter part of the analysis has indicated that these evaluative receipts are not limited to particular 'instructional' settings, but appear to occur pervasively in ordinary child–adult conversations. They demonstrate that a child's utterances can be treated by the adult, not as sequentially located contributions to an exchange, but as articulatory objects which are being dealt with on linguistic terms. A child's utterances are thus awarded the status of linguistic displays, and the role of monitor over their correctness is explicitly taken by the adult. One could argue that the most important kind of 'feedback' that children are getting here is the very fact that they are getting linguistic feedback at all. That is, the particular kind of adult–child relationship in which such linguistic pedagogy is relevant is constituted by the very structure of this talk, and built on the intersubjective understandings which the talk affords.

A number of directions for future research are suggested by the research presented here. First, the latter part of the analysis focussed on affirmatory adult responses rather than corrective ones. A similar investigation into instances of reparative adult responses of various kinds could make a direct contribution to the 'no negative evidence' debate discussed in the Introduction. Second, the terms of reference for the study reported here were set by an analysis of picture-labelling interactions which deal (for this age group, at least) predominantly with single word utterances on the part of the child. Hence, consideration was limited to lexical and phonetic matters, rather than syntactic ones. A very similar analytic approach, however, could be brought to bear on grammatical aspects of children's utterances. Again, the findings of such an investigation might directly inform the 'no negative evidence' debate. Third, it would be of interest to pursue this line of investigation with conversational data from older age groups, to get a sense of how far the phenomena reported here are characteristic of early stages of development. Finally, the kind of linguistic monitoring by adults of children's utterances evidenced here may have important implications for the development of self repair skills in young children – an important area which is as yet under-researched. In sum, we have a long way to go in understanding the various ways in which young children glean linguistic information from the conversations in which they engage, but it is clear that in order to do this we must refine our understanding of how conversational interaction works. It is hoped that the analytic procedures employed here offer a promising way forward on this path.

Acknowledgements

With grateful thanks to Clare's parents Peter and Margaret Tarplee for the permission to publish their daughter's work. Thanks too to John Local (University of York) for his advice on phonetic transcription and Lily Donlan for help with updating the manuscript.

References

Atkinson, J.M. and Heritage, J. (eds) (1984) *Structures of social action: Studies in conversation analysis*. Cambridge: Cambridge University Press.

Bohannon, J.N. III and Stanowicz, L. (1988) The issue of negative evidence: Adult responses to children's language errors. *Developmental Psychology*, **24** (5), 684–689.

Brown, R. and Hanlon, C. (1970) Derivational complexity and order of acquisition in child speech. In J. Hayes (ed.), *Cognition and the development of language*. New York: Wiley.

Demetras, M.J., Post, K.N. and Snow, C.E. (1986) Feedback to first language learners: The role of repetitions and clarification questions. *Journal of Child Language*, **13**, 275–292.

Drew, P. (1990) Conversation analysis. In R.E. Asher (ed.), *The encyclopedia of language and linguistics*. Edinburgh: Pergamon Press and Aberdeen University Press.

Farrar, M.J. (1992) Negative evidence and grammatical morpheme acquisition. *Developmental Psychology*, **28** (1), 90–98.

Furrow, D., Baillie, C. and McLaren, J. (1993) Differential responding to two- and three-year-olds' utterances: the roles of grammaticality and ambiguity. *Journal of Child Language* 20, 363–375.

Gallaway, C. and Richards, B.J. (eds) (1994) *Input and interaction in language acquisition*. Cambridge: Cambridge University Press.

Harris, M. (1992) *Language experience and early language development: From input to uptake*. Hove: Lawrence Erlbaum Associates.

Heritage, J. (1984a) *Garfinkel and ethnomethodology*. Cambridge: Polity Press.

Heritage, J. (1984b) A change of state token and aspects of its sequential placement. In J.M. Atkinson and J. Heritage (eds), *Structures of social action: Studies in conversation analysis*. Cambridge: Cambridge University Press.

Hirsh-Pasek, K., Treiman, R. and Schneiderman, M. (1984) Brown and Hanlon revisited: Mothers' sensitivity to ungrammatical forms. *Journal of Child Language*, **11**, 81–88.

Huttenlocher, J., Haight, W., Bryk, A., Seltzer, M. and Lyons, T. (1991) Early vocabulary growth: Relation to language input and gender. *Developmental Psychology*, **27** (2), 236–248.

Lerner, G. (1995) Turn design and the organisation of participation in instructional activities. *Discourse Processes*, **19**, 111–131.

Levinson, S. (1983) *Pragmatics*. Cambridge: Cambridge University Press.

Local, J. (1992) Continuing and restarting. In P. Auer and A. Di Luzio (eds), *The contextualisation of language*. Amsterdam: John Benjamins Publishing Co.

Marcus, G.F. (1993) Negative evidence in language acquisition. *Cognition*, **46**, 53–85.

McHoul, A. (1978) The organisation of turns at formal talk in the classroom. *Language in Society*, 7, 183–213.

Mehan, H. (1979) *Learning lessons: Social organisation in the classroom.* Cambridge, MA: Harvard University Press.

Moerk, E. (1991) Positive evidence for negative evidence. *First Language*, **11**, 219–251.

Morgan, J.L. and Travis, L.L. (1989) Limits on negative information in language input. *Journal of Child Language*, **16**, 531–552.

Morgan, J.L., Bonamo, K.M. and Travis, L.L. (1995) Negative evidence on negative evidence. *Developmental Psychology*, **31** (2), 180–197.

Nelson, K.E., Camarata, S.M., Welsh, J., Butkovsky, L. and Camarata, M. (1996) Effects of imitative and conversational recasting treatment on the acquisition of grammar in children with specific language impairment and younger language-normal children. *Journal of Speech and Hearing Research*, **39**, 850–859.

Penner, S.G. (1997) Parental responses to grammatical and ungrammatical child utterances. *Child Development*, **58**, 376–384.

Pine, J.M. (1994) The language of primary caregivers. In C. Gallaway and B.J. Richards (eds), *Input and interaction in language acquisition*. Cambridge: Cambridge University Press.

Sacks, H. (1995) Lecture 4, Winter 1970. Greetings: adjacency pairs: sequential implicativeness; the integrative function of public tragedy. In G. Jefferson (ed.), *Lectures on conversation*. Cambridge, MA: Blackwell.

Sacks, H. (1995) Lecture 4, Spring 1972. The relating power of adjacency; Next position. In G. Jefferson (ed.), *Lectures on conversation*. Cambridge, MA: Blackwell.

Saxton, M. (1993) Does negative input work? In J. Clibbens and B. Pendleton (eds), *CLS 93: Proceedings of the Child Language Seminar 1993*. Department of Psychology, University of Plymouth.

Saxton, M. (1997) The contrast theory of negative input. *Journal of Child Language*, **24**, 139–161.

Schegloff, E.A. (1972) Sequencing in conversational openings. In J. Gumperz and D. Hymes (eds), *Directions in sociolinguistics*. New York: Holt, Rhinehart & Winston.

Schegloff, E.A. and Sacks, H. (1973) Opening up closings. *Semiotica*, **7**, 289–327.

Schegloff, E.A., Jefferson, G. and Sacks, H. (1977) The preference for self-correction in the organisation of repair in conversation. *Language*, **53**, 361–382.

Searle, J.R. (1969) *Speech acts*. Cambridge: Cambridge University Press.

Sinclair, J.M. and Coulthard, R.M. (1975) *Towards an analysis of discourse*. Oxford: Oxford University Press.

Snow, C.E. (1994) Beginning from baby talk: Twenty years of research on input in interaction. In C. Gallaway and B.J. Richards (eds), *Input and interaction in language acquisition*. Cambridge: Cambridge University Press.

Tarplee, C. (1993) *Working on talk: The collaborative shaping of linguistic skills within child–adult interaction*. Unpublished DPhil thesis, Dept of Language and Linguistic Science, University of York, UK.

Tarplee, C. (1996) Working on young children's utterances: Prosodic aspects of repetition during picture labelling. In E. Couper-Kuhlen and M. Selting (eds), *Prosody in conversation*. Cambridge: Cambridge University Press.

Wootton, A.J. (1989) Remarks on the methodology of conversation analysis. In D. Roger and P. Bull (eds), *Conversation: An interdisciplinary perspective*. Clevedon: Multilingual Matters.

Chapter 2

Hm? What? Maternal repair and early child talk

JULIETTE CORRIN

Introduction

In adult conversation, open-class repair initiators such as hm? or what? provide a default response to troubles of hearing or understanding the prior speaker's turn without seeming to locate the trouble-source within it. It is left open to the prior speaker to assess the nature of the possible trouble and, accordingly, produce a repair that in some way repeats or reformulates the turn. In contrast to other forms of other-repair initiation that target a repeat or reformulation of a specific element(s) of the prior turn, minimal forms such as hm? and what? are thought to have limited conversational power (Schegloff *et al.* 1977).

Seen within the field of childhood conversation, the concept of conversational power has educational connotations. The capacity of the adult repair-initiating turn to locate the source of the trouble in the child's prior turn – and hence facilitate the necessary linguistic repair – is seen not only as an effective resolution of a local trouble, but also as an educational stimulus that shapes the child's learning of the adult language (Norrick 1991; Saxton 2005). Perhaps, for this reason, research has concerned itself primarily with forms of adult repair initiation that provide the child with linguistically specific 'feedback', such as the understanding check or recast (Saxton 2000), and explored the therepeutic potential of such repair initiations for children with speech and language disorder (Conti-Ramsden 1990; Chouinard and Clark 2003; Fey *et al.* 2003). Conversational power, then, is taken to equate to the specificity of adult feedback in locating the trouble-source within the child's prior turn. In this sense, open-class adult repair initiators such as hm? or what? have been viewed as inefficient devices (Langford 1981). For example, in Extract 2.1 the child (R) and the mother (M) are talking about telephones – both a real one visible on the other side of the room, and the toy one the child has in his hand.

Extract 2.1 *'your phone'*

```
1        R:    ((looks across room, points with extended arm))
               [əˈwɛːjəʊ] .    (a hello)
```

2   (0.6)

3   M: ((*turns to follow R's point, turns back to look at toy phone that R is holding in his lap*))
            that's my phone isn't it . (.) that's mummy's phone up there . (1.1) is
            somebody on <u>your</u> phone ?

4   (.)

5   →   R: ((*takes receiver of toy phone in his RH in upward movement, LH touching the
            phone base*))
            [jə'fəʊː].   (your phone)

6   (1.0)

7   →   M: hm?

8   (0.4)

9   →   R: ((*continues same actions with his hands, as above, but sits forward momentarily
            and looks up across the room towards his mother's phone*))
            [ɪsjɔ'fəʊː].   (I(t)'s your phone)

10   (0.8)

11 →   M: that's <u>my</u> phone .

The four-part sequence (lines 5–11) is organised as other-initiated self-repair:

> Position 1: a child turn treated by the adult as a trouble-source ('your phone')
> Position 2: an adult turn initiating open-class repair (' hm?')
> Position 3: a child turn that effects self-repair ('i(t)'s your phone')
> Position 4: an adult turn that receipts the self-repair ('that's <u>my</u> phone')

On the surface, the mother's use of hm? appears to prompt a mundane moment of self-repair for the child that passes off smoothly. He receives conversational feedback that his prior turn was problematic, but no linguistic feedback in the repair-initiating turn – either as to the nature of the trouble she experienced in understanding him or any candidate wording that might be a resource for designing the repair turn (Tarplee, this volume). And yet, there is evidence of language change. Note how the repair turn is reformulated from 'your phone' to 'i(t)'s your phone'.

Open-class repair-initiation sequences have been well documented in child–adult interaction as a social practice that is bound up with language learning in important ways. It was shown to be prevalent among Western families (Ochs 1988) and the second most common type of clarification after requests for confirmation (Gallagher 1981). Furthermore, children as young as one year of age have been found to respond to these moments of interactional accountability by producing repairs that systematically reflect their emerging language skills, both revising the trouble-source turn as illustrated in Extract 2.1, and also repeating it (Gallagher 1977; Garvey 1977; Anselmi *et al.* 1986; Corrin, forthcoming).

However, this body of research has developed in large part from experimental methods where young children are presented with contrived adult repair initiations (e.g. 'what?' spoken 20 times in one hour) during the course of play interaction. As a result, we know little about the natural occurrence of these sequences. More recently, this need has been addressed by conversation analytic work that explores the nature of other-initiated repairs experienced by children of 3 years of age (Soininen 2005; Soininen and Laakso, submitted), and traces change in the sequential character of the child's response to other-initiated repair forms across the early pre-school years (Forrester 2008).

Alongside these broader studies, the motivation of this report is to provide a specific focus on open-class repair initiation at an early stage of language development. The analysis considers why the child's turn becomes a source of trouble in the local moment of conversation. In Extract 2.1, for example, one questions why, in a context rich with established visual and linguistic reference (lines 1–4), the mother should find the child's turn 'your phone' (line 5) troublesome. Furthermore, the analysis considers the manner in which the child draws upon a variety of vocal and non-vocal resources to design a response that is sequentially sensitive as a next-turn following hm? or what?. In this respect, Extract 2.1 illustrates how, at line 9, the child evidently alters not only the linguistic design of his utterance 'i(t)'s your phone' but delivers it with a synchronous shift in eye gaze towards the 'phone in question. Researching such moments when the child is relied upon to 'talk the interaction out of trouble' promises to provide a valuable insight into the interdependence and reciprocity between learning about talk-in-interaction and learning about language.

Data

The single case described in this study, Robin, was the first-born, typically developing child of socio-economically advantaged parents from the South-East of England, living in a community where Standard English dialect was typical. His data forms part of a research corpus of seven similar children.[1] A weekly maternal diary of Robin's expressive language was kept over a 4-month period from c.a. 1;4 to 1;8. This inventory facilitated subsequent interpretation of spontaneous speech recordings. Between c.a. 1;7.8 and 1;9.3 the author-researcher videorecorded the dyad weekly, yielding 8 half-hour films. The video films sampled the mother and Robin playing with his customary range of toys in their home environment.

Transcripts were made of the turn-by-turn dialogue and play action between Robin and his mother for each video/audio recording. Through repeated video viewing all sequences of conversation were identified in which the mother had produced a next-turn repair initiation such as hm? or what? that invited Robin to produce a self-repair of his prior turn (Schegloff *et al.* 1977). These were transcribed in fine-grained detail using a combination of conversation analytic and IPA (IPA-SAM phonetic fonts 1996) systems of notation as witnessed in the work of Tarplee (1996) and Gardner (2006). A collection of 87 sequences were analysed in this way. For ease of interpretation, a lexical gloss is provided for Robin's turns within the extract transcriptions.

---

[1] This study was supported by a Postdoctoral Fellowship Award from the Economic and Social Research Council (ESRC): PTA- 026-27-0060.

Analysis

The occasioning of open-class repairs

While past literature has documented the existence and nature of open-class repair in adult–child talk, it has taken for granted the occasioning – in effect, why such moments become a relevant next action for the mother. Given the highly coordinated nature of object play and the strategies available to the mother for other-initiated repair by way of an understanding check or request to clarify, it becomes intriguing to consider what details of context could conspire to bring her to such a momentary standstill in intersubjectivity – that she, of apparent necessity, treats Robin's turn as being a non-usable next increment in the shared reality they are co-constructing through talk and play (Schegloff 1992).

The early stage of child development makes intelligibility an obvious candidate for analysis – that these are moments when the mother cannot make lexical sense of what she has heard the child say. In Robin's data, while this factor is contributory both in terms of phonological and syntactic/semantic turn construction, it does not provide a general account of the data; many turns are linguistically intelligible and yet are still met with open-repair initiation by the mother. In Extract 2.2, for example, Robin is completing a puzzle with his mother's help. His phrase 'go there?' at line 2 is one of his stock phrases for asking whether his intended placement of a puzzle piece is correct. Intelligibility is clearly not an issue. On finer inspection of the collection it transpires that a more subtle interplay between factors is at work involving turn sequencing and turn design; it is not simply a matter of what Robin says, but whether she can make sense of what his turn is 'doing' as a next action in the unfolding sequence of their interaction. These are the issues that are addressed in the analysis to follow.

Extract 2.2 *'piece go there'*

1			((*M extends LH slightly, holding a next puzzle piece*))
2	→	R:	((*takes an existing piece off the puzzle board*)) go there ?
3			(0.7)
4	→	M:	h:m: ?
5			(3.3)
6		R:	((*holding original puzzle piece in RH, reaches for puzzle piece that M is offering with LH*)) °piece (.) piece° ? (1.0) piece ?
7			(0.4)
8		M:	you want that piece ?
9			(0.5)
10		R:	((*places M's puzzle piece on the board*)) piece ?

11   (0.5)

12   M: it goes <u>the:re</u> do you think ?

With respect to turn sequencing, it is of interest that more than three-quarters of instances in the collection arise where Robin's trouble-source turn is produced as an *initiation*. Further, these initiations become problematic despite the fact that his mother is, in all but a small minority of cases, listening attentively and not speaking. In Extract 2.2, as in the data generally, the case for initiation is straightforward – Robin starts out with a turn that sets up a trajectory for a sequential response from his mother in next-turn position. In other less commonly occurring instances, the initiation is sequentially misplaced. In Extract 2.3 Robin and his mother have just engaged their attention with a picture book. On first inspection, Robin's trouble-source turn at line 4 has the sequential status of a response to his mother's prior question at line 2, 'what's in this book (1.1) what can you see'. However, closer inspection shows it to be an initiation in its own right. While the mother has finished with the business of seating and now turns her attention to the book's pictures, Robin is not settled. His trouble-source turn 'a read a book?' initiates a question of where he should best be seated for the book's reading; he wants to sit not on the floor but on her lap – and does so.

Extract 2.3 'read a book'

1   ((*M seated cross-legged on floor; R seated in front of M, holding book, turns to pass book to M behind him*))

2   M: ((*holds out closed book for R to view*))
              °what's in this book°. (1.1) °what can you see° .

3   (1.5)

4 → R: ((*takes book from M's hand, turns, gives book back to M*))
              a read a book ?

5   (1.0)

6   M: hm ?

7   (1.5)

8   R: ((*stands up; reverses onto M's lap*))
              go there ?

9   (1.6)

10   M: >°'ts it °<(.) sit down ,

In such instances the source of the mother's trouble with Robin's turn becomes clear. She expects a response to her question in next position – in this case for him to point to or name pictures he can see in the book – but instead is met with a somewhat tangential initiation 'a read a book?' where his forthcoming line of action in re-seating himself is not available as contextual interpretation. Yet these tangential initiations are very much the minority. To return to the canonical instance exemplified in earlier Extract 2.2 'go there?', there is no *prima facie* reason why sequentially well-positioned initiations such as this should prove to be a problematic turn action for the mother – unless, perhaps, it has something to do with the interactive work they accomplish.

In this respect, the analysis shows that Robin's initiating trouble-source turns are closely bound up with topic work. While the analysis of topic within mundane talk-in-interaction is notoriously complex (Atkinson and Heritage 1984), the physical situated-ness of early child–mother object play lends a degree of confidence to the interpretation: by and large, topic is what is being said about what is being done with toys in the here-and-now, and is therefore analytically transparent. In this way, the data suggests that Robin's initiations are prone to intersubjective vulnerability because they attempt a degree of topic progression, introducing new thematic elements to the current co-construction of meaning. In Extract 2.2 we noted how he shifts their line of joint action from the previous to a next relevant puzzle piece, asking his mother where this now topically proposed piece should go. And countless other instances fall into this canonical pattern: for example, he initiates talk about related aspects of the same piece of toy (e.g. from naming the puzzle piece to talk of its location), or contextually related pieces of the same toy (e.g. from the red key to the yellow key of a posting box) or contextually unrel-ated aspects of the same toy (e.g. from naming his soft toy tiger to talk of his action of bouncing on it). These can be likened to what are termed stepwise shifts (Jefferson 1984; Sacks 1992) in mundane adult talk where the new topic grows seamlessly from the old without an obvious boundary, but here, for the child, supported through the stepwise progression of play action that serves as a shared visual trajectory of topic development.

This point is taken to extreme in the few instances involving boundaried topic move-ment (Button and Casey 1984) where there is an unrelated shift. In fact one of the earli-est instances of open-repair in the data set arises when, quite without contextual forewarning, Robin suspends play to talk about the microphone that is recording his speech, which from his visual vantage point seems to be a ball shape. Note in Extract 2.4 how, despite the fact that his referential pointing gesture has succeeded in shifting top-ical focus at line 1, his turn at line 4 nevertheless becomes a source of trouble as he attempts to name the microphone lexically as 'ball', articulating it without the final 'l'. Here, then, we see how lexical/phonological issues may interact with topic shift to bring about problematic initiation.

Extract 2.4 *'ball'*

1		((*R points to microphone while looking at M*))
2	M:	don't worry about that .
3		(0.7)
4	→ R:	((*continues pointing to microphone, looks at microphone*)) [bɔː] . (ball)
5		((*continues pointing to microphone, looks to M*)) (1.2)
6	M:	((*tilts her head downward towards R*)) what?
7		(0.4)

| 8 | R: | ((*continues pointing to microphone, looks at microphone*)) |
| | | [bɔ:] .   (ball) |

| 9 | | (0.8)   ((*M looks across to microphone*)) |

| 10 | M: | ((*R's pointing gesture fades*)) |
| | | °> well is sort of<° does look a bit like a ball on the end hhhh . |

To review, the suggestion so far is that an interplay between linguistic intelligibility, sequence initiation and topic progression are contributory in explaining why, of Robin's turns, particular ones become a source of trouble sufficient to motivate an open-repair such as hm? or what? from his mother. But testing out this account across the data set shows it to be lacking in differentiation. Reconsidering Extract 2.2, 'go there?', will show that other important details of temporal alignment are interactionally relevant to the argument. A finer analytical lens uncovers a lack of temporal synchrony between the lines of action for talk and play.

In moments preceding line 1 Robin has noticed that his mother is holding a next possible piece of puzzle in her hand, balanced in a subtle gesture of proffering as she rests her wrist on her folded knee. His turn at line 2, 'go there?', is temporally synchronous with his play action of removing a puzzle piece from the board, but turns out not to be 'about' that piece. Rather, his turn refers to his *future* play action of positioning the piece that she is proffering, and that he is yet to take from her. What he appears to mean is: 'does that piece you are holding go there somewhere?'. It is the mis-coordination of talk and play that becomes a source of trouble for the mother's sense-making: she hears him say 'go there?' as he does just the opposite, not locating a piece within the puzzle but removing it. The trouble becomes resolved through his action of saying 'piece' several times while reaching for the piece that his mother proffers; now she understands that it is *her* piece of the puzzle that Robin's 'go there?' refers to and so she says 'you want that piece?' and later still 'you think it goes there?'. Note how this differs from Robin's temporally well-synchronised use of 'go there?' in Extract 2.5, allowing talk to progress smoothly.

Extract 2.5 *'go box'*

| 1 | M: | You can put it all in the box . |

| 2 | → R: | ((*holding puzzle piece poised over open box*)) |
| | | go there ? |

| 3 | M: | yup (.) in there . |

A further instance of temporal asynchrony becomes apparent on reviewing Extract 2.3 in which Robin and his mother are settling to a picture book. At line 1 he passes the book to his mother, indicating that she 'read' it to him, prompting her question at line 2 'what's in this book . what can you see'. His next turn 'a read a book?' is spoken as he takes the book and unexpectedly passes it back to her, leading to an obvious problem in her sense-making: he appears to be asking his mother to read a book he has already asked to be read, and been offered to be read. Once again, the source of trouble lies in the temporal coordination of talk and non-vocal action. His turn 'a read a book?' refers not to the book itself, but to the future action of reseating himself – in effect, about *where* the book is to be read. Had he said 'a read a book' while already partway through the non-vocal action of reseating himself on her lap, his locative meaning would have become contextually transparent. Note how his self-repair 'go there?' at line 8 is responsive to this locative issue.

By way of final example, this section is concluded by looking at Extract 2.6, which illustrates similar temporal asynchrony in design.

Extract 2.6 *'a go keys'*

1		((R touches blue posting house door))

2   →   R: ((*leans forward to pick up bunch of keys for posting house, briefly touches yellow one*))
             > [ədəgədəgəˈdiːs] < ?   (xxxxx keys)

3   (0.7)

4   M: h:m: ?

5   (0.4)

6   →   R: ((*picks up pink key, turns to posting house*))
             [əˈgəʊːdis] ?   (a go keys)

7   (0.6)

8   M: ((*turns posting house to bring pink door into view*))
             wh – what's the next colour .

9   (1.6)

10   R: ((*tries pink key in green door*))
             go there .

Robin is playing with a posting house in which each coloured door is opened with a corresponding colour of key. The posting house is oriented to face him so that his mother does not see him briefly touch the blue door (line 1). He then reaches for the bunch of keys that lie on the floor in an action of selecting the one that would fit. In synchrony he produces the turn [ədəgədəgəˈdiːs], which combines a pattern of syllables centred around 'go' and ends with the word 'keys'. Intelligibility is undoubtedly contributory here, but it is also apparent that sense-making is complicated by the lack of synchrony between his play and talk: this turn fits not with the current play action of moving to pick up the keys, but with his *next* play action of bringing the key up to the door in an anticipated action of opening it – the turn is a locative action. Note how his self-repair at line 6 simplifies and repeats the key lexical elements 'go' and 'keys' which, this time, are appropriately synchronous with the play action they narrate as he aligns the key and the key hole.

In summary, this section has revealed that the occasioning of open-repair initiation by the mother is responsive to a subtle combination of the child's turn features. Typically, these are turns where Robin initiates a sequence of talk to effect a degree of topic movement that weaves new thematic elements into their co-constructed meaning, with the additional vulnerability of producing a linguistically intelligible construction that is timed to afford his mother a meaningful temporal alignment between his actions of play and talk as a basis for her contextual sense-making. The interactional upshot is that their intersubjectivity is brought to a momentary standstill. Without maternal help to identify the source of the problem with his prior turn or a solution, these are true moments of other-initiated *self*-repair. It is up to Robin to 'talk the interaction out of trouble'. The following section examines his response.

The child's response to open-repair initiation

Two issues characterise the portrayal of the young child's response to maternal open-class repair initiation in the child language literature. The first of these is the reliability with which the child produces a repair response in next-turn position. The second concerns the nature of the self-repair where repeats of the trouble-source turn are contrasted with structural revisions. In this section, these same questions are reviewed, bringing to the surface details of non-vocal interaction that enrich the analysis.

Robin's data accords with past studies (Anselmi *et al.* 1986; Fagan 2008; Gallagher 1981; Garvey 1977; Wilcox and Webster 1980) in that he fulfils his social obligation to produce a spoken self-repair in next-turn position with moderate reliability, i.e. more than two-thirds of the time, the remainder being superseded by the dynamic flow of play without apparent interactional consequence. The yardstick for what counts as a child's response to open-repair initiation is traditionally taken to be a turn at talk – that the child says something in next-turn position which is, as far as the data can reveal, both designed and treated as a self-repair. Nor is this analytic focus surprising given our adult-centric perspective; we look for talk. Yet the non-verbal events of play are an equally important resource and line of action for the young child constructing a turn; in fact, in Robin's data the relationship is sometimes inverted such that the ongoing stream of play interaction is punctuated by bursts of talk, rather than the other way around. This casts an interesting light on instances classed in the child language literature as 'no repair response'. Consider Extract 2.7, for example.

Extract 2.7 'key go there'

1		((M reaches for posting house, puts it down in front of R, repositions herself))
2	R:	((R leaning over the posting house toy, trying to fit red key into key hole of red door))
		<u>a:</u> go there ? ('a' = pronominal referent for 'key')
3		(0.6)
4	M:	((R continues fitting key into key hole . . .))
		huh ?
5		((R's action continues . . .))
		(0.6)
6 →		((M leans forward to get a closer look))
		that's right that's the red one in the red door . (.) °well done° .

This is a familiar 'posting house' scene, taken in the moments preceding Extract 2.6 when the activity has just begun. Robin asks a question 'a: go there?' at line 2 as he leans forward trying to fit the red key into the red door lock. In this context his emphasised and prolonged 'a:' is a non-specific syllable that appears to carry pronominal reference for 'key', i.e. key go there? Although visually attentive, his mother cannot see his precise action from her position on the floor and she treats his turn as problematic, leaning forward to take a closer look. Unlike his temporally discrete burst of speech, Robin's play actions are continuous and provide an ongoing resource for the mother's contextual interpretation. There is no indication whatever that Robin redesigns his line of play action for the mother's recipiency *as* a self-repair; he simply continues the play action of turning the key without so much as eye contact. The importance lies, however, in how she treats it. Her two-part response 'that's right that's the red one in the red door (.) well done' orients not only to his play action as a solution to the trouble – 'that's the red one in the red door (.) well done' – but additionally to his prior trouble-source question 'a: go there?' for which she now provides an answer, 'that's right'. Despite the lack of verbal response as self-repair, Robin is very likely to be learning the interactional implications of having his actions treated as sequentially implicative within an other-initiated self-repair design. This is salutary in showing how our analytic attention to 'no response' instances can reveal the child's opportunities for learning: it is the mother's treatment of the unfolding course of action that is key.

The focus now turns to instances where the child does produce a spoken response in next-turn position. Here the literature has taken a linguistic stance in portraying self-repair as being either 'a repeat' or 'a revision' of the trouble-source turn. Of these two types, greater analytical attention has been given to structural revisions of the self-repair turn which provide insight into the child's early grammatical patterns; not unexpectedly, lexical repeats have held little interest for the linguist. However, as becomes apparent in the analysis to follow, lexical repeats may involve the re-doing of phonetic and non-vocal turn features relevant to the action of repair that raise their profile of interactional importance.

Repeat repairs

In Extract 2.8, Robin and his mother are looking at the shapes from his shape-sorting box. At line 1 he names the current shape as 'fish' and his mother acknowledges this at line 3 'that's right that's a fish'. The trouble-source in this instance comes at line 5 when Robin says 'more fish?'. Note that the spoken words are accompanied by eye gaze to his mother and a simultaneous and rapid gesture of his right hand, which reaches outwards and slightly behind his body as if to signal that another 'fish' might be found elsewhere in the room/house. In response to huh? he repeats the words 'more fish?' but re-does other aspects of the design: his right hand holds its outward posture to signal the ongoing engagement with the search for another 'fish', while his eye gaze shifts downward to his toys on the floor and his head makes a slight side-to-side searching movement. Additionally, there are phonetic changes. The first speaking of 'more fish?' is clearly articulated at a loudness that matches surrounding talk, ending with a marked pitch rise on 'fish'; the second speaking is a comparative downgrade with diminished loudness, incomplete frication of 'sh' in 'fish' and a less prominent pitch rise. The self-repair is successful, allowing the mother to produce a more facilitative type of other-initiated repair in the form of an understanding check 'you want another fish?'.

In moving the analysis beyond a linguistic focus in this way, it becomes clear that lexical repeats are the same words but by no means the same turn – by virtue of a unique sequential position each is a distinct social object in the interaction. We witness how phonetic aspects of articulation combine with posture, eye gaze and gesture as resources for Robin's construction of self-repair. In adult talk, it has been found that sequentially well-fitted repeat repairs are systematically produced as a phonetic upgrade of the trouble-source turn (Curl 2004). In Robin's data, however, there is no indication of such orderliness; phonetic features are variable within the dynamic mix of resources and, as in Extract 2.8, may be downgraded.

Extract 2.8 *'more fish'*

1		R:	((*takes shape out of posting box, extends LH to show M*)) fi:sh .
2			(0.4)
3		M:	(hhh) that's (hh) right (hh) that's a fish . (h)
4			((*holding fish LH, looks down-left to floor*)) (1.6)
5	→	R:	((*looks up to M + gestures outward and behind with RH*)) <u>mo:re</u> fish ?
6			(0.4)
7		M:	((*leans in toward R, tilts head up*)) huh?
8			(0.7)
9	→		((*looks down at posting box, slight scanning head movement, R and L arms held open and outward*)) °<u>more</u> fish°?
10			(.)
11		M:	you want <u>another</u> fish ?
12			(.)
13		R:	yis .
14			=
15		M:	yeah I don't know where I've got anymore fishes .

Revision repairs

While repeats occur in Robin's data, revisions are more common. The issue of why children tend to repeat or revise in response to other-initiated repair has been debated in the child language literature. One approach has been to relate the type of self-repair response to the type of other-repair initiation. Anselmi *et al.* (1986), for example, report that neutral queries such as 'what?' (here called open-class repair) typically elicit repeats while specific queries (*C: doll A: doll where?*) elicit revisions, this being taken to indicate the child's sensitivity to the possible nature of the listener's trouble in understanding the prior turn. Another perspective has been to consider the type of self-repair response to be an either/or choice, both of which might potentially help the child to pursue this goal within a social context: '. . . naïve speakers might try either strategy available to them' (Fagan 2008: 65). Interestingly, these studies have presented the child with contrived repair initiations. As the following analysis of Robin's data suggests, our understanding of which trouble-source turns get repeated and which get revised promises to come from analysing the occasioning of the mother's spontaneous repair initiations – a context where we witness the outcome to be a locally governed response for the child, rather than the deployment of some general conversational strategy.

Further, there has been considerable interest in the linguistic nature of self-repair in terms of the comparative frequency with which the child uses the available patterns of revision (e.g. addition, omission, replacement or re-ordering) and with which constituent elements become revised (e.g. verb, noun, adjective) – these outcomes being taken as reflective of the child's emerging structural knowledge of the language (Gallagher 1981). For Robin, however, it is the sequential context of the self-repair that appears to shape his linguistic revision.

In Extract 2.9, for example, Robin is looking at a picture book that has balloons graphically illustrated on its front cover. Robin wants to know whether the balloons can be taken off and so he produces the following succession of single words, 'balloon. uppies. more. off', as one prosodically cohesive turn (Corrin *et al.* 2001). His mother cannot make sense of his meaning. Following her hm?, he produces the turn 'off?', which she accepts as a self-repair, then comes in with her assessment of his proposal 'well those are balloons they're stuck in your book darling (.) they don't come off'. In linguistic terms Robin's self-repair would be counted as an instance of omission: he quite clearly omits the first three elements of the prior turn, leaving only the fourth word 'off' – the preposition that functions to denote the locative action he intends. But this is to assume that, for Robin at this local moment of interaction, omission is in some way an equivalent revision option alongside addition, re-ordering and replacement. Through the lens of conversation analysis, this is shown not to be the case.

The sequence begins after a prolonged silence during which Robin has selected the book and seated himself on the floor. His mother is seated adjacent and faces him, watching his actions. At this point Robin's succession of single words begins (lines 1–7). Note how Robin begins to finger the balloon with his left thumb at line 3 'uppies', and how his mother leans in to take a closer look at his actions at line 5 while his turn is still in progress. Then at line 7, note how Robin looks up to his mother to mark and visually direct the moment of turn completion with the final word of the succession 'off'. He further solicits her response by continuing to thumb the picture, indicating the as-yet-incomplete nature of things.

Extract 2.9 *'balloon up'*

```
1       R:   ((holding book))
             balloon ,
```

2		(.)
3		((*L thumb fingering the balloon picture*)) uppies , (up)
4		(.)
5		((*M leans forward, looking at book cover*)) more ,
6		(.)
7		((*continues action of L thumb + looks to M*)) off ?
8		(.)
9	M:	hm ?
10		=
11 →	R:	((*continues rubbing action and holds gaze to M*)) off ?
12		(.)
13	M:	((*R and M looking down at book cover*)) well those are balloons they're stuck in your book darling (0.7) they don't come off .

During the course of the trouble-source turn some subtle interactional business has already been successfully conducted. Robin has introduced the balloons as a topical focus by saying the word and referencing them with his left thumb. His mother has become posturally attentive and visually engaged with the balloon picture. At line 7, on suddenly looking up at her, Robin witnesses their collaboration – he sees her looking at the picture he is rubbing with his thumb. This is pivotal to the design of his self-repair to follow. For Robin, at this moment, two aspects of meaning become established as inter-subjectively 'given' – firstly, the balloon and, secondly, the intention of some action rela-tive to the balloon – as yet not successfully communicated. Witnessing his mother's sustained visual attention to the balloon and to his gestural action of rubbing it, Robin is now afforded a considerable economy of self-repair – he need say only 'off' to convey what is new in his semantic focus. Evidence for such an interpretation is warranted by noting (a) the adults use of the qualification 'well', (b) explicit reference to 'stuck' that presupposes her understanding of his gestural thumb action and (c) explicit reference not just to 'off' but to 'come off'.

To return to the issue of his options for revision of the trouble-source turn, it becomes apparent that in sequential context Robin's need for self-repair of 'balloon – uppies – more – off' would not be effectively met by the addition, replacement or re-ordering of turn elements. The addition of elements would be tautologous. The re-ordering of ele-ments would not satisfy the required semantic focus; at this age, successive single-word utterances are marked canonically by stress on the turn-final word (Wells and Corrin 2004), thus a re-ordering to produce 'off-<u>balloon</u>' would produce a stress on what is already semantically given, the balloon. Finally, the replacement of elements is not necessary since 'off' is already semantically precise. Following this line of argument suggests a caution in the analytic assumption that omission, addition, replacement and re-ordering operate for the child as equivalent options for revision, in particular where frequency counts of instances across these categories are then taken as an index of grammatical maturity (Gallagher 1977, 1981). How the trouble-source turn gets revised is evidently a matter of local sequential organisation.

Different repairs

In this final section the analysis considers a type of response where Robin does not repeat or revise his trouble-source turn, but rather produces a turn that is linguistically different, albeit semantically related. These were unexpected in the data; indeed, there is no apparent evidence in the literature; understandably, up to now, repair has been synonymous with repetition and revision.

In Extract 2.10 Robin and his mother are completing a familiar puzzle of large pieces. The sequence is simple: he asks whether the piece he has in his hand should go in a particular location; she says 'no' and advises him. The key question analytically is whether Robin would have gone on to say 'a there' anyway, or whether it was produced as a self-repair in response to hm?. In this instance, phonetic detail shows it to be the former: Robin's production of 'da piece' is the first of two increments – 'go there?' being the intended second. However, he presents his mother with a conflicting set of turn-completion cues. Although ending the element [da'pɪsəʔh] with a glottal stop that typically indicates turn-holding (Corrin *et al.* 2001; Local and Kelly 1986) he produces a pitch fall on the final vowel that extends into the post-glottal exhalation. She appears to orient to this prosodic change as indicative of turn-completion (Wells *et al.* 2004) and comes in with 'hm?'.

Extract 2.10 *'that piece'*

```
1  →  R:   ((holding puzzle piece in right hand))
           da piece .        [da'pɪsəʔh]

2            (0.9)

3     M:   ((sitting back; watching R))
           hm?

4            (0.4)

5  →  R:   ((lowers piece towards a position in the puzzle))
           a the:re ?        [ə'daː] ?

6            (0.4)

7     M:   ((leans forward and points to puzzle location))
           n:e :h : : ( .) look that piece goes round there (. ) to fill in that piece (.)
           don't you think ?
```

In this important sense, it cannot be claimed that Robin's next turn, 'a there', was produced *as* a self-repair. With added loudness and a marked pitch rise/fall it is hearable as the semantic focus of his two-part turn and its completion. Yet Robin learns from this interactional moment in two different ways. He experiences the outcome of failing to use mid-pitch for turn-holding by having his mother's premature incoming following his first turn, and the outcome of having his mother treat the sequence as an other-initiated self-repair following his second turn. Note how her response is oriented to both elements of his turn, namely 'the piece' and 'go there' combining these in the phrase 'look that piece goes round there'.

If it is true that young children can pull off self-repair using a linguistically different turn in next-position then there should be evidence that such instances arise by interactional design, not merely by interactional chance, as in Extract 2.10. This is the case in the data. And yet, as will be seen in the final Extract 2.11, the status of these self-repairs remains curious.

Extract 2.11 *'sheep'*

1		M:	((*giving sheep to R*))
			oh no no (.) here we go (3.3) how many sheep have you got now .
2			(0.4)
3	→	R:	((*holding sheep, looks up to M*))
			[əˈpuba:] ? (a 'sheep')
4			(0.5)
5		M:	((*R continues to look at M, holding sheep*))
			hm?
6			(0.7)
7	→	R:	((*points to bag out of which M has just taken sheep*))
			[ɡəʊˈda] ? (go there)
8			(.)
9		M:	no that's definitely it (1.0) that's all the sheep I've got .

Robin and his mother are exploring a bag of farm animal Duplo characters. He is interested in the 'sheep' and refers to them consistently as 'pooh baa' – this being a home-grown combination of 'baa' for sheep and 'pooh' for 'Pooh Bear'. While holding the sheep in his hand he looks up to his mother and says 'a pooh baa?'. This becomes the trouble-source. Following her hm? repair initiation he points to the bag out of which she has just taken the sheep and says 'go there?'. Now she understands that he is asking whether there are any more sheep in her bag. As with Extract 2.10 the key analytical question is whether Robin is going on to say 'go there?' in any event, or whether both 'a pooh baa?' and 'go there?' stand as complete turns that designedly occasion and respond to the mother's hm?. A closer look at the prosodic and non-vocal turn features affirm the latter. In this case it can be argued that 'a pooh baa?' is a complete turn by virtue of (a) a long final vowel with no glottal closure and complete expiration of breath; (b) a steady pitch rise on 'baa'; and (c) sustained transfer of eye gaze to his mother as the turn completes. Note also that Robin is physically and vocally still during the time that his mother responds with hm?. Then comes his next turn 'go there?'. And here there is a twist to the story. While 'go there?' stands as a complete turn with respect to its prosodic contour and gestural point, there is evidence that it is produced *relative to* the prior turn 'a pooh baa?': it is louder and spoken with a higher pitch rise. When heard together, the two are prosodically cohesive and provide a topic and comment structure: 'a pooh baa – go there?'. These same prosodic features systematically define the collection of such instances.

While the evidence is neat, the interpretation poses a challenge. In what sense can we claim 'go there?' to be a self-repair of 'a pooh baa?'? It is positioned as such and treated as such by the mother. From her perspective, then, the sequence is unidimensional – it is straightforwardly an instance of other-initiated self-repair. But for Robin it appears that there is more than one sequential dimension. He pulls off a turn that functions to do relational semantic work typical of unproblematic progressions of talk (Corrin 2002), but places it in self-repair position. At the risk of attributing psychologies, he must there-fore assume that the first topic-delivering turn 'a pooh baa' was both heard and under-stood in context in order to pave the way for the comment-delivering turn to follow 'go there?'. In this sense, it is not the trouble-source turn itself that gets repaired. Rather, 'go there?' repairs the overall semantic framework required for his line of action to become intelligible – and it does so through completion of the sequence – what one might term a 'completion repair'. For young children as yet unable to fluently produce a multi-word turn such as 'a pooh baa go there?' under a single intonation contour, the incremental two-turn structure inadvertently provided by the trouble-source + self-repair sequence might afford a valuable moment for language learning.

Conclusion

This report has aimed to provide an overview of the sequential organisation of open-class repair-initiation sequences in talk-in-interaction between a mother and her typic-ally developing toddler. The density of the sequences within the data set at 87 within 4 hours of footage indicates that it can, at least in some dyads, be an interactional prac-tice contributory in shaping the child's experience of other-initiated self-repair and of language learning at a the age of one-and-a-half to two years. The analysis has made the following key observations:

● The occasioning of open-class repair initiation by the mother is motivated by a subtle interplay of sequencing and design factors within the child's turn. One main source of vulnerability is a sequential move by the child to initiate talk that accomplishes a degree of topic movement. This concurs with CA literature on repair initiation in mundane adult conversation which describes how repair is 'systematically relevant' in first sen-tences in topic-initial turns or in topic shift position (Schegloff 1979). In this sense, the process of learning is self-serving. It seems that to progress talk the child becomes vulnerable to the experience of other-initiated self-repair which is itself a mechanism for the learning of that talk. Additionally, the child's turn is made vulnerable by the temporal misalignment between what is being said in the turn at talk and what is being done with the objects of play. Indeed, it is paradoxical that the physical resources of play, while providing a contextual framework for the mother's sense-making, also complicate the child's task in aligning the temporal unfolding of these concurrent courses of action. Finally, the linguistic intelligibility of the child's turn is contributory.

- The child's response to open-class repair initiation is evidently more than a matter of 'saying something' in next-turn position. Even where there is no vocal response, there remains an opportunity to overcome the trouble presented by the trouble-source turn through recourse to the intelligibility of the unfolding line of play action. This enables the mother to preserve the sequential order of the repair sequence and treat the child's actions as consequential by producing a receipting turn; she honours the preference for self-repair (Schegloff *et al.* 1977) and affords him an apprenticeship in the sequential organisation of this social practice. Where the child does provide a spoken response, repairs are of three types: 'repeat', 'revision' or 'different'.

- Repeat repairs are shown to be somewhat misnamed. Important vocal prosodic and non-vocal changes are implicated in effecting the reparative action of the turn in combination with lexical repetition. It is apparent that these are traded for their dynamic relevance; for instance, the vocal prosodics of the reparative turn may be downgraded while the gestural aspect is upgraded, relative to the originating trouble-source turn. As indicated in the detailed work of Curl (2004), there is a rich line of research that flows from investigation both of prosodic and articulatory aspects of repeat repairs.

- Revision repairs predominate in the data, involving addition, omission, replacement and re-ordering of turn elements. The analysis tells a cautionary tale of sequential organisation. It transpires that, far from being equivalent options for the child, the nature of revision is locally determined. What counts is the relationship between the design of the trouble-source turn and the child's assessment of the mother's sense-making in the sequence thus far. What gets added, omitted, replaced or re-ordered is a matter of local efficiency for the repair of semantic focus. As with repeat repairs, non-vocal aspects of turn design are consequential in that aspects such as gesture and eye gaze may be sustained or themselves revised. For the child, these resources serve to shape the mother's focus of attention during the repair process as well as being actions implicated in the design of the repair turn.

- Different repairs were an unexpected finding arising from inductive inspection of the data. Two scenarios are evident. There are accidental moments in which the child's intended but misprojected increment of talk is treated by the mother as a self-repair following her intrusive hm? or what?. However, there are also well-designed moments in which the mother's repair initiator inadvertently provides the interactional structure required for child to produce a further increment of talk. A similar phenomenon is reported in the smooth progression of talk during the transition from single to multi-word speech where intervening adult turns scaffold the child's build-up of meaning increment by increment (Scollon 1979).

In these respects the report has shown, contrary to indications in the literature (Schegloff *et al.* 1977; Langford 1981), that open-class repair initiation may hold a particular developmental power for the language-learning child. Paradoxically, it is the very fact that the repair initiation does *not* locate the source of the trouble within the child's prior turn that brings this opportunity: open-class initiation gives the child the opportunity for what one might call 'open-class repair'. The child is required to consider the adequacy of his prior turn – to re-process it *as* a trouble-source within prior sequential context, invoking skills such as working memory, turn-tracking and perspective-taking, and 'do' a self-repair that in some way enables the turn to become a next increment of shared understanding in the social reality their playtime collaboratively constructs. This is not true to the same extent in the case of facilitative repair initiations such as understanding checks and clarification requests where the mother's turn delivers a 'trouble' but also a possible corrective solution (Saxton 2000). There would appear to be a principle of evolutionary efficiency at work. It seems that the high interactional demands of self-repair following open-class initiation deliver high learning rewards. The child not only learns about self-repair as a self-righting mechanism for the organisation of language use in social interaction (Schegloff *et al.* 1977) and about the manipulation of speech and language units for turn construction, but most importantly about their interdependency.

References

Anselmi, D., Tomasello, M. and Acunzo, M. (1986) Young children's responses to neutral and specific contingent queries. *Journal of Child Language*, **13**, 135–144.

Atkinson, J. and Heritage, J. (1984) *Structures of social action: Studies in conversation analysis*. Cambridge: Cambridge University Press.

Button, G. and Casey, N. (1984) Generating topic: The use of topic initial elicitors. In J.M.Atkinson and J. Heritage (eds), *Structures of social action: Studies in conversation analysis* (pp. 167–189). Cambridge: Cambridge University Press.

Chouinard, M. and Clark, E. (2003) Adult reformulations of child errors as negative evidence. *Journal of Child Language*, **30**, 637–669.

Conti-Ramsden, G. (1990) Maternal recasts and other contingent replies to language-impaired children. *Journal of Speech and Hearing Disorders*, **55**, 262–274.

Corrin J. (2002) *The emergence of early grammar: A conversation analytic perspective.* Department of Human Communication Science, University College London.

Corrin J. (2009) Maternal repair initiation at MLU Stage I: The developmental power of 'hm?'. *First Language* (Forthcoming).

Corrin J., Tarplee, C. and Wells, B. (2001) Interactional linguistics and language development: A conversation analytic perspective on emergent syntax. In M.Selting and E. Couper-Kuhlen (eds), *Studies in interactional linguistics* (pp. 199–225). Amsterdam: John Benjamins Publishing.

Curl, T. (2004) 'Repetition repairs': The relationship of phonetic structure and sequence organization. In E.Couper-Kuhlen and C.E. Ford (eds), *Sound patterns in interaction* (pp. 273–298). Amsterdam: John Benjamins.

Fagan, M. (2008) Toddlers' persistence when communication fails: Response motivation and goal substitution. *First Language*, **28**, 55–69.

Fey, M., Long, S. and Finestack, L. (2003) Ten principles of grammar facilitation for children with specific language impairments. *Journal of Speech-Language Pathology*, **12**, 3–15.

Forrester, M. (2008) The emergence of self-repair: A case study of one child during the early preschool years. *Research on Language and Social Interaction*, **41**, 99–128.

Gallagher, T. (1977) Revision behaviours in the speech of normal children developing language. *Journal of Speech and Hearing Research*, **20**, 303–318.

Gallagher, T. (1981) Contingent query sequences within adult-child discourse. *Journal of Child Language*, **8**, 51–62.

Gardner, H. (2006) Training others in the art of therapy for speech sound disorders: An interactional approach. *Child Language Teaching and Therapy*, **22**, 27–46.

Garvey, C. (1977) The contingent query: A dependent act in conversation. In M. Lewis and L. Rosenblum (eds), *Interaction, conversation and the development of language* (pp. 63–94). New York: Wiley.

IPA-SAM Phonetic Fonts (1996) International Phonetics Association. http://www.arts.gla.ac.uk/IPA/ipa.html

Jefferson, G. (1984) On stepwise transition from talk about a trouble to inappropriately next-positioned matters. In J.M. Atkinson and J. Heritage (eds), *Structures of social action* (pp. 191–222). Cambridge: Cambridge University Press.

Langford, D. (1981) The clarification request sequence in conversation between mothers and their children. In P. French and M. Maclure (eds), *Adult-child conversation* (pp. 159–174). London: Croom Helm.

Local, J. and Kelly, J. (1986) Projection and 'silences': Notes on phonetic and conversational structure. *Human Studies*, **9**, 185–204.

Norrick, N.R. (1991) On the organization of corrective exchanges in conversation. *Journal of Pragmatics*, **16**, 59–83.

Ochs, E. (1988) *Culture and language development: Language acquisition and language socialization in a Samoan village.* Cambridge: Cambridge University Press.

Sacks, H. (1992) *Lectures on conversation: February* (1971; vol. 1). Oxford: Blackwell.

Saxton, M. (2000) Negative evidence and negative feedback: Immediate effects on the grammaticality of child speech. *First Language*, **20**, 221–252.

Saxton, M. (2005) 'Recast' in a new light: Insights for practice from typical language studies. *Child Language Teaching and Therapy*, **21**, 23–38.

Schegloff, E.A. (1979) The relevance of repair to syntax-for-conversation. *Syntax and Semantics*, **12**, 261–286.

Schegloff, E.A. (1992) Repair after next turn: The last structurally provided defence of intersubjectivity in conversation. *American Journal of Sociology*, **98**, 1295–1345.

Schegloff, E.A., Jefferson, G. and Sacks, H. (1977) The preference for self-correction in the organization of repair in conversation. *Language*, **53**, 361–382.

Scollon, R. (1979) A real early stage: An unzipped condensation of a dissertation on child language. In E.Ochs and B. Schieffelin (eds), *Developmental pragmatics* (pp. 215–227). London: Academic Press.

Soininen, M. (2005) *Three-year-olds problem turns in mother-child interaction: A study of mother-initiated repair sequences.* Department of Speech Sciences, University of Helsinki.

Soininen, M. and Laakso, M. (2009; submitted) Mother-initiated repair sequences in interactions of 3-year-old children. *First Language*.

Tarplee, C. (1996) Working on young children's utterances: Prosodic aspects of repetition during picture labelling. In E.Couper-Kuhlen and M. Selting (eds), *Prosody in conversation: Interactional studies* (pp. 406–435). Cambridge: Cambridge University Press.

Wells, B. and Corrin, J. (2004) Prosodic resources, turn-taking and overlap in children's talk-in-interaction. In E. Couper-Kuhlen and C.E. Ford (eds), *Sound patterns in interaction* (pp. 119–144). Amsterdam: Benjamins.

Wilcox, M. and Webster, E. (1980) Early discourse behaviour: An analysis of children's responses to listener feedback. *Child Development*, **51**, 1120–1125.

Chapter 3

Ethnomethodology and adult–child conversation: Whose development?

MICHAEL FORRESTER

Introduction

In research that adopts a conversation analytic orientation to the study of children's talk-in-interaction, the question of what constitutes an ethnomethodological approach to development remains unexamined. While significant work is beginning to emerge which describes, at a fine-grained level of detail, the skills and competencies that children exhibit when they are learning how to talk, the manner in which such descriptions may or may not presuppose certain theoretical accounts of development has yet to be addressed. As critics within the sociology of childhood indicate, the concept of development, particularly the idea of natural development, can engender an overemphasis on something not being quite right: children exhibiting social practices indicative of a 'developmental lag' and, in some important respects, somehow being deficient in some manner compared to adults. This seems to be particularly the case with children categorised as 'atypical'.

In what follows my first aim is to outline a number of observations regarding the interrelationships between conversation analytic studies of adult–child interaction, notions of development and the question of what constitutes membership in ethmometho-dology. The underlying question being posed is whether the area needs to distinguish between research that employs conversation analysis as a methodology in the service of asking developmental questions, and work that one might call developmentally focused ethmomethodologically informed conversation analysis. In order to understand what might distinguish these two sub-themes of research, my second aim is to highlight the advantages and challenges of adopting a specifically ethnomethodological conversation–analytic approach to the study of adult–child interaction.

Ethnomethodology and conversation analysis

Within psychology, education, sociolinguistics and related areas of applied social and health sciences concerned with understanding naturally occurring talk between adults and children, there are indications that conversation analysis (CA) is becoming one of the main methodologies of choice. Primarily the form adopted is the sequence-focused examination of conversational practices and, less often, membership categorisation analysis – an additional, and some might say complementary, form of analysis outlined in the original work of Harvey Sacks and colleagues during the late 1960s and 1970s (Sacks 1992; Hester and Eglin 1997). Historically it may help to remember that CA was one form of ethnomethodology or, rather, the ethnomethodological project as originally conceived and developed by Garfinkel and his colleagues (Garfinkel 1967; Turner 1974). Ethnomethodology emerged from within sociology and its proponents exhibited a shared sense of dissatisfaction with macro-level explanations of sociological phenomena, particularly proposals that people's everyday behaviours and actions could be linked deterministically to notions of class, race, gender and other similar structural constructs. Central to the ethnomethodological enterprise is the focus on the myriad social actions produced by members of a culture that constitute their sense-making practices locally *in situ*. Simultaneously, macro-theory scepticism is exhibited in the methodological injunction that analytic concerns, interpretations and commentary should not go beyond demonstrable evidence which shows that some participant members display an orientation to whatever orderliness, rule, convention or organisation is said to be in place when members are pursuing their sense-making everyday practices. Commenting on descriptions of ethnomethdology, and the significance of naturally occurring everyday activities, Livingston (1987: 10) notes:

> The activities are reflexive, self-organizing, organized entirely in situ, locally. That organization is not God-given, not determined by the innate properties of mind, and only obfuscated by referring to it as socialized or learned behaviour – as if those terms explained what, in detail, was actually being done and, therefore, what the participants were supposed to know or to have learned.

Leaving aside for now the challenges this perspective raises for attempts at describing or theorising about development within an ethnomethodologically informed CA approach to the study of children's talk, Livingston (1987: 11) provides us with a comprehensive description of ethnomethdology, one that emphasises the inherent reflexivity between the production of practical actions and their independence with members' own recognition of their being accountable for such actions:

> . . . [the] . . . central issue and the central research problem is the examination of the unwitting, without extrinsic motivation, production of the ordinary social object. By finding what the practically accountable social object consists of as a produced object – as the achievement of its local production cohort – the ethnomethodologist simultaneously begins to find what it means to be a member of that cohort – that is, what a member of a production cohort actually is . . . [it is a] massive domain of phenomena – the domain of practical action and practical reasoning. It is this omnipresent domain of *practical methods*, through which and wherein people *make of the things they are doing* the *things that they accountably are*, that the ethnomethodologist seeks to investigate. By examining those methods in the material detail of their always-idiosyncratic embodiments, the ethnomethodologist seeks to understand those methods in and as that same, endlessly diversified, identifying specificity (*emphasis* added).

This is a far-reaching project or enterprise, in fact it is potentially all-encompassing with respect to the study of social interaction. As one form of ethnomethodology, conversation analysis takes to heart the focus on members' methods of sense-making alongside the methodological injunction that analytic criteria should be demonstrably participant-oriented. At the same time, conversation should be seen as dynamic action and not language in the formal linguistic object sense. Heritage (1984: 139) comments that understanding language is not in the first instance a matter of understanding sentences, but actions, 'constructively interpreted in relation to their context'. Additionally, the conversation analyst has to approach the study of conversation or talk-in-interaction with unmotivated attention, otherwise there is considerable danger that analysis becomes distorted by the analyst's preconceived interpretations, failing consistently to focus solely on participant-members' orientations to what constitutes sense-making in context. And it is not simply just a case of showing, for example, that a context such as 'the doctor's surgery' is something that forms part of the general background of an ongoing interaction, but specifically that *this* element bears on the particulars of what is going on. Schegloff (1992: 111) highlights what this issue means for the analyst:

> Even if we can show by analysis of the details of the interaction that some character-ization of the context or the setting in which the talk is going on (such as 'in the hospi-tal') is relevant for the parties, that they are oriented to the setting so characterized, there remains another problem, that is to show how the context or the setting (the local social structure) *in that aspect*, is procedurally consequential to the talk. How does the fact that the talk is being conducted in some setting (e.g. 'the hospital') issue in any consequence for the shape, form, trajectory, content, or character of the interaction that the parties conduct? (*emphasis* added).

Similarly, Wowk (2007) points out that for EM/CA, invocation of 'context' is not theoretically derived but is to be argued from the demonstrably local orientations of members themselves in and through their practical and methodological enquiries. Wowk cites in support, Lynch's (1993) critique of structural (i.e. external) overinterpretation (Wowk 2007: 125):

> Instead of trying to overcome heterogeneity by theoretically postulating an homo-geneous domain . . . ethnomethodologists attempt to investigate a patchwork of 'orderliness' without assuming that any single orderly arrangement reflects or exem-plifies a determinant set of organization laws, historical stages, norms, or paradig-matic orders of meaning. They do not deny the historical and social 'contexts' in which social action and interaction take place; rather, they insist that specification of such contexts is invariably bound to a local context of relevances.

Ethnomethodology and development

For CA work that is both developmentally focused and ethnomethodologically informed such observations present a fairly significant challenge. When explicating the nature of members' methods represented through their spontaneous production of recognisably accountable social objects, in what sense does current adult–child EM/CA work high-light the requirement that the notion, construct or concept of 'development' as a specific participant-member orientation, should demonstrably bear on the interaction?

Sketching out this issue in more detail, we might note that within the sociology of childhood and discursive psychology there are a number of writers and critics who question the value of the concept 'development' and related notions of childhood, stages of development, critical periods and similar constructs (James and Prout 1996; Edwards and Stokoe 2004). Certainly, there is no shortage of competing accounts or discourses of development – the logical–epistemological variety of Piaget; the social–semiotic inter-actionism of Vygotsky; the numerous frameworks found in cognitive science and child language research; the various themes and topics central to psychoanalytic theory; and the socialisation theories favoured in sociology, social policy and sociolinguistics. Burman (1994), however, argues that developmentalism consists of the production of, and reliance on, explanatory statements concerning the regulation of change across the life-span – statements that tend to gloss over the observation that development is always somebody's work and the 'production' of the child and childhood are made through human activity. It is only in the relatively recent past that critiques of developmental discourses are to be found in the social sciences. Among other criticisms, what is often overlooked in the various discourses is that the notion of development itself often presupposes the idea of something 'getting better' or 'becoming more' or being 'qualita-tively richer' and, more often than not something that is natural and just happens.

With reference, then, to the emergent CA on adult–child interaction, we can raise the question of whether there is a need to distinguish between a research focus that is primarily 'developmentally informed' – that is, the methodology of CA is being employed in order to map out or highlight developmental profiles of this or that particular skill – or whether the focus is 'ethnomethodologically informed'. In other words, under what conditions do participant members themselves orient towards the host of constructs, ideas and social practices associated with the social object 'development', 'childhood' or 'stage-of-life'?

Given the observation that most studies fall into the first category above, we can turn instead to the problem of articulating what an ethnomethodologically informed devel-opmental focus might be. We need first to remind ourselves what membership means in ethnomethodology and conversation analysis (EM/CA). There are at least two consider-ations: first, what constitutes being a member of a particular culture and being treated as such by other members; and, second, how do we conceptualise members' skills, com-petencies or abilities? Turning to definitions of membership, Garfinkel and Sacks (1970: 339), in an earlier formulation of the concept, noted:

> The notion of member is the heart of the matter. We do not use the term to refer to a person. It refers instead to mastery of natural language, which we understand in the following way. We offer the observation that persons, because of the fact that they are heard to be speaking in a natural language somehow are heard to be engaged in the objective production and objective display of commonsense knowledge of every-day activities as observable and reportable phenomena.

Childhood and cultural membership

Whatever membership might be, it involves performance, for instance, in doing whatever is understood by others as the production and display of commonsense knowledge of every-day activities as potentially observable phenomena. Displays of commonsense knowledge are closely linked to the mastery of language, i.e. although the concept of member does not necessarily refer to a person, it is associated with whatever is meant by mastery of language (recognisable by others as such). This formulation, taken literally, has some curious implications, the most important here being: it is couched in terms of 'ability'. Thus membership may be tacitly granted or ascribed in virtue of presumptions of ability – in other words, of presumed potential to perform appropriately. For CA studies of adult–child interaction we need to be particularly aware that there is often a certain slippage from description to argumentation, especially when, to paraphrase Livingston (1987), the 'fascination' with children's competencies glosses the implicit presupposition that somehow children's experiences are 'incomplete'. Some years ago, Mackay (1974: 182) noted:

> The terms adult and children are borrowed from the common-sense world by sociologists, but if they are viewed as theoretical formulations, then a very serious problem emerges. That is, to suggest theoretically that there are adults and children is to imply that to pass from one stage to the other is to pass from one ontological order to another. The passage from one ontological order to another is also suggested in the formulation of the world as static and as constituted by discrete stages – childhood and adulthood, incompleteness and completeness, lack of agreement and shared agreement.

Developing this point, Shakespeare (1998) notes that ethnomethodologists see the concepts of 'adult' and 'child' not so much as things with an independent existence but as 'collections of conventions which are used to establish and reinforce non-symmetrical relations between grown-ups and children' (p. 56). Outlining what she calls half or 'less-than-full' membership, Shakespeare argues that because children are not effectively full members, their role in interaction is constructed in terms of them building towards becoming competent individuals where much of their experience is replete with examples from adults concerning how to achieve full membership. If this is indeed the case, then one way of describing or considering the development of membership competencies or skills is to identify the conditions within what Garfinkel and Sacks (1970) term 'glossing practices', and become just that – social objects that are invisible, unnoticeable and unremarkable. Here, glossing practices mean 'assemblages of practices whereby speakers in the situated particulars of speech mean something different from what they can say in just so many words' (p. 342). In other words, is it possible to trace out methodic practices that initially are, or may be, worthy of remark, instruction or comment by full members (typically towards those without full membership) and then indicate how such practices transform or change so that their successful performance elicits no explicit comment or remark?

Therefore, in answer to the question of why membership might arise in some situations and not in others, a participant displays membership through mastery of language, but mastery of language is a concerted accomplishment on occasion precisely because membership is displayed by *not* drawing attention to the fact that one is indeed a member – which is evidenced in the use of the *that* and the *how* of speaking. In other words, one way of displaying membership is to show that knowledge of the etiquette involved in not drawing attention to the fact that another (a child), because of their possible limited use of language, is *not* (yet) a member (see also Forrester and Reason 2006).

Of course, as earlier work in developmental pragmatics indicates (Ochs and Schiefflein 1979), possessing necessary skills and competencies, such as knowing when to repair your own talk or answering a question appropriately, does not necessarily guarantee membership status. There is clearly something in the level of detail regarding those warrantable practices to which people orient with reference to speaker's rights, obligations and related issues germane to adult–child relations. O'Reilly (2006) documents the sophisticated nature of children's interruption strategies and competencies in adult–child talk, highlighting the observation that having such skills can be ignored by adult co-participants. On this point Shakespeare (1998: 56) notes:

> Accepting the role of child means formulating a performance that acknowledges the interactional rights of others. It is part of the interactional work that children do. Yet, depending on the degree of asymmetry they perceive, children may take more or fewer interactional rights (perhaps more with parents and few with adults whom they don't know).

Formulating a performance that displays an orientation to asymmetrical role-relations seems to be of a different order and competence than, say, knowing when to produce a second pair part during talk. In EM/CA, Sacks (1992) alluded to the problematic nature of membership for children when he noted the sophisticated strategy children often employ utilising the fact that when someone is asked an 'open' question (what?) then that person obtains rights regarding participation and holds the floor during talk. This underpins the common observation that often children, who as participants do not necessarily have full speak-at-any-time membership rights, often employ phrases such as 'do you know what, Mummy?', thus initiating the requisite response from the adult, 'What?', and guaranteeing the floor in their next turn.

Given the well-established literature on the complex nature of question–answer sequences within EM/CA (Steensig and Drew 2008) in what follows, the recognition and production of appropriate answers and questions by one child over a two-and-a-half year period will serve as an entry point for highlighting issues surrounding children's conversational skills and membership status. In earlier work on the nature of questions, Sacks (1992) – when discussing what is involved in recognising a question as just that sort of member formulation requiring a response – noted that answering according to the project of the question involves a particular skill or competency, which was presupposed in his comment: 'what you can see that the question wants to find out, is something that controls how you answer it' (p. 56).

The ability or competence to 'see what the question wants to find out' provides us with an example of a methodic practice which a competent member would not, in most circumstances, warrant explicit remark or comment. At the same time, we can say that for a child who is learning 'what you can see', 'what there is "to see"', or indeed that there is something 'to see' at all, indicates that having the ability of 'seeing' presupposes knowledge or familiarity with the boundary conditions for what might constitute an appropriate answer.

In order to elucidate this further, we can turn to this one particular competency in order to identify not only the factors that constitute the membership practices surrounding the asking and answering of questions, but also what a child or any 'less-than-full' member (e.g. a non-native speaker) has to learn so that the set of practices presupposed in the activities involved become unremarkable.

Data

The data resource for the extracts described in this chapter come from a series of video-recordings (31) of the author's daughter, Ella. This child was filmed during mealtimes as she was interacting with her father, mother and older sibling, Eva (aged 8 at the beginning of the recordings). The recordings were first collected when the child was aged 1 year and continued until she was 3 years 5 months. The length of the recordings range from 10 to 45 minutes with the total recording amounting to around 11 hours. The resulting data corpus can be viewed through the web-data feature of the CLAN software (CHILDES 2005). Please see the Endnote on page 57 regarding their particular location in the corpus. Earlier analyses of this child's repair skills have been reported elsewhere (see Forrester 2008).

Analysis

Focusing on what it is a child may or may not be able to 'see' with regard to the project of the question – that is, his or her recognition of the conditions, circumstances, social practices, (i.e. the member's methods in play when engaged in producing questions and answers) – we can examine the earliest example in the data corpus where the child produces an action that appears to be designed as a question, but is initially not treated as such by her co-participant. One question informing the analysis of Extract 3.1, and from the child's point of view, is under what conditions does she learn how an utterance can be taken up as an initiating action – a first pair part – one that requires a response on the part of an addressee.

Extract 3.1 *Child age: 1 year 8 months* [see Endnote on page 57]

Context: The context is mealtime and in this instance the father is moving around the room, taking something out of the fridge. Immediately prior to this extract the child's mother has moved through the room, and gone outside to the garden, to hang up washing. The child has been watching/looking out of the window and has moved her position on her chair to enable her to see outside.

Summary exposition of extract: The issue of what might constitute questioning – or asking a question in one of its earliest forms – is the focus of this extract. The child appears to ask a question that is transformed by the father into a statement, and subsequently a clarification request on his part. There are indications that his failure to respond with an appropriate answer to her question (or statement) produces interactional trouble – and a repair by the child. In response the father takes up her initial topic and they discuss this briefly.

```
1       (24.7)

2   F:  °rounds this somewhere°

3       (0.5)

4   F:  mm:: good (.) eh

5       (1.5)   ((E stands up in chair and looks out of window))

6   E:  bi:::b   (possible reference to 'bib' on washing line outside)

7       (0.4)

8   F:  ↓ba↑by
```

9   (0.7)

10   E: ↓ba↑by ((*E moves back in chair and looks attentively at window*))

11   (0.3)

12   F: what's baby having [now] ?

13   E: [ma::]::m   ((*E sustains look out of window*))

14   (1.0)

15   E: °mummy°?

16   (0.6)

17   F: daddy

18   (0.2)

19   E: MU:::MMY ?=   ((*E turns and looks towards F*))

20   F: = what's she do::in ?   ((*F sits down and looks towards window*))

21   (0.3)

22   E: mummy hanging [the xx]   ((*E looks back towards window*))

23   F: [hanging] the washing up ?

24   (0.3)

25   E: HA:::ni[ng]   ((*turns again towards F*))

26   F: [ve::y] good

27   (0.5)

28   E: bi:: it

29   (0.3)

30   F: biscuit

We begin by noting that, at the start, while the father is moving around the room, the child first looks towards the window, stands up and then, around line 6, utters the word 'bib'. Although it remains unclear, and possible that she is referring to a child's bib being hung on the washing line outside by her mother, the father simply produces a repetition of his mishearing 'baby' to which the child herself subsequently echoes. In the next part of this sequence, he then moves around the kitchen and, using the referent 'baby' form of address, asks the child what she is going to have (to eat) next (line 12). Since line 6, the child has maintained a sustained and close interest in looking towards the window, then overlaps his question by first saying briefly 'mam' (line 13), and produces what appears to be a question – certainly with respect to the rising inflection in the use of the sound (line 15).

The father seems to treat this simply as a statement and in response produces a standard relational pair item (daddy). However, his response is treated as an inadequate response to her question, as evidenced in the observation that the child then produces a repair of her original question (line 19), in answer to which the father then produces an 'open type' question formulation in line 20.

Consider, first, the conversational skills the child exhibits. The question at line 15 is produced in an appropriate fashion, that is, it is placed sequentially as a first pair part; it exhibits intonational inflection indicative of a question, and the child, on finishing, stops speaking (i.e. hands over the floor to her co-participant). However, this is to no avail – the father does not respond, as far as the child is concerned, in an appropriate way. It would be difficult to suggest that this failure on his part has necessarily anything to do with asymmetrical adult–child role relations. Consider next, the skills the child then exhibits with the following question in line 19. Here, she does at least three things additional to the earlier formulation, (i) she increases the volume, (ii) she produces a stretch on the first syllable of the utterance and (iii) as she speaks she turns towards the father establishes eye contact and maintains it as she speaks. This utterance is now recognised as a question formulation. If the child is learning anything, then this appears to be a naturally occurring instructional context where you learn that if you want to ask a successful question (one that is answered in a manner indicative of a question having been asked) then make sure your addressee is attending.

As for 'seeing' what the project of the question(s) wants to find out, in this context we have examples of how the child appears to 'see' what is being asked of her in line 20, and what the father appears to 'see' as regards her question to him at line 19. In the first instance we appear to have a rather unambiguous interdependence with regard to 'seeing' and 'providing information'. In other words, what precedes and follows on from lines 19 to 22 is something akin to the 'open-question' initiation employed by older children (Sacks 1992), where what the child does following line 20 indicates that what she 'sees' is what she expects to see, i.e. her immediate comment when queried by the father. The questions at line 15 and 19 then serve as resources to initiate a mini-narrative interchange between the parties: 'look what mummy is doing outside'.

As for the father, and what he 'sees' the project of the question being designed for, it is noteworthy that as he moves to sit down at lines 19–20, as the child produces her question-repair, he glances towards the window, and simultaneously treats the child's question as if the child wishes to initiate talk about what is going on outside – to tell *him* something, not for him to tell her something. It remains unclear as to why the question is seen in this way by the father; however, it does appear to offer opportunities for the participants to engage in a narrative-like question–answer scenario: 'What's she doing? She's hanging out the washing. Is she really hanging the washing up? Yes, hanging it up! Very good.'

With regard to the child's membership status and the related question of evidence or indices of participant orientation to 'development' or 'childhood', it would seem that the father, at line 12, takes up the opportunity offered by the 'word-imitation' practice across lines 8–10, to then ask the child a question; however, doing so using a 'stage-of-life' membership category term and, although addressing her, referring to her in the third person. Such usage in adult–child talk has been documented elsewhere (Brener 1983). The manner in which this asymmetric referring might be said to have a bearing on the sequence of the interaction is however, if anything, opposite to that indicated by Shakespeare (1998) and O'Reilly (2006). Here we find the child interrupts his turn-at-talk displaying no orientation to his question and proceeds, as we noted, to ask a question herself.

In Extract 3.2, in contrast we find an occasion where the status of the child's member-ship as a fully participating individual is called into question, this time by an older sibling. Also, the extract highlights adult-to-child examples of question–answer prac-tices, typical instructive exemplars which, Shakespeare (1998) suggests, adults provide for children on the road to full membership status.

Extract 3.2 *Child age: 2 years 1 month*

Context: This recording takes place earlier during the recording reported above. Immediately prior to the beginning of the extract, Ella has indicated that she might start crying in response to being told off. The father is out of camera, some distance from a table where Ella is sitting with her older sister Eva (aged 8 at the time of the recording). Throughout the extract the father is asking questions while moving around the kitchen.

Summary exposition of extract: The extract contains more than one example of the father appearing to instruct the child in the practice of 'doing answering'. Additionally, the older child, Eva, displays an orientation to the likelihood that her younger sibling may not know what is being asked of her. The trajectory of the turn-at-talk following this statement might be described as the older siblings subsequent production and performance of the fact that her sister is a 'less-than-full' member.

```
 1   F:    where did mummy and Kirsten go ?

 2         (1.4)

 3   F:    did they [ go ] to see Sophie ?

 4   E:             [a::w]

 5         (0.4)

 6   E:    y:::es

 7         (0.7)

 8   F:    where did they go Ella ?

 9         (1)

10   E:    eh (.) to doctors =

11   F:    = that's right they went to doctors clever girl

12         (.)

13   F:    cause Sophie's in eh hospital?

14         (0.4)

15   E:    ye::a

16         (1)

17   F:    why is she in hospital?          ((E places food in her mouth))

18         (0.7)
```

19	E:	why ?
20		(0.8)
21	EV:	how's <u>she</u> meant to know ? ((*turns around towards F while asking*))
22		(2.1)
23	F:	cause I told ↑her
24		(0.8)
25	E:	why ?
26		(1.8)
27	F:	I'm asking you why
28		(0.3)
29	EV:	why's Sophie in hospital Ella ?
30		(0.8)
31	E:	cause hos ( ) ( ) why ?
32		(0.4)
33	F:	that's right cause she's not well
34		(8.7)

In this extract we find some clear examples of the adult apparently instructing or showing the younger child what is involved in 'doing question/answering'. First we find questions regarding 'where' something happened (line 1), then a 'closed' question referring to a reason why somebody went somewhere (line 3), followed then by a repetition of 'where' (line 8), then a question regarding 'why' (line 19), and then after an interjection from the older sibling, an explicit formulation of the 'doing questioning' that is going on (line 27), followed finally by the child producing a somewhat unintelligible utterance, and then her own question (line 31) which is, curiously, treated by the adult as an appropriate response to the sibling's question in line 29.

A closer examination of the sequence reveals noteworthy indications of what is involved in the child 'seeing' what kinds of project questions are designed for her. First of all, the sequence itself appears to be initiated by the adult as a method or strategy to displace ongoing trouble exhibited by the child immediately prior to the interaction at the start of the extract. In other words, 'questioning' is something adults do on occasion in order to distract children. Second, notice that immediately following his first question, to which the child appears to be a little late in responding (the overlap in line 4), the father, when no answer is forthcoming, then provides a possible 'answer' in a second follow-up 'closed' clarification request. From here, and third, when she produces an appropriate answer, his response is both very quick (fast uptake lines 10–11) and contains an evaluation of what she has just said. To some extent one way of describing this sequence is as an adult-to-child lesson in 'here's what doing answering a question' involves.

At this point, his next question appears to cause problems for both children, for different reasons. At precisely the moment the father speaks (line 17), Ella places food in her mouth and begins to eat, and then as she eats, replies by asking a question herself. Leaving aside the issue of whether or not the child treats father's question as a statement to which she then responds with a question (line 19), immediately following this sequence, the older child then also produces a question addressed to the father. This highlights her evaluation of the appropriateness of her sister being asked to produce an explanation or reason why somebody is in hospital. From an 8-year-old participant's point of view, it would seem that a child of 2 years would not know this kind of thing. We have a specific instance where 'development' influences the trajectory of the sequence of the interaction: whatever the potential or realised membership status of this child as participant, her skills and competencies, as oriented to by a co-participant, are procedurally consequential.

Here, and in response, the father first produces an account of why she *should* know, and then, in response to Ella's repetition of her question of line 19, explicitly articulates the 'doing formulating' which is in place (line 27). In other words, whatever else is going on, the utterance produced by Ella in line 19 is deemed inappropriate – you don't respond to a 'why' question simply with an echo of the phrase. It would seem to be the case that 'seeing' the project of this kind of question calls for an answer of a different kind. Interestingly, in what follows, the child then produces an unintelligible utterance followed again by 'why' in line 31, which this time is treated as indeed an appropriate answer.

Central to the notion of membership is mastery of language, and one indication of this for Garfinkel and Sacks (1970) was 'doing formulating', a practice where 'one finds conversationalists, in the course of a conversation, and as a recognized feature of that conversation, formulating their conversation' (p. 353), saying in so many words what they are doing. Whatever else we think membership might be, it has something to do with showing that you understand, through the *ways* you produce the particulars of speaking, that these particular language practices are always available, as a set of skills, dispositions, or competencies, for further extension, clarification, repair and whatever might constitute being called to account for the manner in which these practices are being produced. Let us turn to Extract 3.3, where it seems that by 3 years of age, a child, when situations demand it, will display an orientation to the formulated 'doing' of talk.

Extract 3.3 *Child age: 3 years*

Context: The child is reading, awaiting breakfast. The father is toasting crumpets, and standing behind the child some distance from where she is sitting.

Summary exposition of extract: The fact that the father keeps talking to the child and asking questions appears to become irritating or annoying for the child. In response, she highlights the kind of action he is repeating and calls him to account.

```
1   E:                              ((lifts up plate, turns towards F and shows it to him))

2   :      (0.2)

3   F:     oh very good I'll make some more then

4   :      (0.4)
```

  5 F: I'll put some on

  6 :   (0.5)

  7 F: one for you and one for me

  8 :   (2.0)

  9 F: have a little read of your book while you're waiting

 10 :   (1.2)

 11 F: miss:::

 12 :   (0.4)

 13 F: is it doctor seuss?

 14 :   (0.4)

 15 E: °yea°

 16 :   (0.9)

 17 F: is he a funny doctor?   ((*E turns back around and looks at her book*))

 18 :   (0.5)

 19 E: yea

 20 :   (0.9)

 21 F: is he a ↑lion?

 22 :   (0.3)

 23 E: N↓::↑O

 24 :   (2.2)

 25 E: he's a person

 26 :   (0.5)

 27 F: a real doctor?

 28 :   (0.5)

 29 E: yea

 30 :   (2.2)

 31 F: not like in eh what's that other story that we've go::t that's [eh]

 32 E: [my day]

 33 :   (0.2)

 34 F: oh my day ↓that's right

 35 :   (3.5)

36	F:	but do you like the my day doctor?
37	:	(0.6)
38	E:	yea
39	:	(1.1)
40	E:	I like him ↑better
41	:	(0.3)
42	F:	>crazy< why d'you like him?
43	:	(0.6)
44	E:	cause I ↑D:::O (.) ↑don't ask me every (.) ↑ti::↓me=
45	F:	=oh ↑all ri::ght
46	:	(1.0)
47	E:	°↑all ri::ght°
48	:	(2.3)
49	E:	a b c count on you

The phenomenon in conversation of doing [the fact that our conversational activities are accountably rational] appears to be one essential skill for becoming or showing that you have become a member or participant. In order to possess the required level of competence for 'doing formulating', members need to be able to exhibit in a methodical way, their recognition that 'doing formulating' is going on, and that they can display to co-participants that they are able to engage in those actions which make such 'formulated doings' possible. Doing formulating appropriately seems to involve having the ability to indicate to others that you recognise that the actions that make conversations possible are reflexively accountable practices.

This extract begins with the father making toast and doing various things around the kitchen (filling the dishwasher) and so on. Around lines 2–3, Ella turns around while still eating and shows him her plate, indicating that she has now finished her pancakes. He then tells her he will make some more and suggests that she could read her book while she waits. Between lines 13 and 42, the father then proceeds to ask her a series of questions; in fact, from the child's point of view, it turns out to be too many questions. (Questions at lines 13, 17, 21, 27, 36, 42.) The questions seem to come faster as the interaction proceeds (note that there is only a 0.5 second pause at line 27, and the question at line 42 hardly gives Ella time to draw breath).

Ella's reply at line 44, and to the question in line 42, is noteworthy and draws our attention to Ella displaying an orientation to (a) the accountable nature of conversation, (b) the particulars of speaking – in this case the asking of questions continuously, and (c) to her recognition that the form of the father's reply – to her calling him to account – is noticeable in some way.

The child's turn-at-talk in line 42 is marked in various ways. Her reply is noticeably louder [I DO], is stretched, is followed immediately with an imperative that the adult should not keep asking her questions, and finishes with a falling/rising intonation on the word 'time' which presupposes annoyance or certainly a display that what he is doing is inappropriate and that he should stop doing it. It also appears to be an attempt at the closing of a topic – discussion about Dr. Seuss – and it would seem that the father's reply (line 45) displays some agreement to the request or demand that the topic is now closed. His reply seems to indicate a co-orientation to the accountable nature of what has been going on (the questioning) and the fact that the child has indicated quite specifically that this should now stop. Notice both the fast uptake and the mirroring or repetition of the intonational contour of the previous utterance (all right . . . with . . . time). It may also be interesting – that is, with respect to the learnability of this 'doing formulating' – that Ella then quietly imitates the reply the father made. Notice that she repeats the phrase 'all right' and does so quietly to herself. Restricting ourselves to the criteria for membership outlined by Garfinkel and Sacks (1970), it would seem that by 3 years of age children are likely to possess the requisite conversational skills indicative of mastery of language, and indicative of possessing membership of a particular culture. One issue, however, is that although members may exhibit a mastery of language (Garfinkel and Sacks 1970: 339), they

> somehow [are] heard to be engaged in the objective production and objective display of commonsense knowledge of everyday activities as observable and reportable phenomena

and as participants in the myriad cultural contexts in which they find themselves, children nonetheless cannot necessarily take up the role or subject position akin to adult membership (O'Reilly 2006).

Concluding comments

We need to recognise that possessing conversational skills indicative of having the ability to produce and recognise reflexively accountable social practices will only be part of the competencies and abilities required for participation. The reason why this is significant for EM/CA work which addresses adult–child interaction specifically, is that the implicit benchmarks of adult competence and/or membership should not be restricted to the performance of talk-in-interaction as 'skills of conversation'. In other words, as a child participant you may possess adult-equivalent performance skills, but nevertheless are not considered a 'full-member'. There is a particular disjunction in equating (external) 'developmental' criteria with 'ethnomethodologically informed' participant criteria. With this in mind, a few concluding comments can be offered.

The recent emergence of CA work focused on adult–child interaction represents research within and across various fields, including developmental psychology, sociolinguistics, child language research, speech and language development work and various related fields often centred on applied problems. One reason for the increase or growth in this work can be traced to the particular advantages of the micro-detailed focus on dynamic naturally occurring interaction. Understanding the fine detail of the process and dynamics of interaction offers an avenue into describing, and possibly explaining, how one or other particular ability develops. There are particular advantages both in the literature, and in this volume, of employing CA as a specific methodology for highlighting significant factors bearing on the everyday interactions of adults and children in naturalistic contexts.

At the same time, it is important to recognise that there are dangers in overlooking the fact that when CA is employed solely as an interdisciplinary 'applications' methodology the significance of the ethnomethodological focus is glossed over or forgotten – that is, the focus on the people's sense-making practices. The brief examination of the extracts above indicates that it might be wise to separate developmental or skills acquisition questions regarding conversational practices from issues surrounding the status of children with respect to participant membership. All too often notions of skill, ability, competence and achievement presupposed in adult–child interaction studies are evaluative analyst-based developmental constructs, not participant-oriented (member) constructs. While such work undoubtedly provides useful parameters for comparisons within and across different interest groups, it is unfortunate that competence or skill also often presupposes deficiency, 'developmental' lag, inability, and associated ideas of something being amiss or missing. One particular problem for work that employs CA in order to map out what and how something develops, is that it is may no longer be 'participant-oriented' development that is under consideration. A related challenge here is that the accounts that document how one particular skill builds on, or rests upon, another might have to articulate how the implicit theory of development (the analysts) maps onto a participant-membership developmental orientation. It can always help to remember that a particular advantage of a specifically participant-oriented developmentally focused EM/CA is that there is not necessarily anything missing or deficient or lacking, or even anything particularly skilful – there is simply what people do, say, accomplish or achieve in their everyday sense-making practices.

Endnote

See http://www.kent.ac.ukzchology/department/people/forresterm/threeQuestionExts.htm for short QuickTime video clips of these extracts. The examples are available for further scrutiny in the data corpus at the CHILDES website (CHILDES 2005). For identification, they can be found at Childes WebData:

Extract 3.1 (week 85)	085.cha lines 906–937
Extract 3.2 (week 108)	108.cha lines 926–960
Extract 3.3 (week 159)	159.cha lines 303–353

References

Brener, R. (1983) Learning the deictic meaning of third person pronouns. *Journal of Psycholinguistic Research* **12**, 235–262.

Burman, E. (1994) *Deconstructing development psychology.* London: Routledge.

CHILDES (2005) *Childes overview system – Basic.* Carnegie Mellon University. Retrieved 2008 from the World Wide Web: http://childes.psy.cmu.edu/media/Eng-UK/Forrester/

Edwards, D. and Stokoe, E.H. (2004) Discursive psychology, focus group interviews and participants' categories. *British Journal of Developmental Psychology*, **22**, 499–507.

Forrester, M.A. (2008) The emergence of self-repair: A case-study of one child during the early preschool years. *Research on Language and Social Interaction*, **41** (1), 97–126.

Forrester, M.A. and Reason, D. (2006) Competency and participation in acquiring a mastery of language: A reconsideration of the idea of membership. *Sociological Review*, **54** (3), 446–466.

Garfinkel, H. (1967) *Studies in ethnomethodology*. Englewood Cliffs, NJ: Prentice-Hall.

Garfinkel, H. and Sacks, H. (1970) On formal structures of practical actions. In J.C.T. McKinney (ed.), *Theoretical sociology: Perspectives and developments*. New York: Appleton-Century-Crofts.

Goffman, E. (1967) *Interaction ritual: Essays on face-to-face behaviour*. New York: Doubleday Anchor.

Heritage, J. (1984) *Garfinkel and ethnomethodology*. Oxford: Polity Press.

Hester, S. and Eglin, P. (eds) (1997) *Culture in action: Studies in membership categorization analysis*. Lanham, MD: International Institute for Ethnomethodology and Conversation Analysis and University Press of America.

James, A. and Prout, A. (eds) (1996) *Constructing and reconstructing childhood*. Basingstoke: Falmer Press.

Livingston, E. (1987) *Making sense of ethnomethodology*. London: Routledge & Kegan Paul.

Lynch, M. (1993) *Scientific practice and ordinary action: Ethnomethodology and social studies of science*. New York: Cambridge University Press.

Mackay, R. (1974) Conceptions of children and models of socialization. In R. Turner (ed.), *Ethnomethodology*. Harmondsworth, UK: Penguin.

Ochs, E. and Schiefflein, B. (1979) *Developmental pragmatics*. London: Academic Press.

O'Reilly, M. (2006) Should children be seen and not heard? An examination of how children's interruptions are treated in family therapy. *Discourse Studies*, **8** (4), 549–566.

Sacks, H. (1992) *Lectures on conversation*. Oxford: Blackwell.

Schegloff, E.S. (1992) On talk and its institutional occasions. In P. Drew and J.C. Heritage (eds), *Talk at work* (pp. 101–134). Cambridge: Cambridge University Press.

Shakespeare, P. (1998) *Aspects of confused speech: A study of verbal interaction between confused and normal speakers*. Mahwah, NJ: Lawrence Erlbaum Associates.

Steensig, J. and Drew, P. (2008) Introduction: Questioning and affiliation/disaffiliation in interaction. *Discourse Studies*, **10** (Special Issue: Questioning), 5–17.

Turner, R. (1974) *Ethnomethodology*. Harmondsworth, UK: Penguin.

Wowk, M.T. (2007) Kitzinger's feminist conversation analysis: Critical observations. *Human Studies*, **30** (2), 131–155.

Chapter 4

'Actually' and the sequential skills of a two-year-old

ANTHONY WOOTTON

Introduction

'Actually' is a word that does not receive much attention in the child language literature. In part this is likely to be because children do not use it very often. In her study of adverbial connectives among children aged 6 to 12, Scott (1984) found that the word was used only twice in a corpus of 17,536 utterances. There is no comparable statistic for younger ages, although it is clear that the word is sometimes used. In her analysis of the dialogue and monologue of one child aged 22–35 months, Feldman (1989) refers to 'actually', treating it as an epistemic adverb along with words like 'maybe' and 'in fact'. But no separate analysis of 'actually' is offered, and within the transcript data cited by Feldman there is no instance of 'actually' and every suggestion that 'maybe' was the most frequent example of this type of adverb. Within the tradition of research on cohesion, prompted by Halliday and Hasan (1976), 'actually' is treated as an adversative conjunction, along with words like 'yet' and 'but' – words which exhibit a recognition that what is being said is contrary to expectation. The most detailed analysis of such conjunctions in the conversation of young children remains that of Bloom et al. (1980). Their analysis was confined to adversative connectives which established a syntactic link with a prior clause (not necessarily spoken by the same speaker), and in practice it was mainly confined to the word 'but', which none of their four children used in this way before the age of 2 years 8 months (2;8). As 'actually' does not qualify as such a syntactic linker, its absence does not necessarily imply that it was not used, but this research again suggests that children's use of adversative constructions is normally quite limited in the first half of their third year.

The impetus for the present study arose from the frequent use of the word 'actually' by a child aged 2 years 3 months (2;3). In the three hours of video recordings made at this age she used this word 59 times, occasionally appearing almost obsessed with it. In prior recordings made at 2;1 there is no sign of the word, while in subsequent recordings of similar duration made at 2;5 she used the word only twice. My focus here is on her usage of this term at 2;3, thus the analysis is mainly cross-sectional in nature. The analysis investigates the role 'actually' plays in this child's turn organization. As language is housed within, and built for, specific moments within the interaction process, then an apt way for identifying the function of 'actually' is through inspection of the particular features of those occasions on which the term is used. These features must minimally include consideration of the sequential position of the turn containing 'actually' and those words that accompany 'actually' within the same turn, and this needs to be done at a level of detail that captures the segmental, prosodic and non-verbal features of potential relevance to the nature of this enquiry. The tradition of research known as conversation analysis (CA) contains the most useful framework for setting about such an exercise, and that framework is adopted here.

When the child, who will be called Emily, was aged 2;3, three hours of naturalistic video-recording were made in her home, mainly of mealtimes and of one or other parent playing with her – no other participants were present. Over the course of two days, three recordings were made, lasting 2 hours, 45 minutes and 15 minutes respectively; on each occasion recording was continuous and was made with a tripod-mounted camera, and on each occasion the word 'actually' was frequently used. At this age the child used 'what' and 'where' questions, although auxiliary verbs were often omitted, as in *Where it gone to daddy?* and *What you reading daddy?* Yes/no answer questions occurred very rarely. Within her request system, for example, there were just two instances of requests formed in this way (both 'Can I have . . . ?') in a corpus of about 170 requests, most of which were in imperative or declarative mode (e.g. *I want some more fish, I like some cheese-cake, Put it back on your plate*). Consequently most yes/no questioning was conveyed through intonational means (e.g. *You like a bit of that cheese daddy?*) (see Wootton 1997: 53–55 for further general details on this child at about this age). The child could use a variety of words in turn-initial position which were reactive to something that had just been said. We shall see that this is a position frequently also occupied by 'actually', and several of these other words could co-occur with 'actually', notably 'oh', 'well' and 'and'. She does not use 'in fact', 'as a matter of fact' or 'maybe', although in turn-final position she could use 'now' in a way that could mark something as in tension with a prior stance taken by either her recipient or herself (e.g. *I want some red medicine now*).

The transcription of the data fragments mainly follows those common in conversation analysis (see Glossary). I have not attempted to preserve many idiosyncratic segmental features of the child's speech production of this age as this would have required a much more extensive use of phonetic transcription. In this sense, many of the child's 'words' as they appear in the transcripts are my glosses of those words; for example, the word 'actually' itself is in fact normally rendered as either /akʃi/ or /akʃli/. Occasionally I have used a schwa sound, /ə/, to represent the centralised vowel which, at this age, this child can use as what is known as a 'filler syllable' (Peters 1995: 471). Non-verbal details that are pertinent to the analysis are noted separately at the bottom of each transcript in a way that allows the reader to place them in relation to the talk. Here, rh and lh indicate right or left hand. Within the text, material appearing in italics forms a direct quotation from talk by the child in question, either from one of the data extracts or from the broader corpus of recordings at this age.

The next section of this chapter details the properties of this child's use of 'actually' which have been revealed by my investigation. The final section develops two themes which are suggested by these findings: the role of sequential understandings in the design of the child's conduct, and the kinds of developmental enquiry towards which this directs us.

Design and uses of 'actually'

Turn position and prosodic design

In adult talk 'actually' can occur in a variety of positions within clauses, these minimally including clause initial, medial and final uses (Quirk *et al.* 1985: 490); similarly they can also occur in a variety of positions within turns (e.g. Tognini-Bonelli 1993; Clift 2001). Within my corpus Emily's use of 'actually' exhibits an affiliation to that position which is both clause, and turn initial. In part this is displayed through the frequency with which this term occupies this position – 65% of the 59 cases occur as turn initial (for the only final position use see Extract 4.4, where it duplicates the 'actually' in initial position). But among the exceptions there are further types of evidence suggesting that such an affiliation continues to be displayed even where other words precede 'actually' in the turn. Cases in which preceding words are the focus of self-repair form one such exception. In Extract 4.1 the child's initial words (*In um:*) are abandoned and the turn restarted; while in Extract 4.2 *>I wa-< m- make a little-* is left incomplete and this component is repackaged in the later part of the turn. In both of these cases the turn is, in effect, re-initiated by the child through the design of her repair, and the word which fronts this re-initiation is 'actually'. Further to this we can also note that although many instances of self-repair by this child at this age involve re-initiation this is not always the case, as is evident in Extract 4.3; but on occasions like this 'actually' is never used in the repair (see Wootton 2007 for a depiction of some of Emily's self-repair techniques at this age). So in these ways the use of 'actually' in self-repair has a distinct association with the initial position of turn components which re-initiate the turn in question:

Extract 4.1 *where the child's* (Ch) *initial words are abandoned and the turn restarted in the course of organising play with her father* (F)

F: Where are we going to make the farmyard.

Ch: (In um:=)↑Ac↓tually /ə/ get all these <u>toys</u> out.

Extract 4.2 *where the child's initial words are left incomplete and the next component started with 'actually'*

Ch: >I wa-< m- make a little- ↑Ac↓tually /ə/ make a little farm↓ya:rd.

Extract 4.3 *where there is no re-initiation in self-repair and 'actually' is not used*

Ch: Doggy .hh wa- <u>don't</u> want to <u>sit</u> the:re

There remain a further 8 extracts in which the 'actually' is preceded by other words within the relevant child turn. In all but one of these the word is a single word – 'oh', 'well' or 'and'. Athough 'actually' is the second word in these cases, it still occurs prior to the main substance of the turn, as in Extracts 4.4 and 4.5.

Extract 4.4 *Referring to a toy animal on the floor; the child reaches for it at turn beginning*

Ch: ↑<u>Oh:</u>. (.) ac↓tually (.) these- (.8) these ones can go .hh on top actually.

Extract 4.5 *Mother is not sitting in the position that the child wants her to sit*

Ch: Well ↑<u>ac</u>↓tually sit (.) (mo:re a bit).

Within the various extracts offered so far we can also see signs of the typical prosodic configuration deployed by Emily across the whole corpus of her uses of 'actually'. In Extracts 4.1, 4.2 and 4.5 the 'actually' begins at a higher pitch than the preceding word(s); in the broader corpus, which mainly consists of turn-initial 'actuallys', the initial syllable of this word is produced at a pitch higher than the child's immediately prior talk and/or higher than her standard pitch on 74% of occasions. Quite often this first syllable is also given stress, and in the vast majority of cases, 97%, there is a sharp pitch drop after this first syllable of the word – as in Extracts 4.1, 4.2, 4.4, 4.5 and most subsequent extracts. In cases such as Extracts 4.1, 4.2 and 4.5 the exploitation of such prosodic resources creates the impression that the word 'actually' has a distinctive role in fronting the words in the turn construction unit.

There is also internal evidence within the wider corpus to suggest that, on occasion, the child herself orients to the salience of one of these prosodic features, high-pitch onset. In Extracts 4.6 and 4.7, for example, she aborts the beginning of the word 'actually' (twice within extract 6), eventually producing it with higher pitch onset:

Extract 4.6 *The child brings a nursery rhyme into the conversation*

Ch: A- a- ↑<u>ac</u>↓tually a master gets his fiddin 'tick an' d- doesn't know what

       te ↑<u>DO</u>::.

Extract 4.7 *Where the pattern of restarting the word is the same as in Extract 4.6*

Ch: A- ↑<u>ac</u>↓tually ↑put it like thi::s.

Within the corpus there are no instances of the reverse pattern to this, that is there are no self-repaired pitch resets to a lower level among the many high-pitch beginnings of 'actually' within the corpus.

Emily's uses of 'actually' are overwhelmingly positioned in the early part of her turn, most commonly in turn-initial position. They also tend to have certain prosodic characteristics, such as high-pitch onset. It is important that these characteristics are not always present as this implies that her production of 'actually' is not done stereotypically, but that its production is sensitive to features of the local environment. The next step is to explore this sensitivity in more detail and to identify what role the word plays within the local environment.

The enactment of departures

In this section I suggest that Emily's use of 'actually' registers some kind of disjuncture with the state of play in the interaction at that point. It registers what, for reasons that will become apparent, I shall call a 'departure' from some understanding as to this existing state of play. Such an understanding can arise in various ways and take various forms, and in this section I shall try to convey a sense of this variety.

Initially it is useful to explore Extract 4.1 (reproduced as Extract 4.8) in more detail.

Extract 4.8 *Father and child both sit on the floor, close to each other. The child has requested to make a farmyard and they both then act in a way as to implement this idea*

F: [a]Where are we going to make the farmyard.

Ch: [b](In um:=)[c]↑Ac↓tually /ə/ get all these <u>toy</u>s out.

[a] Ch looks through toys in an adjacent box, as though searching for relevant figures.
[b] Ch starts lifting some toys from the box.
[c] Ch puts the first of these toys on the floor near her.

Here the child has requested to make a farmyard, and in the course of preparing to do this her father asks *Where are we going to make the farmyard*. The immediate reply to this, *(In um:)*, projects an answer fitted to the 'where' question, but Emily then goes on to re-initiate with a turn less fitted to this question, one that explicates the nature of the non-verbal action, lifting toys from a basket, which in fact has been occupying her from when she first says *(In um:)*. Here, then, 'actually' precedes those words which depart from the fitted response to the question, and the use of 'actually' contributes to the disjunctive sense of these words for this sequential position. Extract 4.9 contains a further example of 'actually' fronting a departure from a locally expectable action. Here Emily's mother is encouraging her to complete sections of a nursery rhyme, successfully so at lines 1 and 2. At line 3 she continues in her efforts, making her expectation clear to the child by features of her voice intonation, by gazing at her and by leaving gaps where she hopes that the child will spontaneously offer the next word(s). At lines 4 and 5 Emily declines to fill these slots and what she does at line 5, taking the book from her mother and shifting their focus to another book, is clearly in tension with what her mother is expecting of her at that point in the sequence:

Extract 4.9 *Mother (M) sits on the floor with the child to her immediate right, kneeling in a child's chair. M holds an open book, the contents of which have touched off the 'Tom, Tom the piper's son' nursery rhyme. M now starts lines of the rhyme, expecting Ch to complete them*

1   M: Stole a pig,[a]

2   Ch: And away he run.

3   M: The pig was (.) eat (0.5) a:nd,[a]

4   (0.7)

5   Ch: [b]Well ↑ac↓tually <u>you</u> might be reading an<u>other</u> one.

6   M: Might I:[c] oh: alright.

[a] M gazes expectantly at Ch during and immediately after both turns.
[b] On *well* Ch moves her hands to hold the arm of her chair; at the beginning of *actually* she starts her rh movement to take the book from M, removing the book during *you*; by *one* the book is discarded on to an adjacent surface.
[c] Ch's rh first touches the pile of books from which she is going to select a new one.

In Extract 4.9 there is also a sense that what the child is doing at line 5 is not just misfitted for the locally operative sequential expectation, but that it is also in tension with the immediate line of action that the parent is trying to get underway. In the other case in which 'well' co-occurs with 'actually' (our earlier Extract 4.5 re-presented below as Extract 4.10), it is clear that Emily's 'actually' turn, at line 7, is again involved in a course of action that is at odds with her mother's preferences, which in this case concern the seating position that her mother has adopted at lines 4–6:

Extract 4.10 *Mother makes to sit by the child, to the child's left*

1   Ch: [a]Come and sit <u>he</u>:re by me.

2   M: Well it's best if I sit this side.

3   (.)

4   M: There's a bit of space here for me to sit.

5   (.)

6   M: See,[b]

7   Ch: [c]Well ↑<u>ac</u>↓tually sit (.) (mo:re a bit).

8   M: Well I <u>am</u> sitting on the floor aren't I?[d]

[a] Ch gesticulates to floor on her right, keeping her rh in that position throughout her turn.
[b] M is now fully seated, to Ch's left; Ch is gazing at M's body, but looks away by the beginning of her next turn.
[c] During the first half of this turn Ch gesticulates to her right, as in line 1; after the micropause she leaves her rh hanging to her right and gazes towards M's body. Immediately subsequent events are consistent with Ch still wanting M to sit on her right.
[d] Here M is innocently or wilfully misinterpreting what Ch is saying at line 7: Ch is not concerned with *whether* her mother is sitting on the floor but with *where* she is sitting.

In both Extracts 4.9 and 4.10 the use of 'well' seems to occur with, and give special marking to, a discrepancy between the parent's immediate preferred line of action and that of the child. But on other occasions, as in Extract 4.11, 'actually' alone can contribute to making such a discrepancy prominent:

Extract 4.11 *Father sits on the sofa, child in front of him on the floor. F has just been given an 'engine' to repair, in fact a stool representing an engine, with one of its legs (in reality) wobbly. F has replaced the stool on the floor, claiming to have mended it. Ch raises again the problem with one of the legs; the stool is still in the position that F placed it on the floor*

1   F: Well its okay if you– if you leave it on thee uh on the floor like tha:t.

2   Ch: ᵃA- ↑ac↓tually ↑put it like thi::s.

3   (1.3)

4   F: Alright then put it like that.

ᵃ Here Ch lifts the stool slightly, then slightly shifts its position on the floor; hands taken off the stool at *this*; doesn't look at F.

So far I've shown how 'actually' can be used by Emily to preface turns which depart from various kinds of locally operative sequential expectation. In another set of cases the departure that is being marked is from an alignment taken up previously by the child herself, where she alters the projectable direction of her own engagement in the situation. In Extract 4.12 the child's initial alignment is explicit – she has just said that she wants to make the farmyard on the floor *by me* (lines 5 and 7), her repeated gesture with her left hand making clear where she means. At line 11, the turn containing 'actually', she is overtly changing her mind about the location of the farm, saying that she now wants to make it on the floor between her legs:

Extract 4.12 *Child and her father sit on the floor, various toys spread about; the topic of farmyards has occurred previously*

1   F: Where are we gonna make this farmya:rd.

2   (2.0)ᵃ

3   F: ºWhich-º

4   (1.2)ᵃ

5   Ch: He : re,ᵇ

6   F: He:re [(   )

7   Ch: [By: me:,ᶜ

8   F: Ri:ght.

9   (.9)

10   F: Oka:y^d=

11   Ch: =^eUm- uma- ↑ac↓tually <u>go</u> <u>through</u> <u>my</u>^f <u>legs</u>?

12   (.)

13   F: Gonna make the farmyard there?

14   Ch: Ye:s.

^a Ch scans the floor to her right, then to her left.
^b Ch slaps the floor to her left with her lh.
^c Repeat of lh slap, in a diminished form.
^d F moves his hand to pieces on floor, as though to start making the farm.
^e Ch starts to move her rh up and down the floor, between her legs.
^f Ch stops her rh gesture and gazes at F.

In other cases the line of engagement from which the child is departing is more implicit. In Extract 4.13, while having her back rubbed, she is holding a book that she and her father have been looking at earlier. At the beginning of line 4, the turn containing 'actually', she disposes of this book then starts to reach for the pile of books near her, extracting one from the bottom, with her father's help, over the course of lines 4–6. Here, then, the departure registered by the 'actually' appears to mark a change from her implicit involvements in the back-rubbing activity and the book that she has been holding, to one centring on the book that she is now seeking:

Extract 4.13   *Child sits between her father's legs on the floor, side on to him; in front of her is a stool with a pile of books on it. She holds an open book that she has been 'reading' to F. F now rubs her back, and this is now being spoken about; M speaks from a standing position nearby*

1   M: Are you liking that?

2   Ch: No:.

3   M: ((*laughs*))

4   Ch: ^a↑<u>Ac</u>↓tually ↑I'm gonna (.) (   ) wanta look /ə/-

5   (.)

6   Ch: ^b↑<u>Ac</u>↓tually I'm gonna look /ə/ <u>tiger</u> one.

7   F: Mm.

^a Just prior to this word Ch closes her book; on *I'm* she places it on top of the pile of books on the chair; she starts to extricate a book from the bottom of the pile at ( ), but slowly and with difficulty; this activity occupies her until the word *gonna*, when the book is removed from the pile. So, both lines 4 and 6 concern the selection of the new book from the bottom of the pile.
^b F's hand goes to steady the pile as the book is being removed.

Line 4 of Extract 4.13 also represents a shift from the immediately prior topic. In this case this shift is, as noted, one which returns to an activity that has earlier been topicalised: her reading of books to her father. Emily's uses of 'actually' are not often involved in the construction of turns which take the interaction in an entirely new topical direction, although this does sometimes happen, as in Extract 4.14.

Extract 4.14 *Father sits on the sofa and child kneels on a low chair nearby. They are talking about foods when an aeroplane flies over. When it has gone the child asks where it has gone*

1   F: [a]It's gone away=I don't know which way its gon:e=[b]its

2   gone- gone away somewhere.

3   (2.8)

4   Ch: [c]↑Ac↓tually ↑I wanta play /ə/ <u>boat</u> today daddy?

5   F: Going to play what?

6   Ch: A boa:t?

[a] Ch gazes at F, appearing nervous of the plane noise.

[b] Ch shifts gaze to her own body and starts to get out of her chair.

[c] Ch reaches F's leg and holds it prior to sitting down between his legs; she has sat down by *boat*. She may here be treating his legs as the *boat*.

In Extract 4.14 the focus at line 4 on playing boats is entirely discontinuous with prior topical material, both in the sense that the immediately prior talk has concerned the aeroplane, and in that playing boats has not formed part of the play agenda that has been underway within the prior play session as a whole (which has then been happening for about one and a half hours). Indeed, the inclusion of the word *today* in the child's request displays her understanding that, irrespective of the unit of time the word *today* represents, playing with the boat now would represent a first occasion – certainly a departure from the overall trajectory of the play that has preceded it. In a few cases such as this, therefore, the inclusion of 'actually' seems sensitive to a more radical shift in topical material being introduced in the turn that this word accompanies, and here it coincides with internal evidence of the child herself treating this new line of talk as discrepant with prior topical material.

Two emergent themes

The analysis has been concerned with one child's use of 'actually' at the age of 2;3. Her usage has a particular association with turn-initial position and the word is typically given a prosodic shape, especially high-pitch onset, that serves to make it contrastive with the shape of her previous or normal talk. As turns fronted by 'actually' are designed to enact departures of various kinds from prior talk/action then this suggests that these features of turn positioning and prosodic shape contribute to, and are consonant with, the contrastive and disjunctive nature of the turn. In this section of the chapter I shall explore two themes which arise from these findings: firstly, the nature of the understandings from which these uses opf 'actually' instigate a departure; and, secondly, the kinds of developmental enquiry that these findings could become part of.

Departures and understandings

To speak of 'departures' is to implicate an action or involvement that is being departed *from* and a 'new' action that is being departed *to*. In Extract 4.9, for example, the departed-from action is that kind of turn which would form a fitted response to her mother's line 3, which in this case might be something like 'Tom went howling down the street'. In Extract 4.12 what is being 'departed from' is the farmyard location on the child's left; the departed-to being the location between the child's legs. One observation that can be made about all of Emily's 'actually' turns is that they overtly address the departed-to rather than the departed from. Thus in Extract 4.9 at line 5 she could have addressed the departed-from action by saying something like 'Actually I'm not doing that . . .', or in Extract 4.12 at line 11 by saying 'actually I'm not making it there . . .'; but these kinds of words do not co-occur with 'actually'. In this connection it is also interesting to find that although 'no' is usable by Emily elsewhere in turn-initial position, 'no' is not a word that co-occurs with 'actually' within her corpus at this age. In these ways Emily avoids constructing her 'actually' turns in ways which overtly reject the departed-from action, even though such a rejection is implicated through the turn design.

At the same time it is also important to note that Emily's 'actually' turn can take up various alignments in relation to the departed-from action. In some cases, as in Extract 4.9, it seems that the new action – the *reading another one*, mentioned at line 5 – precludes her doing what the parent is immediately wanting her to do, completing the nursery rhyme which relates to the book currently being held. In this sense there is an implicit rejection of the departed-from action. And something similar seems to be true of Extract 4.10, where the mother's preferred sitting location, expressed at line 4, is being implicitly rejected in the child's 'actually' turn (also taking into account her non-verbal actions) at line 7. In both Extracts 4.10 and 4.12 the 'actually' is also preceded by 'well', the only such occasions within the corpus, which suggests that 'well' is being used to mark the tension between the kind of parental alignment inscribed in the departed-from action and the child's departed-to action.

Elsewhere the relationship between the 'actually' turn and the departed-from action can take a different form. In Extract 4.12 the action that the child's 'actually' turn is departing from is an alignment that she herself has earlier taken up, her indication of the location to her left at line 5. Through substituting a new location for this earlier one, at line 11, she comes to be recognisable as changing her mind as to where the activity of making the farmyard is to proceed – for practical purposes the old location is now redundant. But in other extracts it is less clearcut whether the departed-from action is being displaced by the departed-to action. For example, in Extract 4.8, the child's interest in getting her toys out, toys which could form part of the farm in question, could be simply postponing rather than cancelling the discussion of where the farm is going to be located. Such a possibility is more clearly articulated in Extract 4.15, where farms are again under discussion.

Extract 4.15 *Child is sitting on her father's knee on the floor, thumb in mouth, holding her comfort blanket. She says she wants to play farmyards; F picks up a toy cow from the floor, saying 'Where shall we make the farmyard'; towards the end of these words she takes her thumb out of her mouth and makes to take the cow from F's hand*

1   F: Shall we make it up [here ((*here* refers to a stool nearby))

2   Ch: [ᵃ(I w-) ↑ac↓tually put the gatesᵇ /ə/ go first daddy?

3   F: Put the gates up first,

4   Ch: Yes.

ᵃ Here Ch takes cow from F, and during the word *actually* throws it to the ground.
ᵇ Here Ch does a new left hand indicating gesture towards the floor, where the gates are; by *daddy* she has the thumb of this same hand back in her mouth.

Although the father's talk is here initially concerned with where the farmyard is to be made, on a nearby stool, Emily is appearing to take issue with the order in which the farm items are to be assembled. The departed-from action is her father's movement of a toy cow towards the surface of the stool; the departed-to action, following the 'actually', is her directive to put the gates in position. Here her wording *put the gates /ə/ go first daddy* makes clear her recognition that other items, like the cow, could be added later.

In these ways it is possible for the child to make use of 'actually' in the composition of turns which take up various kinds of alignment to departed-from actions, the nature of which will hang on the configuration and details of individual sequences. Nevertheless, at this age 'actually' is exploited as a resource by this child so as to exhibit her recognition that across this variety of sequences there is a sense in which what she is now proposing is discordant with a departed-from state of affairs. The generic usability of 'actually' seems to hinge on it playing this kind of interactional role – one which, as Halliday and Hasan (1976) suggest, marks the 'actually' turn as in some way contrary to expectation. Put another way, the child's use of 'actually' registers her recognition of the current sequential relevance of such an expectation, the expectation which makes it available for us to recognise, in each case, a departed-from action. And in registering such a recognition in such a widespread way at this age, what this child is revealing to us is that across many sequences she is able to project an alternative trajectory that the talk and action could be expected to have taken at that specific point in time; her 'actually' usage in this way shows an orientation to the *projectability* of sequences.

From these data it is possible to say something about the procedures drawn on by the child which underpin her capacity to take into account sequence projectability. Some of these clearly hinge on the operation of adjacency pairs, of the child recognising that together with a particular first pair part there is an expectation that recipient, in next position, will produce a fitted second pair part. In Extract 4.8, *Ac↓tually /ə/ get all these toys out.* is not a fitted response to the parent's question, the first pair part; and in Extract 4.9, *Well ↑ac↓tually you might be reading another one* is not a fitted response to her mother's solicit of the end of the rhyme in line 3. In such cases the expectation from which the child's 'actually' marks a departure, seems clearly linked to what is projectable from the prior first pair part. In other cases projectability appears to be underpinned by the child taking into account alignments which either she or her parent have adopted at some earlier point in the interaction. In Extract 4.12 the child herself initially decides on one location in which to make the farm at line 5, but then later at line 11 changes that with ↑ac↓*tually go through my legs?*; in Extract 4.10 in dealing with her mother's choice of a seating position which is at odds with the child's stated preference at line 1, the child uses *Well* ↑ac↓*tually sit (.) (mo:re a bit).* to resist the alignment that has just been taken up by her mother. Elsewhere I have shown that the design of various other actions by this child at about this age is also sensitive to the nature of such alignments that have been adopted in immediately prior interaction. Specifically, the design of her requests is shaped by such matters as whether the child has already indicated that she is going to engage in some course of action and whether what the child is asking for is linked to, and compatible with, what evidence she has of her recipient's action preferences on that occasion (Wootton 1997: ch. 3, also Gerhardt 1991). And it is the breach of such locally operative alignments which lies at the heart of certain episodes in which the child reacts with distress to what the parent is doing (Wootton 1997: ch. 4). The findings on the uses of 'actually' further suggest that an orientation to earlier alignments is of generic relevance to the shape of the child's conduct at this age.

In ways described above, a child of this age can arrive at an expectation of what is expectable in any specific interactional position in any specific interactional sequence. Through her use of 'actually' she is choosing one way of registering a departure from such an expectation, which often, most clearly in cases like Extract 4.9, involves recognising a divergence between the expectation of her co-participant and the line of action in which she wishes to engage. So, through these minutiae of interaction, she is routinely adjusting her verbal conduct in order to display awareness of, and attention to, such divergences. In this respect there are obvious connections with the concerns of those psychologists who, in recent years, have focused on the child's emerging understanding of what other people think and feel, with their 'theory of mind' (for overview see Carpendale and Lewis 2006) – especially for the matter of where and when children recognise that other people can have perspectives on a situation that differ from their own. We've seen that the properties of their interactional practices foster an orientation to such divergences on the part of children, so these practices form a site for the emergence and practise of the kinds of inferential skill highlighted in the theory of mind tradition (for other relevant practices, especially those associated with clarification sequences, see Tomasello 1999).

Developmental implications

Certain kinds of developmental enquiry are suggested by the line of argument above. Central to this has been the claim that Emily's use of 'actually' registers her recognition that some kind of sequential expectation is being breached. An important developmental parameter here, then, is the emergence of such sequential expectations and the child's techniques for displaying some recognition of them. The previous discussion has identified two types of sequential expectation which are of relevance here: ones associated with adjacency pairs, and ones associated with earlier alignments taken into account by the child. Each of these merits careful investigation.

There is now a variety of evidence suggesting that children recognise the constraining power of the first pair parts (FPPs) of adjacency pairs from an early age, certainly the beginning of their second year of life (e.g. Bruner 1983: Griffiths 1985: Filipi 2001). This is especially so regarding sequences in which the child herself produces the FPP; particularly important here is the fact that the child will pursue her first pair part on receiving no second pair part (SPP) from her recipient (Forrester 2008) and that where her recipient appears to misunderstand the FPP the child can employ devices designed to rectify this predicament (Wootton 1994). Much less is known about sequences in which the FPP is produced by the child's carer. The kind of carer FPP that has received most attention has been clarification requests, turns designed to engage in repair on something that the child has just said – and such clarification requests are most often built as insertion sequences after a child FPP. Analysis of the child's early responses to non-clarification FPPs has focused more on whether they are comprehensible to her, and with identifying those features that seem to facilitate this (e.g. Zukow *et al.* 1982). As the child's own production of repair initiations in the form of clarification requests is quite delayed – for example, not in use by Emily until recordings at 2;9 – then this kind of evidence regarding children's grasp of insertion sequence initiation and resolution is not normally available prior to 2 years of age.

We've seen that Emily's use of 'actually' after adult FPPs is associated with turns that can be misfitted in various ways to the FPPs, so her incorporation of 'actually' is a way through which she recognises this misfittedness, and forms one kind of relevant evidence as to the constraints which, for her, are brought into play through an adult FPP. In some cases, such as Extract 4.15, the child's 'actually' turn may be involved in postponing a reply to the adult FPP, in which case the 'actually' turn could be initiating a type of insertion sequence. But other 'actually' turns function in a different way. In Extract 4.9, for example, with *Well ↑ac↓tually you might be reading another one*, at line 5, the child is both recognising the fact that a departure from the carer's current FPP expectation is being enacted, through *Well ↑ac↓tually*, whilst breaking away from the sequence trajectory projected by the prior turn. These kinds of turn are dissimilar to the insertion sequences found in adult talk, as here the child's response to the FPP does not defer the production of the SPP (on adults, see Schegloff 2007: ch. 6), but rather cancels the expectation that such a SPP will be forthcoming. They resist the sequential implications of the prior turn while giving them a perfunctory recognition. Charting the shape and nature of such turns – turns that follow FPPs but are not fitted to those FPPs, and the ways in which their shape alters through time – will form one ingredient of a developmentally oriented conversation analysis.

The majority of Emily's uses of 'actually' do not mark departures from what is expected by a FPP; they orient to various other kinds of alignment taken up either by herself or by her carer in the prior course of action. In registering a departure from such alignments she recognises the accountability of so doing, and that there is some basis upon which it was expectable for her to have acted otherwise. Tracing the ontogenesis of such a sequential orientation – through the ways in which it is displayed – is another task facing a developmentally oriented conversation analysis. Elsewhere I have argued that an important benchmark in this respect is the child's manner of orientation to prohibitions in the second half of her second year, specifically through her use of a new and distinctive form of negation (Wootton 1997: ch. 2). And at later ages it seems clear that configurations of such local alignments connect in systematic ways with the emergence of new request forms and with how the child makes request selections (Wootton 1997: chs 3 and 5; and Wootton 2005).

Another strategy for developmental enquiry would be to examine how the uses of the word 'actually' alter as the child becomes older. In Clift's (2001) findings on adults, for example, this word is not restricted to turn-initial environments, and certain uses of the word in other turn positions by adults do not appear to have an obvious parallel in this child's usage – for example, the inserted forms of self-repair identified by Clift (2001: 274), such as *We were travelling- we were- we'd just left the ashram actually and we were travelling with some Jain women.* Also in the context of self-repair, a further contrast relates to the turn design associated with 'actually' when it is used to restart a turn. Whereas Clift found that in adult usage the words subsequent to the 'actually' differed from the part of the turn that had been earlier abandoned, it appears that Emily can reuse these earlier words in her 'actually' prefaced restart, as in Extract 4.2.

To conclude I want to make two points about this kind of developmental comparison. First, it seems clear that Emily's frequent use of 'actually' at this age is likely to be somewhat idiosyncratic, so in a more general population there would be grounds for examining words other than 'actually' which can appear to perform equivalent discourse functions: obvious candidates here would be words like 'but' 'well' and 'maybe'. In effect, the most useful unit of analysis would be the discourse function rather than any particular word, such as 'actually', involved in the realisation of this function. The second point is that in making age comparisons we also have to take into account the general turn design, the kind of action that 'actually' is part of. In the examples above from Clift, 'actually' is one component of that part of a turn which deals with self-repair. The various techniques involved in self-repair are themselves going to show developmental change; , indeed, it may be that in an example like *Jain women* above, this kind of inserted self-repair is a later developmental phenomenon. In order to establish this one would need to compare the child's repertoire of self-repair skills at different points in time – not, of course, restricting such enquiry to instances containing particular words such as 'actually'. If such inserted self-repair was shown to be a later phenomenon, then it is the evolution of such a self-repair technique that would seem to require primary analytic attention, a technique which makes possible the kind of 'actually' use that we find in *Jain women*. In these various ways this child's use of 'actually' suggests lines of developmental enquiry that extend well beyond the usage of this particular word.

Acknowledgements

An earlier version of this chapter was given at the ESRC seminar on Analysing Interactions in Childhood, held at the University of Sheffield in September 2006. I am especially grateful for helpful comment at that time from Bill Wells and Melissa Wright. I can be contacted at ajwoott@ajwoott.plus.com.

References

Bloom, L., Lahey, M., Hood, L., Lifter, K. and Fiess, K. (1980) Complex sentences: Acquisition of syntactic connectives and the semantic relations they encode. *Journal of Child Language*, 7, 235–261.

Carpendale, J. and Lewis, C. (2006) *How children develop social understanding.* Oxford: Blackwell.

Clift, R. (2001) Meaning in interaction: The case of *actually. Language*, 77, 245–291.

Feldman, C.F. (1989) Monologue as problem-solving narrative. In K. Nelson (ed.), *Narratives from the crib.* Cambridge, MA: Harvard University Press.

Filipi, A. (2001) *The organization of pointing sequences in parent-toddler interaction.* Unpublished doctoral dissertation. Monash University: Australia.

Forrester, M.A. (2008) The emergence of self-repair: A case study of one child during the early preschool years. *Research on Language and Social Interaction*, 41, 99–128.

Gerhardt, J. (1991) The meaning and use of the modals HAFTA, NEEDTA and WANNA in children's speech. *Journal of Pragmatics*, 16, 531–590.

Griffiths, P. (1985) The communicative functions of children's single word speech. In M. Barrett (ed.), *Children's single word speech.* Chichester: Wiley.

Halliday, M.A.K. and Hasan, R. (1976) *Cohesion in English.* London: Longman.

Peters, A.M. (1995) Strategies in the acquisition of syntax. In P. Fletcher and B. MacWhinney (eds), *The handbook of child language.* Oxford: Blackwell.

Quirk, R., Greenbaum, S., Leech, G. and Svartvik, J. (1985) *A comprehensive grammar of the English language.* London: Longman.

Schegloff, E.A. (2007) *Sequence organization in interaction.* Cambridge: Cambridge University Press.

Scott, C.M. (1984) Adverbial connectivity in conversations of children 6 to 12. *Journal of Child Language*, 11, 423–452.

Tognini-Bonelli, E. (1993) Interpretive modes in discourse: *Actual* and *actually.* In M. Baker, G. Francis and E. Tognini-Bonelli (eds), *Text and technology: In honour of John Sinclair.* Amsterdam: Benjamins.

Tomasello, M. (1999) *The cultural origins of human cognition.* Cambridge, MA: Harvard University Press.

Wootton, A.J. (1994) Object transfer, intersubjectivity and third position repair: Early developmental observations of one child. *Journal of Child Language*, 21, 543–564.

Wootton, A.J. (1997) *Interaction and the development of mind.* Cambridge: Cambridge University Press.

Wootton, A.J. (2005) Interactional and sequential configurations informing request format selection in children's speech. In A. Hakulinen and M. Selting (eds), *Syntax and lexis in conversation: Studies in the use of linguistic resources in talk-in-interaction.* Amsterdam: Benjamins.

Wootton, A.J. (2007) A puzzle about 'please': Repair, increments and related matters in the speech of a young child. *Research on Language and Social Interaction*, 40, 171–198.

Zukow, P., Reilly, J. and Greenfield, P.M. (1982) Making the absent present: Facilitating the transition from sensorimotor to linguistic communication. In K. Nelson (ed.), *Children's language*, Volume 3. New Jersey: Erlbaum.

Chapter 5

Children's emerging and developing self-repair practices

MINNA LAAKSO

Introduction

This study investigates the emergence and development of conversational self-repair practices by Finnish children. Repair practices are the main means of solving problems in speaking, hearing and understanding in order to maintain intersubjective understanding between interlocutors; repair is the *'self-righting mechanism for the organization of language uses in social interaction'* (Schegloff *et al*. 1977: 381). Focusing on 1-to-4-year-old children interacting with their parents, the relationship between self-initiated (by the child) and other-initiated (by the parent) self-repair will in particular be studied, as some prior studies suggest that children's self-repair of speech first emerges when the parents other-initiate repair by requesting clarification. The role of repairing activities in the process of learning to use language will also be considered.

It is already widely acknowledged that children acquire language and learn to communicate through participation in meaningful interactions with adults and other children (see, e.g., McTear 1985; Wootton 1997; Chapman 2000; Tomasello 2003); to learn to use language 'children appear to need exposure to language in interactive contexts' (Clark 2003: 28). Parent–child interaction in the early years and peer interaction at a later stage are important arenas of learning and practising language skills. In particular, parents' repairs of their children's early expressions are seen as an essential feedback mechanism for language learning (e.g. Corsaro 1977; Sokolov and Snow 1994; Saxton 2000).

From more child-centred perspectives, the motivation to learn language comes from the need to establish oneself as an agent in the social world, using language to communicate with others and carry out social actions. Repair is, in this perspective, a critical skill used in revising speech errors and in rectifying if one has been misunderstood. In this way, the child's self-repair enhances the mastery of language by making the child's expressions more accurate and understandable to others. Furthermore, the use of repair enhances effective communication in solving problems in mutual understanding.

The most common practice of repair in adults is same-turn self-repair by the speaker who cuts off speaking and modifies the talk in progress. In Finnish, cut-off is not the only means to initiate same-turn self-repair: self-repairs are also indicated with lexical particles such as *eiku* (negation *ei* + particle *ku*, corresponding to some extent to 'no I mean' in English), *tai* ('or') and *siis* (a particle corresponding approximately to 'I mean') (Sorjonen and Laakso 2005). By cutting off and modifying in self-repair, the speaker displays an analysis of his or her ongoing speech. In this way, self-repair opens a window to the developing cognition and to language monitoring in particular, and can thus reflect the ongoing process of language learning. The study of the organisation of repair thus also offers a view of the child's developing skills to monitor the behaviour of oneself and others and to recognise potential failures in interaction.

In ordinary adult conversations there is a preference for self-repair over other-correction, i.e. the speaker of a problematic turn has the first opportunity to repair, and other-corrections rarely occur (Schegloff *et al.* 1977). This means that the recipients of problematic turns do not usually other-correct but only other-initiate repair by requesting clarification, and the original speaker of the problematic turn does the actual self-repair in the third turn after the problem turn. However, it has been suggested that in conversation between children and adults there is no such preference for children's self-repair but rather parents' other-corrections are common and even 'one vehicle for socialization' and 'a device for dealing with those who are still learning [. . .] to operate with a system which requires that they be adequate self-monitors and self-correctors' (Schegloff *et al.* 1977: 381).

Until recently, there has been rather little study on the emerging repair practices of children, and work on Finnish children is particularly scarce (see, however, Leiwo 1991; Jokinen 1998; Laakso 2006; Tykkyläinen 2007). According to observations on children acquiring English, self-repair – i.e. the management of one's own talk – is found to be in use as early as 1;6 to 2 years of age (Clark 1978; McTear 1985; Forrester 2008). Even at an earlier age, children clarify their speaking turns in the third position, i.e. if they have not been understood by the recipients of their talk (Golinkoff 1986; Wootton 1994; Filipi 2002). Children begin to make other-initiations of repair, which occur in connection with problems of hearing or understanding the talk of others, when they are approaching 3 years of age or even younger (Garvey 1977; Forrester and Cherrington 2009). However, even before the age of 3, children respond to other-initiations by others (Schegloff 1989). In English-speaking communities, other-initiations of repair (e.g. *Pardon?*, *What?* and *Hm?* or other questions) are found to be frequently used by adults to get the child to repeat her or his previous turn in a corrected form (Drew 1981; Langford 1981; Corrin, forthcoming, and Chapter 2 this volume). This suggests that children's self-repair may evolve from these kinds of parent–child sequential social routines into same-turn self-repair within the child's own speaking turn. However, in a recent longitudinal case study of an English-speaking child from 1 to 3;6 years of age, the child was observed (almost at all recordings studied) to self-initiate repair more often than respond to the parent's other-initiations (Forrester 2008). Similar quantitative observations on children producing clearly more self- than other-initiated self-repairs have also been made on Finnish 2-year-olds (Jokinen 1998).

Some researchers also claim that parents other-correct more the speech of younger children who make more errors (Corsaro 1977; Chouinard and Clark 2003), whereas other researchers have found that parents correct more their older and linguistically advanced children (see, e.g., Saxton 2000). Furthermore, some researchers claim that parents of younger children more often make other-initiations and encourage their children to self-repair whereas with older children parents are more likely to other-correct

(Vander Woude and Barton 2001). Previous research findings on parents' other-correction and children's self-repair are thus not quite consistent in relation to the age of the child. The proportions of children's self- and other-initiated self-repair may vary during the child's development, although it is not yet clear how.

Aim

The aim of this study is to produce new scientific knowledge about the development of conversational self-repair practices by 1- to 4-year-old Finnish-speaking children. Focusing on parent–child interactions, I will look at when the children's first self-repairs emerge and how the self-repair practices develop during the first years of life. In particular, the relationship between self- (by the child) and other-initiated (by the parent) repair will be examined to see whether children's self-repairs first emerge through parents' initiations (e.g. questions, candidate understandings or other-corrections). Furthermore, I will examine which features of talk and interaction children's first repairs address and discuss how the development of repair relates to the development of language and communication.

From the Finnish language point of view and its repairing practices, the emergence of lexical repair devices (the particles *eiku*, *tai* and *siis* in particular) will be examined. Furthermore, it is not self-evident that the preferences and practices of repair found in English-speaking children and their parents exist in Finnish culture as well. On the basis of the repeated viewing of the Finnish data, the parents' open other-initiations (questions like *Pardon*, *Hm?* and *What?*) appear to be particularly few in number although they regularly occur in English interactions of the same kind (cf. Drew 1981; Corrin, Chapter 2 this volume). Instead of other-initiating, Finnish parents appear to directly other-correct their children's speech.

Data and methods

The data consists of both longitudinal parent–child interactions and cross-sectional parent–child and child–child interactions that were gathered for this study from a larger data base that was collected in a project entitled 'The child's developing language and interaction' during the years 2002–2007. The project (PI Minna Laakso) collected two large corpora: the Helsinki Longitudinal Child language corpus includes about 120 hours of videos of five children who were followed from 10 months until the age of 5; the Helsinki Cross-sectional Child language corpus includes about 150 hours of videos of different interactions (with family and friends) of ten 3-, ten 4- and ten 5-year-olds. All interactions were videotaped at home by a cameraman, except for the latter corpus where the parents also videotaped their children for one week during daily activities.

In the present study the longitudinal corpora consist of the videotapes of four children interacting with one of their parents in a follow-up from 1 up to 3 years of age (see Table 5.1). From the cross-sectional corpus, interactions of three 3-year-olds and two 4-year-olds were selected for the present study. This study thus focuses on the parent–child interactions of four longitudinally followed children: three girls, Helmi, Nuppu, and Vilma, and one boy, Juha. In addition, the interactions of three 3-year-olds

Table 5.1 The children and the number of recordings studied

Child	Sex	Age	Number of recordings (duration)
Helmi	girl	1;0–2;6	10 (8 hours)
Juha	boy	1;0–3;1	10 (9 hours)
Nuppu	girl	1;0–3;1	16 (12 hours)
Vilma	girl	1;0–2;6	9 (8 hours)
Liisa	girl	3;3	4 (2 hours)
Martti	boy	3;3	4 (2 hours)
Selina	girl	3;1	4 (2 hours)
Emma	girl	4;8	4 (2 hours)
Hilma	girl	4;11	4 (2 hours)

(Liisa, Martti and Selina) and two 4-year-olds (Hilma and Emma) from the cross-sectional corpus were studied. Thus, the whole corpus contains parent–child interactions from nine children, altogether about 47 hours of videotape (see Table 5.1).

Conversation analysis (CA) was adopted as the method for this study due to its empirical nature and strong focus on the analysis of sequentially evolving moment-by-moment interaction (Goodwin and Heritage 1990; Schegloff 2007). The method is data driven and it sees the context and identities of the participants as locally produced and interpreted. However, previous CA findings on turn-taking, sequential and repair organizations are used as the basis for observing and identifying the structures and practices of the children's interactions. The videotapes were inspected for the occurrences of children's self-repair, and the potential repairs with their co-occurring context of talk were transcribed following CA notation (see Glossary of Transcript Symbols). In addition to speech, also some relevant aspects of non-verbal communication were marked in the transcript (e.g. gaze direction, hand gesturing, and handling of toys). In the analysed data extracts, the talk of each person is depicted on two lines. The lines are read as follows: the first line shows the original talk in Finnish and the second is the translation into English. Utterances that are in the analytical focus are also provided with a grammatical word-by-word gloss in between the line of original Finnish and the English translation (see Appendix 5.1 for the glossing symbols). When eye gaze is noteworthy in the analysis of the videotaped examples, the speaker's gaze is marked with a line above the spoken utterance; gaze notation is simplified from the transcription convention developed by Goodwin (1981). When of analytical interest, the non-verbal activities are transcribed within double brackets below the spoken utterance, or on a line of its own, if non-verbal action takes place independent of speech. Smiling voice is represented by a £ sign at the beginning and end of the featured utterance where it occurs.

In what follows, I will first concentrate on repairs in the second year of life where children's first self-repairs appear to emerge. Second, I will describe 2-year-olds and their developing repair practices. After this I will look at the repair practices of 3- and 4-year-olds who revise their utterances to match different activities and recipients, using a greater variety of means. Finally, I will discuss the relationship of self- and other-initiated repair and the relevance of the emerging and developing repair practices for language learning and for maintaining intersubjective understanding between the interlocutors.

The emergence of first self-repairs in the second year of life

The following two observations can be made about the interactions of the four children who were studied longitudinally. Firstly, from 1 year of age onwards the children made revised attempts at communicating when their parents misunderstood their prior utterances. Problems in understanding occurred quite frequently, as the children did not yet speak or spoke with multi-modal proto-word expressions in which the proto-word does not yet have a fixed referential meaning. Secondly, the first actual self-initiated self-repairs emerged at the age of 1;8–1;11 (with the age of emergence depending on the child). At the same age the parents also frequently other-corrected their children's speech.

Self-repair after parent's misunderstanding

Below we can see how a child and mother communicate when the child does not yet speak but uses gesturing and word-like vocalisations (proto-words) to express her intentions. Proto-words are the first articulated word-like structures that usually consist of one articulatory movement (such as the closure of the airway with the tongue) during phonation (Menn 1983). Interestingly, it is often the child who initiates the conversation using the pointing gesture and vocalisation, and the mother then verbally interprets the child's expression as if offering it to the child for confirmation. In Extract 5.1 the mother is feeding Nuppu (1;0) in the kitchen. Nuppu sits in her highchair with the mother beside her. As the mother offers her porridge, Nuppu does not take it but produces a proto-word [ættæ] and points at a flower on the table in front of her (line 2). The mother names the targeted object: *se on kukka* 'it is a flower' (line 3) and the feeding continues. (The two-part sequence is marked in bold face in the transcript.) Later the mother also brings the flower closer so that Nuppu can see it better. However, she does not give it to Nuppu but keeps it out of her reach.

Extract 5.1 *Nuppu (girl; age 1;0) and her mother*

1   Mother: M::hym?
            ((*the mother offers Nuppu a spoonful of porridge*))

2   Nuppu: Ät::↑tä,
            ((***Nuppu points to a flower on the table***))

3   Mother: Se on ku̲kka.
            It is a flower.

4   (7.0) ((*The mother feeds the spoonful to Nuppu*))

5   Mother: °(Täytyy) ottaa° ↑kukka °vähän° (2.0) tännepäin
            °(Let's) take° the ↑flower °a bit° (2.0) closer here

6   ja ka̲tsella sitä.
            and (let's) look at it.
            ((*the mother stands up, reaches the flower and takes it closer on the table*))

7   (2.0) Kaunis kukka.
            (2.0) A beautiful flower.
            ((*the mother sits down*))

After this the child's early efforts to repair come into play (see Extract 5.2 where the interaction continues). Nuppu is not satisfied with the label 'flower' but repeats her proto-word expression in revised form (see line 8). Again, the mother names the flower (line 9). After the mother's labelling response Nuppu extends her body further towards the flower, rubs her ear and rejects the spoon of porridge that the mother offers. Furthermore, she displays her dissatisfaction by crying a bit when saying her proto-word (line 11 marked with an arrow). This clearly is an attempt to reject the mother's response as a misunderstanding of Nuppu's intention. Thus, potentially, here is a problem in the intersubjective understanding concerning what Nuppu's pointing/reaching action and proto-word mean: the mother has interpreted Nuppu's initiating action as requesting a label for an object, whereas Nuppu herself revises here her prior turn by reaching more clearly for the object (as if she wants to touch it and inspect it more closely; see Extract 5.2). After this the mother produces a vocalization with rising intonation (*M::mhym?*, line 12) with which she minimally requests Nuppu to continue. Nuppu then repeats her proto-word utterance, again accompanied with a pointing gesture towards the flower (line 13). This time the mother responds by naming the flower with a rising intonation, as a try-mark, as if offering the flower for confirmation (line 14). Simultaneously the mother also turns the flower a bit so that Nuppu can see it better, but still keeps the poisonous flower out of Nuppu's reach. Nuppu responds to the mother's action of turning the flower pot with more distress (she moves restlessly in her chair and also cries longer; lines 15–16). At this point, the mother offers Nuppu a spoon obviously in an attempt to move Nuppu's attention away from the flower (line 17), which indicates that she may have understood what Nuppu was after. However, the spoon does not interest Nuppu. Instead, Nuppu re-introduces, for the fourth time and now with clearly emphasised prosody, her proto-word expression and pointing towards the flower (line 19; see Figure 5.1). As the mother again only names the flower, Nuppu starts to cry (lines 22 and 24), and finally the mother moves on to give Nuppu some vitamins.

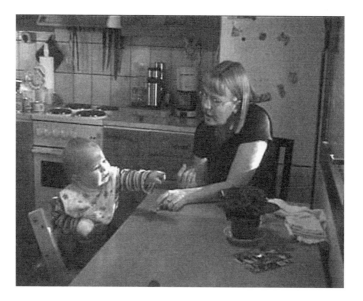

Figure 5.1 Nuppu is reaching for the flower. Used with parental permission.

Extract 5.2   *Nuppu (girl; age 1;0) and her mother* (continued from Extract 5.1)

8   Nuppu: Ät:ti.
((*Nuppu extends her hand and reaches for the flower*))

9   Mother: Kukka.
A flower.

10   Nuppu: →   (15.0) ((*Nuppu looks at the flower, drops the sippy cup from her hand, extends her body towards the flower, rubs her ear, and rejects the spoon the mother offers her*))

11   Nuppu: →   Ättbbhhh.=

12   Mother: = M::mhym?

13   Nuppu: Ät::↑tä,
((*Nuppu reaches forward and points towards the flower*))

14   Mother: Kukka? (2.6) No:i.
A flower? (2.6) So:.
((*the mother turns the flower pot*))

15   Nuppu: →   (6.0) ((*Nuppu rubs her ear and moves restlessly in the chair*))

16   →   ↑ÄÄÄÄhHÄÄÄÄHHHÄÄÄ

17   Mother: =Toss oli sun oma lusikka.
=There was your own spoon.
((*The mother puts a spoon on the table in front of Nuppu*))

18   (2.5)

19   Nuppu: ↑Ät:::::↑tä,
((*Nuppu reaches forward and points to the flower, Figure 5.1*))

20   Mother: Kukka?
A flower?
((*the mother looks at Nuppu*))

21   (2.0)

22   Nuppu: →   (K)hhbbhybhybhy.
((*Nuppu looks down, the mother takes Nuppu's spoon from the table and puts it to her hand*))

23   Mother: Mmm[:h.
                     [
24   Nuppu: →   [(k)bbhybhybhy,

25   Mother: Tossa lusikka. (1.0) Ai niin meijän piti ottaa noi
There's the spoon. (1.0) Oh yes we should take those
((*the mother stands up and leaves to fetch*

(.) vitamii°nitipat.°
(.) vitami°n drops.°
the vitamin bottle))

It is noteworthy that prior to this sequence the mother has given the sippy cup to Nuppu after she produced a similar expression of a proto-word and a pointing gesture at the cup. Here Nuppu obviously tries to get the mother to give her the flower, and thus keeps on repeating her request in a revised and emphasised form to clarify her intention to the mother. It is also remarkable that the child insists on revising her expression for so long (lines 10, 13 and 19) and rejects the mother's labelling responses by crying (lines 11, 16, 22 and 24), until the mother changes the activity. Thus it is clearly observable in Extract 5.2 that even a child who does not yet speak can attempt to clarify her expression if she is misunderstood by her interlocutor. This finding is in line with the observations of slightly older children doing revisions after parental misunderstanding (Golinkoff 1986; Marcos 1991; Wootton 1994) as well as with the more recent experimental studies on repeated pointing gestures by 1-year-olds (Liszkowski *et al.* 2007), and supports the claim that the ability to repair communicative breakdowns develops before speech, at the same time as intentional communication, with gestures being integral parts of these 'preconversational' repairs (cf. Alexander *et al.* 1997).

The emergence of children's first self-initiated self-repairs of speech in same turn

The children's first same-turn self-repairs within their own speaking turns were lexical or phonological revisions of prior speech initiated with a cut-off. In the present data, these abruptly cut-off utterances emerged in the speech of the four longitudinally followed children (Helmi, Juha, Nuppu, and Vilma) at the ages of 1;8–1;11. After cutting off, the children accomplished self-repair within the same turn by replacing the cut-off word with another or by revising the pronunciation of the word. Words and their pronunciation, i.e. basic lexicon and phonology, were also the aspects of language the children were currently acquiring at this age, before the age of 2 years. However, the instances of same-turn self-repair were still rare. The following extracts exemplify some early self-initiated self-repairs of speech within the same speaking turn by Nuppu (1;10) and Juha (1;11).

In Extracts 5.3 and 5.4 Nuppu and her mother are sitting on the floor and inspecting toys that are in a string bag. In this extract the mother frequently asks Nuppu to name the toys she finds in the bag. However, Nuppu is inspecting the toys and playing with them and frequently answers the mother only with a deictic term, the pronominal adjective *tommonen* (that kind of + adjective ending; 'one like that'). Nuppu also requests her mother's help in getting one of the toys, a plastic banana, out of the bag, and is more focused on her own agenda of finding the banana than in replying to her mother. Nuppu's self-repairs emerge in lines 15 (Extract 5.3) and 42 (Extract 5.4). In both cases she abruptly cuts off the word she is producing and revises her speech.

Extract 5.3 *Nuppu (girl; age 1;10) and her mother*

1   Nuppu: Hiinä hommonen. ((*hommonen* is a child form of *tommonen*))
                There one.like.that.
                ((*Nuppu pulls a plastic lemon fruit from the string bag*))

2   Mother: Mikäs se ↑on,
                What is ↑it.

3   Nuppu: No hommonen. ((child form))
                Well one.like.that.
                ((*Nuppu flings the lemon to the floor*))

4   Mother: Mikäs se on.
                What is it.

5   Nuppu: Manani. ((a child form of *banaani* 'a banana'))
                A banana.

6   Mother: Teil oli tänään tämmönen pikkunen ku mummin kanssa tulitte kotiin.
                You had today such a little one when you and granny came home.
                ((*the mother shows the lemon to Nuppu*))

7   (.)

8   Mother: Mikäs se on.
                What is it.
                ((*the mother shows the lemon to Nuppu*))

9   Nuppu: No homm↑monen? ((child form))
                Well one↑.like.that?
                ((*Nuppu shows an egg to her mother*))

10 Mother: Hedelmä?
                A fruit?

11 Nuppu: Hememmä? ((child form of *hedelmä*, 'fruit'))
                A fruit?

12 Mother: Tää on sitruuna.
                This is a lemon.

13   (2.0) ((*Nuppu searches the bag for a new toy*))

14 Mother: Ja tämä, (1.8) mikä [tä-
                And this, (1.8) what [thi-
                                    [

15 Nuppu: →   **[Manen- (.) banaani.**
                                    [Manen- (.) banana.
                                    ((*Nuppu searches the bag*))

16   (.) onnoonoo (7.5) banaani. (2.0) Homm↑onen?
                (.) onnoonoo (7.5) a banana. (2.0) One↑.like.that?
                ((*Nuppu searches the bag, finds a plastic giraffe and gives it to the mother*))

17	Mother:	Mikäs tää on?
		What is this?
		((*the mother shows the giraffe to Nuppu*))

18	Nuppu:	Banaani. (10.5) BANAANI,
		Banana. (10.5) BANANA,
		((*Nuppu searches the bag*))

19	Mother:	Joo:?
		Yea:h?

20	Nuppu:	MANAANI TU(O)LTA MANAANI,
		banana there.from banana
		BANANA FROM THERE BANANA,

21	Mother:	Siinä. (.) Banaani (.) noin,
		There. (.) A banana (.) so,
		((*the mother takes the banana from the bag and gives it to Nuppu*))

22		(3.0) ((*Nuppu plays as if eating the banana*))

23	Mother:	£Nam nam nam?£ (2.8) Leikkibanaani.
		£Yum-yum yum?£ (2.8) A toy banana.

As can be seen above, in line 16, Nuppu is searching for the banana in the bag when she starts saying *manen-* (a child form of banana) which she then cuts off. After the cut-off she revises the word phonologically to *banaani*, the Finnish word for banana. Her self-repair demonstrates her orientation to the phonological detail of the word she is producing. Interestingly, Nuppu's cut-off utterance overlaps her mother's request to name another toy (line 15). Both the mother and Nuppu are initiating new interactive sequences here; the mother initiates a labelling sequence (cf. Tarplee 1996), whereas Nuppu starts the activity of searching for the banana. Thus, instead of naming things, Nuppu is oriented to her own interest in finding the banana, and finally does so with the help of her mother (line 21).

The second self-repair in line 42 is a lexical replacement (see Extract 5.4 below). Nuppu finds a toy apple in the bag and starts to name it *omen-* (*omena* is apple) but cuts off and produces the word *banaani* ('banana'). With her self-repair she actually mis-names the fruit, replacing the name of the fruit she is holding in her hand (an apple) with another (a banana). However, in doing self-initiated self-repair Nuppu already shows awareness that there are different names for different types of fruit. Furthermore, her subsequent actions show that she is actively trying to recover those names: after naming the apple as a banana she starts looking around and searching for the toy banana (line 42). Her mother joins the activity and labels the fruit Nuppu is holding as an apple (line 44) and then takes the banana from the floor and shows it to Nuppu (line 46) who then names it correctly as a banana (line 47). The mother confirms this and they start playing as if eating the banana. Thus in Extract 5.4 the labels of the fruit inspected are negotiated jointly as the result of the child's self-repair.

Extract 5.4   *Nuppu (girl; age 1;10) and her mother* (continued from Extract 5.3)

((18 lines of playing with a toy egg and pear omitted))

41   Nuppu: (9.5) ((*Nuppu takes a tiny toy apple in her hand and inspects it*))

                    ((looks at the apple))

42   Nuppu: →   **OMEN- u:::m::: b̲a̲naani.**
                    Appl(e)   banana
                    appl- u:::m::: b̲a̲nana.
                    ((Nuppu holds the apple in her hand))

                    ((Nuppu starts to look around searching))
43   (2.0) ((*Nuppu turns her head from side to side*))

44   Mother: O̲me̲na se °on.°
                    apple   it   is
                    It is an a̲pp̲le.

45   (.)((*Nuppu looks at the banana that lies on the floor*))

46   Mother: Ja tääl [on-
                    And here is-
                    ((the mother takes the banana from the floor))

                         [
47   Nuppu   [Manaani=
                    [A banana=
                    [((*Nuppu takes the banana from her mother's hand*))

48   Mother: =Siin on banaani.
                    =There is a banana.

49   Nuppu: .mt .mt .mt
                    ((Nuppu 'eats' the banana))

50   Nuppu: Äiti,
                    Mother,
                    ((Nuppu offers the banana to the mother))

51   Mother: .mt .mt Kiitti?
                    .mt .mt Thanks?
                    ((the mother 'eats' the banana from Nuppu's hand))

52   Nuppu: ((*Nuppu turns to the banana in her left hand*))

53   Nuppu: .mt .mt .mt .mt .mt .mt .mt [.mt .mt
                    ((Nuppu turns to the apple in her right hand and 'eats' it))

                                [
54   Mother: [Onko h̲y̲vää. (.) nam ↑nam ↑nam?
                          [Is it good (.) yum ↑yum ↑yum?
                          [((*the mother turns towards Nuppu*))

55   Nuppu: ((*Nuppu puts the toy apple in her mouth and bites it*))

It is noteworthy here in Extracts 5.3 and 5.4 that self-repairs occur in places where the child and the parent have different orientations to the activity they are engaged in. The child's self-repaired one-word utterances initiate new interactive sequences of joint focus in the interaction. The repair stops the speech flow and simultaneously the parent starts to orient to the activity the child is engaged in. Consequently, some mutual play with the inspected toys emerges. In Extract 5.3 Nuppu plays as if eating the toy banana and the mother comments on this with a smile (lines 22 and 23) and, in Extract 5.4 Nuppu 'eats' the toy banana herself and also offers it to the mother who plays as if eating it. In these moments there is playfulness and mutual gazing at one another.

Similarly, in Extracts 5.5 and 5.6 Juha and his mother are sitting on the floor and inspecting cardboard pictures that lie there. The pictures describe different objects and are shaped in the forms of these objects (e.g. in the form of a spoon, a hammer and a guitar). Also here the mother is requesting Juha to name the pictures but Juha himself is more oriented to inspecting the pictures and exploring their uses. Juha makes two self-initiated self-repairs in lines 9 and 28. Interestingly, both self-repairs emerge in an address term when Juha addresses his mother. Juha starts to say *mummi* ('grand-mother') and then replaces it with the address term *äiti* ('mother'). In both cases, the disfluency of the self-repair intensifies the effect of the address term in directing the mother's gaze and orientation to the activity Juha is engaged in. Before the self-repair in line 9 Juha has been trying to put the cardboard spoon under his heel while the mother has been asking him to name a picture of a hammer. After the self-repaired address term, the mother says '*mmh?*' (line 10) and Juha shows the mother what he is doing with the spoon (line 11). The mother asks Juha if it is a shoehorn (in Finnish shoehorn is *kenkälusikka* 'shoe spoon') and Juha confirms this (lines 12–14). They both smile.

Extract 5.5 *Juha (boy, age 1;11) and his mother*

		((*Looks to the floor*))
1	Juha:	Tonne, tonne,
		there.to there.to
		To there, there,
2		(0.7)
3	Juha:	No ni,
		Well so,
4	Juha:	((*Juha takes a cardboard spoon and* [*pushes it to his heel*))
		[
5	Mother:	[Ti<u>e</u>dätkö sä mikä t<u>ä</u>mä on.
		[Do you know what this is.
		[((*the mother shows a hammer*))
6	Juha:	((*Juha glances at the picture of a hammer and continues to push the spoon under his heel*))
7	Juha:	Noi,
		So,
8		(0.2)

```
                         ((Juha glances at mother))
  9   Juha: →     Mum-     Äiti?
                         Gran(ny) mummy
                         Gran-    Mummy?
                         ((Juha turns towards the mother))

                         J___
 10   Mother:    mmh?

 11   Juha:       ((Juha pushes the spoon to his heel))

 12   Mother:    Onks se ↑kenkälusikka, £hhhh£
                         Is it a ↑shoehorn, £hhhh£

                         M_____X
 13   Juha:       ((Juha smiles))

 14   Juha:       °(on)°
                         ° (it is) °
```

In the other self-repair in line 28 Juha also addresses his mother and similarly first produces the beginning of the word *mummi* ('grandmother') (see Extract 5.6). Again, the mother responds to this with *mm* as a signal to go ahead, and Juha shows her how he uses the cardboard spoon as a shoehorn (lines 29–30). The mother and Juha look at each other, both smiling and laughing about Juha's action with the spoon. After this, the mother verbalises Juha's action by asking whether he is putting his shoes on (line 33). In line 34 Juha does not answer the mother's question but asks 'where'. This one-word utterance is in this sequential place difficult to interpret and it launches a repair sequence where the mother other-initiates repair; first with a question, '*Ai mikä*' ('you mean what (is where)', line 35) and then with a polar question with two candidate answers, shoe and shoehorn (line 36). Juha responds non-verbally by nodding (line 37) and the mother provides the answer to Juha's original question by explaining the location of the shoehorn (line 39). However, now Juha rejects his mother's answer by saying *ei* ('no') and shaking his head which displays that the mother has not satisfactorily answered his question and there is a potential misunderstanding (line 40). The mother then offers the other alternative, the shoe, as the object which Juha is trying to locate, and Juha confirms this by nodding (lines 41–42), and, finally, the mother is able to answer the question Juha asked in line 34. Therefore besides self-initiated self-repairs, sequential construction of mutual understanding is also taking place, as it did with 1-year-olds (cf. Extract 5.1).

Extract 5.6 *Juha (boy, age 1;11) and his mother* (Extract 5.5 continued)

```
 15   Mother:    Tää on vasara. (0.5) kop kop kop [kop kop.
                         This is a hammer. (0.5) knock knock knock
                         ((the mother hits the floor with the picture of a hammer))
                                                                              [

 16   Juha:                                              [((Juha takes the hammer))
```

17 Juha: kaakka, hakka, kaakka. ((potentially child forms of *hakkaa* 'hits'))
         hit,   hit,   hit.

18 Juha: hmh, hmh,
         ((*Juha puts away the hammer and bends down to look at the pictures*))

19 Juha: Tää.
         This.
         ((*Juha takes the picture of a guitar*))

20 Mother: ↑Kitara.
         A ↑guitar.

21 Juha: ((*Juha hits the floor with the cardboard guitar*))

22 Mother: £E(h)ei se mikään hakattava ole.£
         £No(h)o it is not something to hit with.£

23 Juha: Tää,
         This,
         ((*Juha shows the hammer to his mother*))

24 Mother: Sillä voi hakata, se on kato vähän sama juttu ku siinä sun-
         With that you can hit, it is y'see a little bit like the same thing as your-
         ((*the mother turns to dig into the toy basket behind her potentially in order to find a
         toy she is talking about*))

25 Juha: (aa-ha tä [hä)
                    [

26 Mother: [Siinä ku sä löit niitä< (0.5) p<u>a</u>likoita tai niitä (0.2) n<u>a</u>ppeja.
                    [When you hit those< (0.5) blocks or those (0.2) buttons.
                    ((*the mother digs into the toy basket behind her*))

27   (0.7) ((*the mother turns back towards Juha who studies the pictures on the floor;
                    Juha takes the cardboard picture of a spoon*))

28 Juha: → **Mum- <u>ä</u>iti,**
         Gran- m<u>u</u>mmy,

29 Mother: mm,

30 Juha: ((*Juha puts the spoon to his heel*))

         J_____ X
31 Mother: [he he he
         [

         [M_____X
32 Juha: [((*Juha smiles*))

33 Mother: Laitat sä sillä kengät jalkaan.
         Do you put shoes on with that.

34 Juha: Missä, (0.5) missä.
         Where, (0.5) where.

35   Mother: Ai   mikä?
                 PRT what-PAR
                 You mean what? (is where)

36   Mother: Kenkäkö, vai   kenkälusik[ka.
                 shoe-Q   or   shoe spoon
                 Do you mean shoe, or shoeh[orn.
                                          [

37   Juha: [((*Juha nods*))

38   (0.2)

39   Mother: Kenkälusikka on siel samassa kaapissa kuin imuri.
                 The shoehorn is there in the same closet as the vacuum cleaner.

40   Juha: Ei.
                 No.
                 ((*Juha shakes his head*))

41   Mother: Kenkä niinkö?
                 shoe   PRT-Q
                 Do you mean shoe?

42   Juha: .ehh
                 ((*Juha nods*))

43   Mother: Kengät on eteisessä.
                 Shoes are in the hall.

44   Juha: (iissi) ((*Juha stands up and walks to the hall*))

As can be seen from both Juha's and Nuppu's extracts above, self-repairs interestingly occur in places where the child and the parent have different orientations to the activity at hand. Furthermore, the children's self-repaired utterances initiate new interactive sequences of joint attention, and after the self-repaired utterance the parent starts to orient to the activity the child is engaged in and some mutual play emerges concerning things and their uses. In Extracts 5.3 and 5.4 Nuppu and her mother play as if eating the banana, and in Extracts 5.5 and 5.6 Juha shows his mother how to use the spoon as a shoehorn. In both cases there is playfulness that is shown in mutual eye contact, smiling and laughter. This observation is in line with Goodwin (1980) who showed that restarts (such as children's cut-off utterances here) are a powerful tool in directing the recipient's gaze and orientation to the speaker. Thus, besides repairing by replacement, the children are learning to use self-repairs interactively for directing the recipients' attention to their own doings. As the child after the first self-repair gets the parent into the joint play frame the child soon reintroduces a new self-repair with the same effect and can be seen to be learning the interactive usage of restarting (see lines 15 and 42 in Nuppu's Extracts 5.3 and 5.4 and lines 9 and 28 in Juha's Extracts 5.5 and 5.6).

In sum, the self-repairs that have been inspected in Extracts 5.2–5.6 have been self-initiated by the children themselves. Self-repairs that are launched after a co-participant's misunderstanding (Extract 5.2) emerge early by preverbal children. However, self-initiated same-turn self-repairs (Extracts 5.3–5.6) also emerge as soon as the children are using single words, well before 2 years of age. At this age, same-turn self-repairs are initiated by cutting off the word in progress and are completed by replacing the cut-off word or some phonemes in it.

Parents' other-corrections: the child self-repairs in third turn

At the same time as first self-initiated repairs emerged in the children's speech the parents also frequently made other-corrections where they revised their children's prior expressions. Parents' other-corrections were very common in all interactions studied. Other-correction often took the form of a corrective repetition of the child's prior single-word utterance. After the parent's correction, the children imitated it and thus self-repaired their initial production in the following third turn. These cases can be considered as sequentially constructed self-repair. Appendix 5.2 presents the frequencies of both children's self-initiated same-turn self-repairs (similar to Extracts 5.3–5.6) and of parent-initiated sequentially constructed self-repairs (see Extracts 5.7 and 5.8).

Similarly as was the case with the children's self-initiated self-repairs in Extracts 5.3–5.6 the parents' other-corrections also focused on phonological aspects and lexical choice. In particular, corrective repetitions occurred when the child and the parent were looking at picture books. Book sharing has been observed to be a common context for labelling objects in pictures (Tarplee 1996). The following two extracts exemplify how the mother other-corrects Nuppu's speech after Nuppu has labelled a picture in the book. In both cases Nuppu imitates the form corrected by the mother and thus orients to revising her speech both phonologically (7) and lexically (8).

Extract 5.7 *Nuppu (girl; age 1;10) and her mother looking at the picture book*

1		(1.0)
2	Mother:	Entäs täällä And what about here ((*the mother points at a picture of a carrot*))
3		(0.8)
4	Nuppu:	No pookkana.((child form of *porkkana* 'carrot')) Well a carrot.
5	Mother:	Joo:o? Yea:h? ((*the mother points at a picture of a rake*))
6	Nuppu:	**Hevava.** ((child form of *harava* 'rake'))
7	Mother:	**Harava?** **A rake?**
8	Nuppu: →	**Havava?** ((child form))
9	Mother:	Joo? (0.7) Entäs täällä? Yeah? (0.7) And here?

Extract 5.8 *Nuppu (girl; age 1;10) and her mother looking at a picture book*

1 Nuppu: **Mmm (kh)aapanen.** ((child form of *kärpänen* 'fly'))
Mmm a fly.
((*Nuppu is pointing at a picture of a wasp*))

2 Mother: **Se on ↑ampiainen,**
It is a ↑wasp,

3 Nuppu: → **Ampinen?** ((child form of *ampiainen* 'wasp'))
Wasp?

In both extracts above a three-part sequence emerges where (1) the child labels something in the book, (2) the parent other-corrects, and (3) the child imitates the correction and simultaneously self-repairs the original label. In Extract 5.7 the mother is pointing at a picture of a rake (*harava* in Finnish), which Nuppu names as a rake but the phonological production the word is still immature (*hevava*, line 6). The mother corrects (*harava*, line 7) and Nuppu imitates the correction (*havava*, line 8). In Extract 5.8 pointing at the book, Nuppu names a picture of a bug as a fly (line 1) and the mother corrects: 'it is a wasp' (line 2), and Nuppu imitates the corrected word (line 3). Although the child still produces simplified forms of the words, the imitated self-repairs, after the parent's other-correction, already adequately approximate the Finnish adult equivalents of these words.

Before the age of 2, all the children studied did imitate their parents' corrections and thus produced sequentially constructed self-repairs. Similar corrective repetitions by parents have been observed in the interactions of English-speaking children and their carers (Langford 1981; Tarplee 1996, this volume). Consistently with the findings of Tarplee (1996), parents' corrective repetitions were often prosodically marked. In my data the prosodic emphasis was done either with a pitch rise before the word (see Extract 5.8) or after the word as a final rise (see Extract 5.7). As the children regularly improved their pronunciation or lexical choice in their sequentially constructed self-repairs, parents' other-corrections appear to emerge as a means of corrective feedback that enables language learning (cf. Saxton 2000).

In sum, as can be seen from the Extracts 5.3–5.8 both self-initiated (by the child) and other-initiated (by the parent) repairs working on the child's prior speech emerge in parent–child interactions when the children are approaching 2 years of age. At this age parent-initiated self-repairs are still more common than self-initiated self-repairs (see the respective frequencies at age point I in Appendix 5.2). However, it is noteworthy that children who use single-word utterances for communicating are already able to monitor their own speech and even cut off when they notice some trouble. In these repairs, the children are also able to revise their utterances either lexically or phonologically. When other-correcting their children the parents did not use lexical repair markers such as *eiku* (negation particle *ei* + particle *ku*), although it is used in other-repairs in Finnish conversation. The parents' other-corrections were in the form of corrective repetition and thus not lexically marked as corrections. Nor did *eiku*, or other lexical initiators, occur in the children's self-initiated self-repairs at this age.

The development of self-repair practices by 2-year-olds

Same-turn self-repairs become more common than parent-initiated self-repairs

As the children passed 2 years of age, the more routinely they revised their speech quickly in the same turn. Simultaneously, the proportion of children's sequentially constructed self-repair clearly diminished (see age point II in Appendix 5.2). In this way, self-repairs reflected the children's developing linguistic skills and the monitoring of their own speech. In Extract 5.9 Helmi and her father are looking at pictures in a book and Helmi is engaged in pointing to and labelling the pictures. In line 3 she quickly revises her speech phonologically by replacing the phonologically less accurate label *kapeli* with *kameli* ('camel'):

Extract 5.9 *Helmi (girl; age 2;2) and her father looking at a picture book*

1 Helmi: ((*Helmi turns the pages quickly*))

2 Father: £S(h)ä muistat nää ulk(h)oo,£
            £Y(h)ou remember these by hea(h)rt£

3 Helmi: →   **Kapeli- ka̱meli.**
            Capel- ca̱mel.
            ((*Helmi points to a picture of a camel*))

4 Father: £O(h)oota.£
            £W(h)ait.£

Helmi's revision of her own speech already resembles self-repair by adult speakers of Finnish. However, she does not cut off in the midst of the word but immediately after it. Similar swift phonological revisions have been reported by English-speaking children over 2 years of age. Furthermore, the observation of regular same-turn self-repairs by 2-year-olds and at the same time diminishing other-corrections by the parents, is in line with prior findings on Finnish children aged 2;0 who were found to make more self- than other-initiated repairs in their play interactions with the parents (Jokinen 1998).

New types of same-turn self-repair emerge in 2-year-olds

Besides making swift and successful phonological revisions and lexical replacements, soon after 2 years of age the children studied also started to produce new and more complex types of same-turn self-repairs by adding to and abandoning elements in their speech. The emergence of new types of self-repair was possible as the children began to produce multi-word utterances once they passed the age of 2. Soon after 2 years the children studied started to recycle their multi-word utterances and add words to them. This kind of repair has been reported to emerge quite late, by 5 years of age with children learning English (Evans 1985). In Extract 5.10 Vilma makes an addition to her utterance (line 1):

Extract 5.10   *Vilma (girl; age 2;2) and her mother are playing with toy animals*

1   Vilma: →   **Syö   tota- (1.0) mun kivahvi syö (.) t<u>ä</u>tä.**
              eat-3 that   my   giraffe eat-3   this-PAR
              Eats that- (1.0) my giraffe eats (.) this.
              ((*Vilma moves the giraffe as if it were eating a piece of a jigsaw puzzle that lies on the floor*))

2   Mother: Ai mitä se syö.
              PRT what it eat-3
              What do you mean it eats.

3   Vilma: Oho. (.) tää liukastui.
              PRT   this slip-3
              Oops. (.) This one slipped. ((*Vilma's giraffe slips on the floor*))

In line 1 Vilma starts her turn with *syö tota-* ('eats that'), but cuts off and adds a subject to her clause: *mun kivahvi syö tätä* ('my giraffe eats this'). Thus she orients to the grammatical completeness of her utterance and shows an ability to monitor those aspects of language she is acquiring, as she has just begun to use multi-word utterances. On the other hand, by describing her actions more precisely she also orients towards maintaining mutual understanding with her mother who then may better follow the course of the play. However, the object of eating is not well defined. Vilma uses deictic terms 'that' and 'this' and, consequently, the mother requests clarification (line 2). For requesting clarification Vilma's mother uses the Finnish turn-initial particle *ai*, which indicates that in the prior talk something was new to its recipient (Hakulinen and Sorjonen 1986). Here the clarification request may even display doubt or disbelief (cf. Schegloff 1996) about the giraffe-eating jigsaw puzzle, but it may well be an attempt to clarify what the pieces of jigsaw might represent in the world of their play. It is noteworthy that Vilma does not reply to this other-initiation of repair.

Besides additions, after 2 years of age the children also started changing the type of utterance or action they were about to produce. In Extract 5.11 Vilma starts an utterance as a comment but then abandons it and changes the wording into a question. Simultaneously, the action she is performing changes from telling to asking.

Extract 5.11   *Vilma (girl; age 2;2) and her mother are playing with toy animals*

1   Vilma: Tää menee työmään.
              This goes to eat.
              ((*Vilma shows a toy giraffe to her mother*))

2   Mother: £Taas menee syömään niink(h)ö.hh£
              again go-3   eat-inf   yeah-q
              £Again goes to eat, doe(h)s it .hh£

3   (4.2) ((*Vilma holds the giraffe eating on the sofa*))

4   Vilma: →   **Se mene- (.) m̲inne menee tää.**
            it go-3   where go-3   this
            It goe-   (.) wh̲ere does this one go.

5   (1.8) ((*Vilma turns to her mother*))

6   Vilma: Nyt (0.8) kivahvi menee tänne.
                Now (0.8) the giraffe goes here.
                ((*Vilma puts the giraffe to her mother's ear*))

7   Mother: £Ai(h)i hi hi hi .hh jos se meneeki syömään korvan takaa jotain herkkusia.
                £Ou(h)ch hi hi hi .hh if it goes after all to eat some goodies from behind
                the ear.

Speech development from single words to multi-word utterances is immediately reflected in self-repairs that change syntactic constructions. With English-speaking children syntactic self-repairs have been reported to emerge later in 3-year-old or even older children (Clark 1982; McTear 1985: 190–195). Furthermore, besides the development of language and repair practices, one can see how the interaction between the parent and the child becomes more versatile: besides inspecting things and naming them, the 2-year-old children and their parents engage more and more in mutual play where they use language in various ways.

Repair organisation in 3- and 4-year-old children's interactions

For 3-year-olds, self-repair practices were already quite well developed except that lexical particles were still not used for marking same-turn self-repair. Furthermore, instead of making corrective repetitions to the speech of their 3-year-old children, the parents other-initiated repair with more varied kinds of specific questions and by offering their candidate understandings (see Laakso and Soininen, in press). The parents' questions as repair initiations gave the child more responsibility in maintaining the intersubjective understanding than the prior practice of direct corrective repetition.

When the children were approaching 5 years of age they had developed repair practices that were quite similar to those of adults speaking Finnish. The issues that were dealt with in the repair sequences also became more complicated. This aspect also reflects the developing nature of parent–child interaction towards more elaborate mutual imaginary play. In Extract 5.12 Emma (4;8) is revising her own speech in the midst of the activity of agreeing upon the names (and who will decide the names) of the dolls she and her mother are playing with. In line 4 Emma cuts off her emerging multi-unit utterance after *sinä* 'you' when she has just said that she will decide the name of one of the dolls they are planning to play with. The subordinate clause beginning with 'you' projects what Emma has planned for her mother to decide upon. The cut-off, however, abandons this emerging clause and a self-repair and reformulation of the prior utterance follows. Furthermore, in initiating self-repair Emma uses the particle *eiku* (approx. 'no I mean') to indicate that she is cancelling her cut-off utterance and replacing it with a new formulation.

Extract 5.12   *Emma (girl, age 4;8) and her mother are playing with dolls on the floor*

1   Emma: u- Sovitaan nyt että tää on vaikka [Lotta   tää on Lott[a   leikisti.
                       settle-PAS-4 now that this is PRT 1NAMEF this is 1NAMEF as.in.play
                       u- Let's settle now that this is for example Lotta, tending this is Lotta.

                                                                    [[
2   Mother: [(coughs) ai   [joo.
                                                  [oh   [yes
                                                  [oh   [okay.

3   Mother: Joo.
                       Okay.

4   Emma: →   Tää on Tuo[mas **mä päätän tän toisen näistä, sä- eiku mä päätän**=
                       this is 1NAMEM I decide-1 this other these-ELA you PRT I decide-1
                       This is Tuo[mas **I decide this other one, you- no I mean I decide**=
                                        [
5   Mother: [joo
                                   [okay

6   Emma: →   =**jooko** [**tän? ni päätä**]   **sä   toi yks poika**=
                       PRT   this so decide-IMP you that one boy
                       =**this okay? so you] decide that boy**=
7   Mother: [(- --)]

8   Emma: =vaik   mä en   täl   puhukkaa,
                       although I   V-NEG this-ADE speak-CLI
                       =although I don't speak with this one,

It is noteworthy that Emma uses the Finnish agreement-pursuing question particle *jooko* (approx. 'is it okay', see Tykkyläinen and Laakso, forthcoming) in her reformulation of how she and her mother should decide upon the names of the dolls they will play with. The utterance Emma was about to produce before the cut-off is, in its form, a simple ordering of what her mother should be doing. After the cut-off she changes her utterance into a more persuasive form by asking her mother whether she would agree with her about the arrangement she suggests. This reflects the fact that older children use self-repairs for similar interactive ends as adults, i.e. for making socially more appropriate formulations of their speaking turns that take into consideration the recipient's point of view.

Conclusions

What can we now say about the developing repair practices and the relationship between the children's self-initiated (by the child) and other-initiated (by the parent) self-repair and the links of the conversational repair routines to learning language use? In this data, misunderstandings of requests of objects were repaired early by preverbal

1-year-old children. Thus, from very early on children are able to recognise potential failures in their communication. The children's first same-turn self-repairs emerged already at the single-word stage before the age of 2, which is also in accordance with prior studies (e.g. Clark 1982; Forrester 2008). At the same time, when the children were approaching the age of 2 the parents frequently other-corrected them, which may have enhanced the emergence of the first self-initiated self-repairs by the children. The three-part sequences of the child's word, the parent's corrective repetition, and the child's imitation that approached more closely the adult equivalent word, were the routine basis on which the children receive a remodel of their first language and can practise it. This observation suggests that some of the basic interactive processes by which proficiency of early language is achieved are other-correction and imitation. By the age of 2 years, parents' direct other-correcting of their children's speech rapidly diminished.

As related to language development, it seems that children (and their parents) repair things the children are currently acquiring. At first, repairs focus on individual words. Repair operations are mainly lexical replacements or phonological revisions. As children start to produce multi-word utterances, new types of repair are possible. Children begin to abandon emerging syntactic constructions and add elements to their utterances. However, in children's first self-repairs, lexical repair initiators typical of Finnish are not yet used. At the other end of the continuum, 4-year-olds are skilful in repairing their utterances for various social-interactive purposes using similar linguistic devices to adult speakers of Finnish (such as using the initiator *eiku*).

The findings of the present study are, at least in part, in accordance with the previous notions that in children's interaction parents' repair is a device for dealing with those who are still learning to be adequate self-monitors and self-correctors (Schegloff *et al.* 1977). As children grow older they seem to develop more advanced linguistic practices for making self-repairs. However, even before children can actually talk they attempt to clarify their intentions to reach mutual understanding. Consistent with Schegloff *et al.* (1977), parents use repair-initiating and other-correction practices to highlight some aspects of their children's prior talk and action. Furthermore, in some cases the adults' repair practices are not necessarily used for restoring intersubjective understanding as such: this is most evident in parental other-correction in picture book sharing where the referents are quite obvious (and often pointed to). The parent-initiated repair sequences there seem to have the capacity to enable the development of children's language and cognition. At the same time, for the most part in this data, the driving force for initiating repair was to restore and maintain intersubjective understanding between the interlocutors. The data strongly suggests that the children from an early stage are able to monitor both their speech and its effect on the interlocutors. However, the interdependence of parental other-correction and the emergence of the child's self-initiated self-repair needs to be studied more closely.

References

Alexander, D., Wetherby, A. and Prizant, B. (1997) The emergence of repair strategies in infants and toddlers. *Seminars in Speech and Language* **18**, 197–212.

Chapman, R.S. (2000) Children's language learning: An interactionist perspective. *Journal of Child Psychology and Psychiatry*, **41**, 33–54.

Chouinard, M.M. and Clark, E.V. (2003) Adult reformulations of child errors as nega- tive evidence. *Journal of Child Language*, **30**, 637–669.

Clark, E.V. (1978) Awareness of language: Some evidence from what children say and do. In A. Sinclair, R.J. Jarvella and W.J.M. Levelt (eds), *The child's conception of lan- guage*. New York: Springer.

Clark, E.V. (1982) Language change during language acquisition. In M. Lamb and A. Brown (eds), *Advances in developmental psychology*, Vol. 2. (pp. 171–195). Hillsdale, NJ: Erlbaum.

Clark, E.V. (2003) *First language acquisition*. Cambridge: Cambridge University Press.

Corrin, J. (forthcoming) Hm? Mother-initiated toddler-repair at MLU stage I: Emergence in conversation. *First Language*.

Corsaro, W. (1977) The clarification request as a feature of adult-interactive styles with young children. *Language in Society*, **6**, 183–207.

Drew, P. (1981) Adults' corrections of children's mistakes: A response to Wells and Montgomery. In P. French and M. McClure (eds), *Adult and child conversation: Adult-child interaction at home and at school* [conference] (pp. 244–267). London: Croom Helm.

Evans, M.A. (1985) Self-initiated speech repairs: A reflection of communicative moni- toring in young children. *Developmental Psychology*, **21**, 365–371.

Filipi, A. (2002) *Before speech: the design of early repair in pointing sequences*. Paper read at the International Conference on Conversation Analysis, Copenhagen, 17–21 May.

Forrester, M.A. (2008) The emergence of self-repair: A case study of one child during the early preschool years. *Research on Language and Social Interaction*, **41**, 99–128.

Forrester, M.A. and Cherrington, S.M. (2009). The development of other-related con- versational skills: A case study of conversational repair during the early years. *First Language*, **29**, 166–191.

Garvey, C. (1977) The contingent query: A dependent act in conversation. In M. Lewis and L.A. Rosenblum (eds), *Interaction, conversation and the development of lan- guage* (pp. 63–93). New York: John Wiley and Sons.

Golinkoff, R. (1986) 'I beg your pardon?': The preverbal negotiation of failed messages. *Journal of Child Language*, **13**, 455–476.

Goodwin, C. (1980) Restarts, pauses, and the achievement of a state of mutual gaze at turn-beginning. *Sociological Inquiry*, **50**, 272–302.

Goodwin, C. (1981) *Conversational organization. Interaction between speakers and hearers*. New York: Academic press.

Goodwin, C. and Heritage, J. (1990) Conversation analysis. *Annual Reviews of Anthropology*, **19**, 283–307.

Hakulinen, A. and Sorjonen, M.-L. (1986) *Palautteen asema diskursissa* [Feedback in discourse]. In P. Leino and J. Kalliokoski (eds), *Kieli*, **1**, 39–72.

Jokinen, S. (1998) Two-year-old children's self-repairs of speech in the mother-child interaction. In K. Heinänen and M. Lehtihalmes (eds), *Proceedings of the seventh Nordic child language symposium* (pp. 38–42). Publications of the department of Finnish, Saami, and Logopedics 13. Oulu: University of Oulu.

Laakso, M. (2006) Kaksivuotiaiden lasten oman puheen korjaukset keskustelussa [Self-repair of speech by two-year-old children in conversation]. *Puhe ja kieli*, **26**, 123–136.

Laakso, M. and Soininen, M. (in press) Mother-initiated repair sequences in interactions of three-year-old children. *First Language*.

Langford, D. (1981) The clarification request sequence in conversation between mothers and their children. In P. French and M. MacLure (eds), *Adult-child conversation: Adult-child interaction at home and at school* [conference] (pp. 159–174). London: Croom Helm.

Leiwo, M. (1991) Self-repairs in the discussion between language-disordered child and adult. In R. Aulanko and M. Leiwo (eds), *Studies in Logopedics and Phonetics*, **2**, 107–121. Publications of the department of phonetics, series B: Phonetics, Logopedics and Speech Communication. Helsinki: University of Helsinki.

Liszkowski, U., Carpenter, M. and Tomasello, M. (2007) Reference and attitude in infant pointing. *Journal of Child Language*, **34**, 1–20.

Marcos, H. (1991) Reformulating requests at 18 months: gestures, vocalizations and words. *First Language*, **11**, 361–375.

McTear, M. (1985) *Children's conversation*. Oxford: Blackwell.

Menn, L. (1983) Development of articulatory, phonetic, and phonological capabilities. In B. Butterworth (ed.), *Language production*, Volume 2: Development, writing and other language processes (pp. 3–50). London: Academic Press.

Saxton, M. (2000) Negative evidence and negative feedback: Immediate effects on the grammaticality of child speech. *First Language*, **20**, 221–252.

Schegloff, E.A. (1989) Reflections on language, development, and the interactional character of talk-in-interaction. In M. Bornstein and J.S. Bruner (eds), *Interaction in human development* (pp. 139–153). Hillsdale, NJ: Lawrence Erlbaum.

Schegloff, E.A. (1996) Practices and actions: Boundary cases of other-initiated repair. *Discourse Processes*, **23**, 499–545.

Schegloff, E.A. (2007) *Sequence organization in interaction*. Cambridge: Cambridge University Press.

Schegloff, E.A., Jefferson, G. and Sacks, H. (1977) The preference for self-correction in the organization of repair in conversation. *Language*, **53**, 361–382.

Sokolov, J.L. and Snow, C.E. (1994) The changing role of negative evidence in theories of language development. In C. Gallaway and B. Richards (eds), *Input and interaction in language acquisition* (pp. 38–55). London: Cambridge University Press.

Sorjonen, M.-L. and Laakso, M. (2005) Katko vai *eiku*? Itsekorjauksen aloitustavat ja vuorovaikutustehtävät [Cut-off or particle *eiku*? Ways of initiating self-repair and its functions in interaction]. *Virittäjä*, **109**, 244–270.

Tarplee, C. (1996) Working on young children's utterances: prosodic aspects of repetition during picture labelling. In E. Couper-Kuhlen and M. Selting (eds), *Prosody in conversation* (pp. 406–435). Cambridge: Cambridge University Press.

Tomasello, M. (2003) *Constructing a language: A usage-based theory of language acquisition*. Cambridge, MA: Harvard University Press.

Tykkyläinen, T. (2007) Kielihäiriöinen lapsi keskinäisen ymmärtämisen vaalijana [How language-impaired children attempt to verify their understanding and make themselves understood]. *Virittäjä*, **111**, 182–200.

Tykkyläinen, T. and Laakso, M. (in press) Five-year-old girls negotiating pretend play: Proposals with Finnish agreement pursuing particle *jooko*. *Journal of Pragmatics*.

Vander Woude, J. and Barton, E. (2001) Specialized corrective repair sequences: Shared book reading with children with histories of specific language impairment. *Discourse Processes*, **32**, 1–27.

Wootton, A. (1994) Object transfer, intersubjectivity and third position repair: Early developmental observations of one child. *Journal of Child Language*, **21**, 543–564.

Wootton, A. (1997) *Interaction and the development of mind*. Cambridge: Cambridge University Press.

Appendix 5.1 Principles and abbreviations used in glossing

In the gloss, a minus sign (–) separates the morphemes from the root word. The following have been treated as unmarked forms, not indicated in the glosses:

– nominative case
– singular
– 3rd person singular
– active voice
– present tense
– 2nd person singular imperative

The different infinitives and participial verb forms have not been specified.
    The abbreviations used in the glosses refer to the following endings:

1 1st person
2 2nd person
3 3rd person
4 passive

The case endings are referred to with the following abbreviations:

Case	Abbreviation	Approximate meaning
Nominative	NOM	subject
Accusative	ACC	object
Genitive	GEN	possession
Partitive	PAR	partitiveness
Inessive	INE	'in'
Elative	ELA	'out of'
Illative	ILL	'into'
Adessive	ADE	'at, on' (owner of something)
Ablative	ABL	'from'
Allative	ALL	'to'
Essive	ESS	'as'
Translative	TRA	'to', 'becoming' 'into'
Instructive	INS	(various)
Comitative	COM	'with'

Other abbreviations:

CLI	clitic	PPC	past participle
PRON	pronoun	PRT	particle
PST	past tense	Q	interrogative

In the transcribed data extracts, the speech of each person is depicted in three lines to be read as follows: the first line is the original Finnish talk, the second is the English word-by-word gloss, and the third the free translation into English. Outside the analytic focus, and if the grammar of the original Finnish and the free English translation do not differ significantly, only two lines were used – that is, the gloss line was omitted.

Appendix 5.2

To explore more thoroughly the relationship between self-initiated and sequentially constructed self-repair, their frequencies were gathered at three different points: (1) in the recording where the first self-repairs emerged, (2) three months later, and (3) at the age of 2;6 more than six months after the emergence of the first self-initiated self-repairs. Although both forms emerged at the same time, there is a clear tendency from parent-initiated (sequentially constructed self-repair) towards same-turn self-repair: before the age of 2 there are more sequentially constructed self-repairs and only few same-turn self-repairs, whereas three months later the proportions are reversed (see Table 5.2).

Furthermore, at the age of 2;6 parents made very few corrective repetitions and the frequency of sequentially constructed self-repairs declined. Children mostly made same-turn self-repairs.

Table 5.2 Proportions of children's same-turn self-repair and sequentially constructed self-repair in the third turn after parent's corrective repetition

Age point (I, II or III)	Type of self-repair	
	Same-turn	Sequential
I	28%	72%
II	70%	30%
III	95%	5%

I = the recording where first self-repairs appeared (child is 1;8–1;11)
II = the recording three months after first self-repairs (child is 1;11–2;2)
III = the recording at age 2;6

Section 2

Childhood interactions in a wider social world

Chapter 6

Questioning repeats in the talk of four-year-old children

JACK SIDNELL

Introduction

In the Sacks archive at the UCLA library there is a folder marked 'NTRI' and contained therein a stack of notes, transcripts, and drafts of papers bearing on the topic of other-initiated repair. One draft begins with the following passage (abbreviated for current purposes):

> While it is obviously quite impossible to assess the universality of the OI (other-initiated) constructions, some thoughts on the matter are as follows: . . . It is one sort of thing if repeat is a universal operation type for turn building another sort of thing if an operation type like that gets assigned to use by repair. Now, consider this that it is remarked on as something of a universal that young children imitate, mimic, repeat. That might then involve that this basic institution of repair can get secured by using very basic operations and skills for its makings, as it uses very basic sequence construction techniques. I am saying that to adapt the operation type at which children are distinctly skilled for repair seems distinctly a rational sort of thing given a deep importance for repair, and for it early too. The connection between mimicry, imitation, repetition and repair seems to bear on the virtue of the sort of strategy repair organisation involves.

Here Sacks notes that enlisting repetition in the service of repair seems a distinctly 'rational sort of thing'. It seems that there is also something 'distinctly rational' in enlisting repair in the service of other actions. It is to this set of connections between repetition, repair and other actions in the talk of young children to which the following analysis is directed.

Consider, then, that one of the ways some participant, other than the speaker of the trouble source, can initiate repair is through a repeat of some or all of a previous turn as in Extract 6.1, 6.2 and 6.3 (see Jefferson 1972; Schegloff *et al.* 1977):

Extract 6.1

| 1 | | ((*click*)) |
| 2 | Anita: | Hello: ¿ |

3	Ben:	hHello, <u>Ma</u>:ry?
4	Anita:	(0.2) ((*kids speaking*)) <u>No:</u>
5		(0.3)
6	Ben:	No, not Ma:ry? hh
7	Anita:	No, it's not <u>Ma</u>:ry=there's no Mary he:re (.) I don' think: hh
8		(3.0)
9	Ben:	Th' tax la<u>dy</u>:
10		(0.2)
11	Anita: →	The ^<u>tax</u> <u>lad(h)y</u>::?
12	Ben:	Ya hhh=
13	Anita:	=Nop-. <u>Wha</u> number were you callin'.

Extract 6.2

1	Ken:	Hey (.) the <u>first</u> ti:me they <u>stopped</u> me from selling
2		<u>c</u>igarettes was this morning.
3		(1.0)
4	Lou:	From <u>s</u>elling cigarettes?
5	Ken:	Or <u>buy</u>ing cigarettes.

Extract 6.3

0		((*telephone rings*))
1	Amy:	What do you want me to pick up?
2	Betty:	Nothi<u>:</u>ng but I want to know how you boil an egg.
3		(1.0)
4		(h)hard boil.
5	Amy:	Oh oka::y and I just read this you know
6		because I always let the water boil but
7		you're not supposed to (.hh) put it in and
8		you (.hh) bring it to a boil (.) but then
9		turn it down 'cause you're really not
10		supposed to boil the <u>e</u>::gg
11		(0.4)

12		you let it (.) uh simmer or you know on me:dium,
13	Betty:	Ri:ght
14	Amy:	fo:r [t w] elve minutes.
15	Betty:	[((*sniff*))]
16	Betty: →	Twelve minutes?
17	Amy:	Well I always do it faster than th(h)at (hh)
18	Betty:	okay=
19	Amy:	=I just boil the shit out of it [but]
20	Betty:	[How]
21		do you know when it's done?

Now although, as Schegloff *et al.* note, a questioning repeat such as 'the tax lady?', 'Twelve minutes?' or 'From selling cigarettes?' quite precisely locates the trouble source in a previous turn, it does not convey what *kind of problem* is being identified. It is, in principle, at least possible that the problem in any particular case might result from incorrect pronunciation, a mis-speaking, a malapropism or, alternatively, from the use of a word that the recipient simply does not know. It is surely significant that despite this *in principle* 'selection problem', participants rarely seem to encounter difficulty in determining the actual nature of the problem. Jefferson (1972: 312) suggests that selection may be 'controlled by the ongoing activity' and cites some suggestive examples. Still, exactly how participants are consistently able to solve what I have elsewhere described (see Sidnell 2006) as 'the other-initiated repair problem' remains something of a mystery.

These extracts have been selected to show the range of responses an initiation of repair via a questioning repeat may engender. In Extract 6.1, 'the tax lady' elicits a simple confirmation 'ya'. In Extract 6.2, Ken responds to Lou's 'From selling cigarettes' with a correction – 'Or buying cigarettes'. And in Extract 6.3, when Betty initiates repair of 'twelve minutes', Amy is encouraged to significantly modify her advice. This range of responses is suggestive of the various different actions a trouble-source speaker may understand a questioning repeat to embody – from a request for confirmation in Extract 6.1, to an invitation to self-correct in Extract 6.3, to an expression of scepticism or a challenge to the accuracy of some prior assertion as in Extract 6.2. This is consistent with what we know about the organisation of repair from the many studies of adult conversation (see, most relevantly in the present context, Schegloff *et al.* 1977 and Jefferson 1987).

Methods and data

This study is based on recordings of 4-year-old children taken from a larger corpus of recordings of children between the ages of 4 and 8. Children were taken from their classes during regular school hours to a special room in which a camera was already set up. There, they were presented with various play things, including blocks for building, plastic toy animals, duplo and so on. They were told only that they should 'play together'. No further instruction was given and the children generally played with minimal intervention from the one adult in the room. Sessions lasted from between 25 minutes and 1 hour. The corpus for 4-year-olds consists of nine sessions amounting to about 8 hours of videorecorded interaction. From these data, all instances of OIR were collected. This resulted in a collection of 42 cases. This included 14 instances of repair being initiated by a questioning repeat.

An initial comparison of the 4- and 5-year data

The distribution of the various formats of repair initiation in the 4- and 5-year-old data (see Figure 6.1) reveals some striking differences between the two groups.

This simple graph seems to indicate a much greater reliance by 4-year-olds on the questioning repeat format. The 5-year-olds, by comparison, show a more evenly distributed pattern involving a significant use of all formats, including those classified as 'complex constructions' (On repetition in children's talk see Keenan 1974, 1976, 1983; Tarplee 1996; Brown 1998).

4-year-old use of questioning repeats – an overview

Figure 6.1 shows a robust use of questioning repeats by both 4-year-olds and 5-year-olds. At the same time, 4-year-olds use this format twice as often as the 5-year-olds. What is going on here? One possibility is that questioning repeats are simpler and less cognitively demanding than other more complex formats and thus more available to children of this age. If we accept this premise, we might suppose that the lower rate of

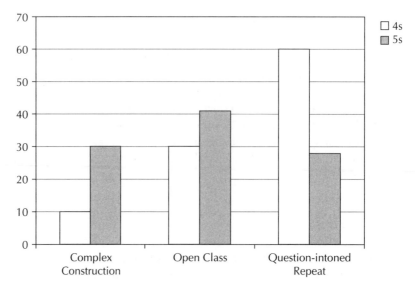

Figure 6.1 Distribution of three OI-formats (expressed as a percentage of the total for each age group (4s total N = 30, 5s total N = 46).

usage among 5-year-olds is a symptom of greater cognitive sophistication – as children mature they tend to rely less on this simple device and more on other more complex turn designs. Virtually all previous studies of repair in children's talk (also known as 'clarification requests' or 'contingent queries') either implicitly or explicitly adopt a developmental perspective of this kind – see, for instance, Garvey (1977), Gallagher (1981), McTear (1985), Tomasello *et al.* (1990). As Mike Forrester points out, this is true across significant differences of theoretical orientation (e.g. Piagetian, Functional and so on). For overviews of the developmental perspective, see Ochs and Schieffelin (1979, 1983), McTear (1985) or Tomasello (1999, 2003). For a slightly different perspective see Ochs (1984), and for a radical alternative consonant in many respects with the position developed in this chapter, see Wootton (1997).

A second possible explanation is that 4-year-olds more often find themselves confronting those specific interactional problems and contingencies which questioning repeats are particularly designed to solve – that is, the difference may stem from more general properties of their interactions. In studies of children's language use, explanations of the first kind are clearly favoured. Indeed, it would not, I think, be inaccurate to say that developmental explanations are maintained with hegemonic force. This 'developmentalist hegemony' – the tendency to see any and all changes in the behaviour of children as reflecting the gradual approximation of more adult-like behaviour, norms, competence – is not only pervasive but also naturalised and deeply entrenched in our ordinary and scholarly ways of thinking. While there is, of course, much to recommend the developmental viewpoint, in this chapter I hope to question that hegemony to some extent and at least raise the question of whether there might be alternative ways in which changes in children's talk might be explained. I see this as consistent with many of Sacks' arguments about children and childhood, and especially his analysis of beginnings such as 'You know what?' (see also Forrester, Chapter 3 this volume and Hutchby, Chapter 8 this volume). Sacks (1974: 229) writes:

> Kids around the age of three go through a period when some of them have an almost universal way of beginning any piece of talk they make to adults. They use things like: 'You know what, Daddy?' or 'You know something, Mommy?'.

Sacks then shows that such beginnings routinely elicit from recipients open invitations to talk on any topic with responses such as 'what?'. He then (1974: 231) goes on to write:

> We may take it that kids take it that they have restricted rights which consist of a right to begin, to make a first statement and not much more. Thereafter they proceed only if requested to. And if that is their situation as they see it, they surely have evolved a nice solution to it . . . we can see whether the beginnings of stories. . . . Might be seen to be beginnings by virtue of the special situation which kids have *vis-à-vis* beginning to talk.

So Sacks eschews a developmental explanation here. Rather, he understands kids beginning their talk with items such as 'you know what, daddy?' and so on as a practice adapted to the particular contingencies of childhood. In this case the practice is fitted to a situation in which children take it that they have restricted rights to talk. In a similar way I do not presume that 4-year-olds use of the questioning repeat format should be explained in developmental terms.

In what follows I will show that all instances of questioning repeats in the talk of 4-year-old children fall into one of three categories. Firstly, there are cases in which repair is initiated in response to genuine problems of hearing on the part of the recipient. Secondly, there are cases in which the questioning repeat is used to highlight the use of an incorrect word or an inadequate pronunciation. And, thirdly, there are instances in which the questioning repeat is the vehicle for a challenge to something done or said in a previous turn.

What is a repeat?

In order for some bit of talk to come off as a repeat of what someone has just said, the speaker must do more than just use the same words. (For discussion of various uses of repetition in conversation see, inter alia, Tannen 1987, Brown 1998. For discussions of repetition in child language acquisition, see Keenan 1976, Ninio and Bruner 1978, Slobin 1985, Bloom 1991.) Consider Extract 6.4 – a selection from Extract 6.10 on page 113 – in which the children are talking about a specific kind of camel.

Extract 6.4

```
19  M:      Yeah are they scary for you?
20  W:      no. (0.4) they're scar:y- all of-
21          every people are scared of these ones.
22  M: →    an- no but not me::
23  W: →    not me::
```

Here, in line 23, Walt uses precisely the same words as Michael has just used – indeed, as the transcription suggests he says 'not me::', also with much the same prosody. However, Walt does not say this *as a repeat* of what Michael has said but rather on his own behalf – he, like Michael, is claiming – in a magnificent reversal of what he has just stated – that he is also not afraid of these camels.

A repeat, then, at least as it is understood here, is not defined on the basis of form alone. Rather this a practice that is constituted in part by the sequential context in which it is embedded. I now turn to consider such repeats and the various actions that they implement in the talk of 4-year-old children.

Repairing a partial or uncertain hearing

With a questioning repeat of part or all of a previous turn, a participant may attempt to repair a partial or uncertain hearing of the repeated portion of the talk. In the following extract, Tim, Michael and Walt are pretending to be a family consisting of a father (Michael), grandfather (Walt) and son (Tim). The boys are pretending that a box on the table is a TV and decide that both sides of it are projecting an image. At line 1, after Michael has turned on the pretend TV, Tim begins a turn in which he mentions the news. Tim has been assigned the role of 'son' in this family drama and his mention of the news is perhaps hearable as inconsistent with that role. Michael appears to hear Tim as on his way to saying that the news is about to start and corrects him saying 'the news started you know. Son.' Tim initiates repair with a questioning repeat and Michael subsequently corrects the mishearing this embodies.

Extract 6.5

```
1   T:     Oh- oh oh the news is- is a- is about (its-)

2          (0.6)

3   M:     [the news started you know. Son.

4   T:     [(    )

5          (1.0)

6   T: →   The news didn't start?

7          (0.2)

8   M:     it started. Already.
```

In contrast to other extracts described below, the problem here appears to be the product of Tim's genuine failure to adequately hear what Michael is saying. Some of the same children also feature in Extract 6.6. Here at line 1, in overlap with something Michael is saying to Walt, Jake says something difficult to discern but apparently ending with the word 'bike'. Then, in the clear as Michael has stopped speaking, Jake says 'I need duh bug'. After a substantial silence, Michael initiates repair with a questioning attempt at repetition, saying 'book?'. Michael's candidate hearing is rejected and Jake corrects with 'dih bike'. Michael initiates repair again with a questioning repeat – offering 'bike' as a candidate hearing. Jake confirms this in line 8.

Extract 6.6

```
1   J:     (havin a bike)

2          I need duh bug

3          (0.8)

4   M: →   book?

5          (0.4)

6   J:     dih bike

7   M: →   Bike?

8   J:     yeah.

9          (.) ([ )

10  M:        [uhm: I been tryin' to fix it.
```

Again the problem to which repair is directed in this extract appears to develop rather straightforwardly out of a failure to properly hear what is being said. Although there is undoubtedly more going on in these extracts, they appear to involve a recipient checking a hearing via a candidate repetition of some portion of a prior turn.

Rejecting a word or pronunciation

Consider now the rather different situation exemplified by Extract 6.7. Here, the children are playing with blocks and small plastic figurines – the latter have taken on various personalities including grandmother, uncle and so on. A few seconds before this fragment begins, Matty announces 'I found my grandfather' and Hanna responds with 'I found my grandmata'. The grandmother is animated and thanked for 'the great soup' and Hanna then turns to Matty saying 'I found your uncle'. In line 6, Matty is apparently reciprocating by picking up one of the figurines, handing it to Hanna and saying 'I found your whybee'.

Extract 6.7

```
 1   H:   I foun' ja- ak- I foun' jur-
 2        (0.2)
 3        uncle: (.) he heh heh ha
 4   M:   Uncle. Thank yo:.
 5   H:   Hello. (I dry a-off)
 6   M:   I fa- I found your whybee
 7        (.)
 8   H:   Whybee:z?
 9        (0.4)
10   H:   (the-heh) no such thing as whybeez.
```

Hanna initiates repair with a questioning repeat of 'whybee' and subsequently rejects this as nonce word saying 'there's no such thing as whybeez'. Interestingly, there is no uncertainty about Hanna's hearing here – she does not as, others did in the previous extracts, seem concerned that she may have misheard what Matty is saying. Moreover, Hanna does not entertain the possibility that 'whybee' is in fact a real word that she does not know. Instead, she rejects the word, saying 'no such thing as whybeez'.

Extract 6.8 presents a rather more complicated case. Here the children are playing with blocks called 'kapla'. This is a generic name for the toy like 'Lego' and thus does not take a singular specific form as in 'a kapla' or a plural form as in 'kaplas'. In line 1, AJ announces 'we need more klapas'. Nora initiates repair with a two-part initiator – first repeating the problematic item and then saying 'what are kapaluz?'.

Extract 6.8

```
 1   AJ:      An' we need more klapas °huh°

 2   Nora:    Kapluz what are kapaluz?

 3   AJ:      These are klapas.

 4            (0.2)

 5            [(an' these, an' these)

 6   Nora:    [You said ka- .hh [(AJ-

 7   AJ:                        [not blocks

 6   Nora:    AJ sa- said kla-pluz.

 8   AJ:      he heh these are klapas. Klapas.

 9            (0.2)

10            .hh heh heh heh heh .hh .hh .hh

11            .hh this is funny.

12   Nora:    How do you say Klap-

13   Cathy:   Echo::: (.) [Echo:?

14   Nora:                [(How-)

15   AJ:      Kla- Kh  [ a : p :     [(.) la:

16   Nora:             [Howdoyou [say-

17            How do you say kapla?

18   AJ:      Yea:h ((Turns to adult))

19   Adult:   Kapla.

20   AJ:      Kapla?

21   Adult:   Ka[pla

22   AJ:        [ah hah huh huh he=

23   Nora:    We know how to say kapla the

24            right way.

25   AJ:      Kapla.
```

Notice then that at line 3 AJ attempts to repair the problem via an ostensive demonstra-
tion saying 'these are klapas' retaining the original form of the word in line 1. There are
two possible problems with AJ's 'klapas'. Firstly, as noted, this word does not generally
take an –*s* plural (the correct form would be 'we need more kapla'). Secondly, AJ has
pronounced the word 'klapas'. It is not clear which possible error Nora means to be

highlighting by initiating repair. Notice, though, that she initially addresses her complaint to AJ – the trouble-source speaker – but subsequently turns to Cathy saying 'AJ sa- said kla-pluz'. After Cathy does not respond, Nora turns to the supervising adult asking, at line 17, 'How do you say kapla?'. After having the adult confirm that AJ's pronunciation is an error, Nora remarks 'We know how to say kapla the right way'. Note that Cathy's 'Echo!' in line 13 is not responsive to the talk directed at her. By pursuing a quite independent line of activity (testing the acoustics of the room), Cathy can be seen to be specifically disattending what Nora is saying to her.

In these extracts the problem to which repair is addressed does not appear to be the product of partial or uncertain hearing. In the first case, Hanna provides a position after the questioning repeat in which Matty might have responded – in which he might have corrected or accepted the candidate hearing that the questioning repeat proposed. When he does not do this, Hanna treats the hearing as confirmed and proceeds by rejecting 'whybees' on the grounds that it is not real word. In the second case, Nora does not provide AJ any such opportunity to accept or reject the candidate hearing proposed by the questioning repeat. Instead she launches directly into a turn in which she disclaims knowledge of the word used.

Challenging a prior turn

The final set of instances have, in common with those we have just considered, a dimension of challenge. Here, however, the object of the challenge is not a pronunciation or a word selection – not a manifestation of linguistic incompetence – but rather a claim. Consider Extract 6.9.

Extract 6.9

```
 1  E:       Ju::de: yer makin' (me) knock it dow:n.

 2           (0.4)

 3           be more careful next time.

 4  J:       I̲: wi:ll:. I we:ll, I will, I will.

 5  T:       He sounds like a (actin) hhh

 6           kinda like (ss) (0.2) ba:(h):by,

 7           (0.8)

 8  J: →     Ba::by?

 9           (0.4)

10  T:       he he ha ha oh .hhhh

11  J:       sshhh.

12           (0.2)

13           You sound like a baby (to adult)
```

Here Erica complains that Jude is, by shaking the table, making her knock down the structure she is building. She enjoins him to 'be more careful next time'. To this Jude responds with 'I: wi:ll:. I we:ll, I will, I will'. Now although he thereby acquiesces and essentially accepts responsibility for 'not being careful', the manner in which he says this – multiple repetition, a whining intonation, etc. – suggests also that he is treating the complaint as less than completely serious. Tina picks up on this in her talk at lines 5–6 saying that Jude 'sounds like – kinda like a baby.' You can imagine, I think, how children of this age might respond to being called a 'baby' or to having their behaviour characterised as 'like a baby' (see Forrester 2001). At 4 years of age, these children have really only just stopped being 'babies'. Moreover, although they are no longer infants, much of their behaviour is in fact very 'baby-like'. So Tina's turn at lines 5–6 which she produces with considerable hesitation is hearable, I think, as a rather grave insult. And notice the very subtle hint of laughter that she introduces into the word. When Jude initiates repair with a questioning repeat Tina withdraws the seriousness of the insult with laughter – thereby treating her own talk and perhaps also Jude's at line 4 as a joke. This is a point to which I'll return later. However, note here that neither hearing nor the form of the word seems to be at issue. Rather the questioning repeat appears to convey a challenge to Tina's claim that Jude sounds like a baby.

In Extract 6.10, Walt and Michael are playing with wooden blocks and plastic animal figurines. The blocks are being used to build pens for the animals which, the boys have decided, are 'very wild'. Just before this segment begins, Walt has suggested 'Camels are so wild you know', to which Michael has responded with 'Yeah, they are'. When Walt then upgrades the assessment 'Camels are rilly wild', Michael responds with less than complete agreement, saying 'Not- not all of them though'. Recognising that not all camels are extremely wild, Walt then attempts to establish that the one he is holding *is*. At lines 6 to 10 Walt proposes that the ones with black humps – like the one he is holding – are particularly scary, indeed, the scariest. Michael, picking up on this recharacterisation of the camel as scary, first says something partially inaudible before claiming 'the real ones like that are not scary to me'. This prompts Walt to offer further evidence in favour of his argument that the camel in question is particularly scary, saying 'bu- bu- (.) he has red eyes'. Michael, however, does not back down from his asserted position and responds 'yeah bu' they're not scary still'. Walt then initiates repair with 'Sti:ll? (0.2) not scary?'.

Extract 6.10

1	W:	un- camels are so wild you know.
2	M:	Yeah, they <u>a</u>re.
3	W:	Camels are ri:lly wild.
4	M:	Not- not all of them though
5		(0.2)
6	W:	I know. But this: camels- the one: oops
7		the sa- um the one with black (thumbs/humps)
8		and black down here:, (.) an' black there are th-
9		are the- are the- are the- are the- are thuh-

10		are the scary (0.2) ist. An' this is the scariest.
11		(0.6)
12	M:	(Do [ ]) scarier.
13	W:	[( )
14	M:	The rea:l ones (th-) like that are not scary to me.
15	W:	Bu- bu- (.) he has red ey:es.
16	M:	Yeah bu' they're not scary still
17		(0.4)
18	W: →	Sti:ll? (0.2) not scary?
19	M:	Yeah are they scary for you?
20	W:	no. (0.4) they're scar:y- all of-
21		every people are scared of these ones.
22	M:	an- no but not me::
23	W:	not me::

Here then the questioning repeat occurs in an environment of disagreement and disaffiliation. Walt has produced an extreme assessment of the camel and Michael has refused to go along with this. Michael first claims that the camels in question are not scary to him, and then at line 16 when he suggests that 'they're not scary still', his disagreement is more direct. This turn at line 16 embodies a claim to be unimpressed by a particular kind of camel and it is this claim which Walt seeks to challenge with his two-part questioning repeat in line 18.

A further extract of a questioning repeat used to challenge something in a prior turn is shown in Extract 6.11. Once again the repair sequence occurs in an environment of disagreement. This fragment – and the tape – begins with Matty challenging a prior claim which was unfortunately not recorded. When Matty asserts that there are 'no ponies inside farms', Tina replies 'Ye:s. so:me'. After a short pause she continues by grounding her claim in prior experience by saying 'I went to a real farm before'. At lines 5–6, Grace begins a turn in which she proposes 'an' once (.) I: rode on a pony'. When this receives no uptake from the other children, Grace turns to the adult in the room saying 'I really did'. The adult produces a minimal acknowledgement token and Grace continues by providing the name of the place where she rode on the pony – Centre Island. Tina picks up on this mention of Centre Island saying something partially inaudible which is confirmed by Grace with 'yes' at line 15. Matty then initiates repair with a questioning repeat of 'Centre Island?' and Grace repairs with a confirmation. This 'I've been there' appears to be particularly oriented to the challenge which Matty's questioning repeat is heard to embody. It is clear that part of Grace's claim involves her having been to Centre Island – if this is where she rode on a pony, then she surely must have been there. In responding to Matty's questioning repeat with 'Yes. I've been there' Grace then seems oriented to a possible challenge to the veracity of her claim.

Extract 6.11

```
1   M:      There's no ponies inside fa:r:ms.=

2   T:      Ye:s. so:me.

3           (0.2)

4           I went to a real farm bef[ore

5   G:                              [an' once (.)

6           I: rode on a pony.

7           (0.2)

8           I really did. ((looks to adult))

9   L:      (mhm)

10  G:      At centre island I rode on a pony.

11          (0.8)

12  M:      (how [  )

13  T:           [( ) centre island?

14          (0.4)

15  G:      yes.

16          (0.6)

17  M: →    centre island?

18  G:      yes. I've been there. (.) On: a ferry.

19          (0.8)

20          a ferry boat.
```

A similar orientation can be seen in Extract 6.12. Here Nora proposes that the group could make – from Kapla – a 'karate class'. When AJ initiates repair with a questioning repeat of 'Karate class' Cathy responds with a confirmation plus defence not unlike G's 'yes. I've been there' in the previous extract. Here Cathy's defence is somewhat more explicitly given as a reason for making a karate class, although this is also complicated by a substitution of 'karate' by 'tae-kwan-do'.

Extract 6.12

```
1   Cathy:  Now I'm making di stairs I (ha' to) go ( ) my class.

2           (0.4)

3           (mm [Nora)

4   Nora:       [okay.

5           (0.2)
```

6	Nora:	(make) How bou' (.) they could have a a karate
7		(0.2)
8		class.
9	Cathy:	Oh my go(hh)
10	AJ: →	Karate class?
11	Cathy:	Yes I go to Tae-Kwan-Do so I'm making a Tae-Kwan-Do building.
12		(0.7)
13	AJ:	What buil[ding.
14	Cathy:	[That's what I'm making.A Tae-<u>Kw</u>an-Do building.
15	Nora:	Cathy:?
16	Cathy:	mhm hm, [(what)
17	Nora:	[Do you wanna make a whole village?

What we see in these extracts then is that a questioning repeat is hearable as a challenge to a claim in the prior turn. In Extracts 6.9 (baby) and 6.10 (not scary) the challenge is to something face-threatening. In Extract 6.9, Tina's has likened Jude to a baby, in Extract 6.10, Michael has disagreed with Walt about whether camels are scary and in so doing has recast Walt's prior assessment in a somewhat negative light. In Extracts 6.11 and 6.12, participants appear to treat the challenge as targeting the epistemic grounds of the claim. Thus in Extract 6.11, Marty's initiation of repair with 'centre island' prompts Grace's assertion 'yes. I've been there'. And in Extract 6.12, AJ's 'Karate class?' elicits from Cathy a fully formed defence in terms of her own participation in 'Tae-Kwan-Do'.

Observation: Items in turn-final position are structurally vulnerable to OIR in next-turn position

Jefferson (1972) notes that items in turn-final position are structurally vulnerable, by virtue of their position in the turn, to repair initiation via a questioning repeat. This is particularly apparent in the 4-year-old data. In all clear cases the repeat targeted the final components of the turn. This includes cases such as Extract 6.13, where the final component is a single word, as well as those such as Extract 6.14 in which the final component is a phrase:

Extract 6.13

1	J:	(havin a bike)
2		I need duh bug
3		(0.8)
4	M: →	book?

Extract 6.14

1 T: I made an- A: for ap- (0.2) apka::

2 Adult: ah o::h,

3   (0.4)

4 E: →   For E:rica:?

Evidence of this structural vulnerability is provided by Extract 6.10, the relevant part of which is reproduced as Extract 6.15. Recall that in this extract Walt has assessed a camel as the scariest and Michael has disagreed saying 'the rea:l ones (th-) like that are not scary to me'. When Michael reasserts that he does not find the camels scary in spite of their red eyes, Walt initiates repair with 'Still? (0.2) not scary?' Notice that the trouble source features a rather odd (slightly marked) word order in which 'still' – which is specifically responsive to Walt's 'red eyes' addition – is post-posed. There are two ways in which Walt might have targeted word final items in his questioning repeat. One option would have been to repeat 'not scary still?'. What Walt does though is to break the repair initiation into two parts – first repeating 'still?' and then 'not scary?'.

Extract 6.15

14 M: The rea:l ones (th-) like that are not scary to me.

15 W: Bu- bu- (.) he has red ey:es.

16 M: Yeah bu' they're not scary still

17   (0.4)

18 W: → Sti:ll? (0.2) not scary?

19 M: Yeah are they scary for you?

In this way Walt is able to initiate repair of Michael's 'not scary still?' and target the final items in the turn.

Observation: Laughter is routinely used to exit from or to transform an OIR sequence

Jefferson distinguishes questioning repeats from what she describes as 'laugh token' repeats 'whereby one demonstrates "appreciation", "enjoyment", etc., of the product-item; where laugh tokens alternate with syllables of the repeat' (1972: 299). She gives the examples reproduced here as Extracts 6.16 and 6.17.

Extract 6.16

1 Al: Then th'r gonna dismantle the frame

2   'n see if the frame's still there.

3 Lou: hh[heh heh heh!

4 Al: →   [Got <u>ter</u>mites.

```
5              (0.6)

6   Ken: →    'T(hh)er(h)mite(h)s' hhh

7   Lou:      Well y'know we-n- fallout. Who knows

8             what they'll eat now.

9             (0.6)

10  Ken:      hhhh

11            (1.5)

13            hh hh

14            (1.0)
```

Extract 6.17

```
1   Roger:    He's a politician.

2   Al:       Yes. I'm a politician.

3             I think I'm greater than all of you.

4             (1.0)

5   Ken:      [I think yer out of yer fuckin mind heh

6   Roger: →  [I beg to differ with you,

7   Al: →     hehh heh hhh 'I b(h)eg to differ with you.'

8   (?):      ((sniff))

9   (?):      ((cough))

10  Roger:    Yer better'n most of 'em. Cept me.

11            (4.0)
```

Jefferson (1972: 300) goes on to suggest that:

> the 'laugh token' repeat differs from the 'questioning' repeat not only in that they do not 'mean' the same thing (for example, that the former demonstrates some sort of approval and the latter demonstrates some sort of disapproval), but in that they do not do the same work. Laugh tokens in general are regularly associated with termination of talk and it can be proposed that the laugh token repeat is regularly associated with termination of talk with reference to its product-item.

The proper way for a recipient to handle a laugh token repeat, according to Jefferson, is to 'ignore it, since, if it is heard as an object signalling appreciation via laughter, then it is a terminator' (1972: 301). However, Jefferson also notes that a laugh token repeat can 'converge' with a questioning repeat 'if it is found to be possibly non-appreciative; that is, it may then call for some remedial work'. I want to briefly consider this convergence in the 4-year-old data. Specifically, I want to raise the possibility that laughter may be introduced into a questioning repeat sequence, either by the trouble-source speaker or the repair-initiator, in such a way as to significantly alter its course or close it down. Firstly, it is useful to begin by observing that straightforward laugh token repeats do occur in the 4-year-old data (Extract 6.18).

Extract 6.18

1   Nora: My dad is a doctor and my mom is a professor

2   Cathy: A professor(h) ha ha ha ha ha

3   Nora: heh hah hah

Here when Nora announces that her dad is a doctor and her mom a professor, Cathy repeats 'a professor' with inserted laugh tokens. It is not obvious here whether Cathy's repeat is meant to be appreciative or not – this ambiguity deriving from the fact that Nora's announcement was not designed to be heard as a joke. Nora handles this by joining in the laughter and thereby treating her own earlier talk as funny (Jefferson 1979). In the next extract, Emma hands Matty some blocks and Matty thanks her using a made-up name – 'Bagda'. Hanna then produces a laugh token repeat of the made-up name, thereby showing appreciation of it. As Jefferson suggests, the laugh token repeat is closing implicative and terminates this sequence.

Extract 6.19

1   E: ka:: ( ) ((*passes some kapala*))

2   M: thank you: Bagda:

3   (0.4)

4   H: ha ha (h)B̲a:ga:?

5   (you're a helpa::)

A trouble-source speaker may also introduce laughter into the questioning repeat sequence. Recall Extract 6.9 (reproduced here as Extract 6.20):

Extract 6.20

1   E: Ju::de: yer makin' (me) knock it dow:n.

2   (0.4)

3   be more careful next time.

4   J: I̲: wi:ll:. I we:ll, I will, I will.

5   T: He sounds like a (actin) hhh

6   kinda like (ss) (0.2) ba:(h):by,

7   (0.8)

8   J: → Ba::by?

```
9              (0.4)

10   T:        he he ha ha oh .hhhh

11   J:        sshhh.

12             (0.2)

13             You sound like a baby (to adult)
```

Here, in response to Jude's problematisation of 'Baby', Tina laughs in this way trans-forming what had looked like a possible complaint and insult into a joke. And notice further that Jude accepts and participates in this transformation, first by laughing along with Tina and subsequently by reusing Tina's joke but now directing it at the adult in the room. By applying the same words 'You sound like a baby' to the adult, Jude also high-lights its status as a joke, as non-serious, as not a literal description.

Participants other than trouble-source speaker and repair initiator may also intro-duce laughter into these sequences. Consider Extract 6.21.

Extract 6.21

```
1    T:        I made an- A: for ap- (0.2) apka::

2    Adult:    ah o::h,

3              (0.4)

4    E: →      For E:rica:?

5              (0.2)

6    T:        E:rica:?

7              (0.2)

8    J:        Erica, whereika, derika, sarika (.) hh eh hh

9    E:        Juda~ duuga~ luuga~ Luke.

10             (0.4)

11   J:        (h)s(h)p(h)hhhhh

12   E:        heh heh ha ha

13   T:        Luke Sky::wal::ker?

14   J:        ah:::: da my real name, Luke Skywalker.

15   E:        No::.

16   J:        Ah hah hah hah.
```

Here Tina announces that she has made something for 'Apka::' – It would appear that she was on her way to 'Apple' but after producing the first syllable of this word decided to change course to 'Erica'. At line 4, Erica initiates repair via a question-ing repeat – 'For Erica?'. Tina then repeats 'Erica' in line 6 and Jude subsequently transforms the activity by creating a string of rhyming words. In her matching response to this, Erica ends with the name/word 'Luke' and, after, Jude and Erica laugh, this becomes a target for repair initiation by Tina, who says 'Luke Skywalker?' Here, then, we have a game built out of the practice of questioning repeats. The game seems to work along the following lines: in listening to a speaker's talk, attend to words that sound like something other than they are – repeat these with question intonation in next-turn position. In this way, Tina transforms Erica's 'Luke' into 'Luke Skywalker' just as Erica had transformed 'for Apka' into 'for Erica?'. It is also possible, however, that Tina specifically designed 'for Apka' to provide for it being heard as a disguised version of 'for Erica'. If this is the case, then it would appear that at line 1 Tina, in speaking the way she does, is actually proposing to start the game.

At this point it may be worth returning to Extract 6.8 with these kinds of transformation via laughter in mind. Recall that, in that case, Nora initiates repair of AJ's 'klapas'. Notice that at lines 6–8, Nora initially continues to direct her talk to AJ, but eventually self-repairs, turns to Cathy and says 'AJ sa- said kla-pluz'. At this point then she abandons the repair sequence in favour of ridiculing AJ's pronunciation to Cathy. In response, AJ repeats his pronunciation and breaks into a vigorous bout of laughter apparently in an effort to transform the 'trouble source' into a joke which might be appreciated as something funny. AJ's laughter does not, however, effect a closing of this sequence. Rather Nora pursues the matter by asking the adult 'How do you say Klap-' (line 12) and 'How do you say kapla?' (line 17).

Extract 6.22

```
 1  AJ:     An' we need more klapas °huh°
 2  Nora:   Kapluz what are kapaluz?
 3  AJ:     These are klapas.
 4          (0.2)
 5          [(an' these, an' these)
 6  Nora:   [You said ka- .hh [(AJ-
 7  AJ:                        [not blocks
 6  Nora:   AJ sa- said kla-pluz.
 8  AJ:     he heh these are klapas. Klapas.
 9          (0.2)
10          .hh heh heh heh heh .hh .hh .hh
11  AJ:     .hh this is funny.
12  Nora:   How do you say Klap-
13  Cathy:  Echo::: (.) [Echo:?
14  Nora:               [(How-)
```

```
15  AJ:      Kla- Kh [ a : p :      [(.) la:

16  Nora:              [Howdoyou [say-

17           How do you say kapla?

18  AJ:      Yea:h ((turns to adult))

19  Adult:   Kapla.

20  AJ:      Kapla?

21  Adult:   Ka[pla

22  AJ:         [ah hah huh huh he=

23  Nora:    We know how to say kapla the

24           right way.

25  AJ:      Kapla.
```

After enlisting the authority of the adult as we saw earlier, there is a second sequence initiated by a questioning repeat. When the adult responds to the inquiry – 'how do you say kapla?' – AJ produces a questioning repeat followed by vigorous laughter (lines 20 and 22). In this he again attempts to recast this as something funny and worthy of appreciation. Nora, however, resists this by treating the issue as one of correct versus incorrect pronunciation saying 'We know how to say kapla the right way'.

Conclusion

It has long been recognised that repetition and imitation play a critical role in language acquisition at just about every stage. While this is widely recognised, researchers have often been uncertain about how to understand and study such utterances. Because these studies have been concerned primarily with what these children are 'learning' as opposed to what they are 'doing', in many cases at least, researchers have not distinguished between different kinds of repeats (those produced with questioning intonation as opposed to those inflected by laughter for example). As Ninio and Snow (1996: 62) write:

> Many investigators have failed to distinguish *the speech act of imitating* (which is probably only used in normal populations by persons engaged in learning a first or second language, as a means of language practice) from repetitions of a previous utterance used *to carry out a communicative intent*, for example, agreeing or disagreeing with a proposition, answering in the affirmative to a yes/no question, answering a restricted alternatives question, agreeing to do as requeseted, acknowledging the interlocutor's utterance, and so on (see Keenan 1977).

Indeed, in some approaches to child language, repetitions are separated from other utterances and treated as a special type with immature characteristics (Bates 1979). Some researchers even go as far as to suggest that repetitions/imitations do not qualify as truly meaningful utterances because they can be performed without comprehension (e.g. Greenfield and Smith 1976).

My approach has been rather different – rather than focusing on repetition for what it might say about something else (learning, language, grammar, etc.), I've been concerned, first and foremost, with what these children accomplish via these repeats themselves. The preceding analysis shows that children use questioning repeats both to maintain intersubjectivity and to challenge talk and conduct they find in some way problematic. The challenges these questioning repeats embody can be seen as a part of the mechanism by which children set standards and police norms for one another's conduct – and in particular their use of language. That is, questioning repeats are used where one child's pronunciation of a word does not meet a certain standard, where a child uses a word which another recognises as 'nonce', or where a child makes a claim that another finds in someway problematic.

Questioning repeats can thus be seen as a mechanism of peer-socialisation. It is notable, however, that children have various ways of handling the challenge that a questioning repeat embodies – in a number of extracts we saw children standing their ground in the face of challenge, in others they acquiesce and in others they attempt to transform the activity by introducing laughter into it. The availability of multiple ways of responding makes this a particularly dynamic mechanism – not so much unidirectional social control or socialisation but ongoing, mutual regulation – a web of accountability (Heritage 1984; Drew 1987).

Returning to the distributional patterns cited at the beginning of this chapter, I want to suggest that the prevalence of questioning repeats in the talk of 4-year-old children is explainable by reference to the special concerns of children of this age. Specifically, these children exhibit a pervasive concern with the conduct of others and specifically the degree to which it meets invocable standards of pronunciation, grammar, precision, accuracy and so on. In the 5-year-old corpus, by comparison, very few other-initiated repairs are addressed to problems of this sort. Rather, among the 5-years-olds, problems which promote the use of repair are often the result of recipient design errors – an overextension of the principle 'over-suppose, under-tell'. The following extracts illustrate this type of problem:

Extract 6.23

1 C: This is a type that attaches, onto **the biggie.**

2 A: → Onto the biggie?=

3 C: =Yeah like this,

Extract 6.24

1 B: No I want one of **tho:se pie:ces.**

2 C: → What,

3 B: Tho::se pieces.

4   (0.4)

5 C: One o::f the fla:t (.) ones?

6 B: No the long- (.) these-

7   (0.2)

8   no

9   (0.4)

10   the::se.

11   (0.2)

12 C: Tho::se? ((*looks in Lego bin*))

Extract 6.25

1 A: ((*looks at door*)) Maybe R–, maybe you can move **it,**

2 C: →   °Move what.°

3 A: Move that thing that('s in the lock)/(yo- in the door).

4 C: Okay.

Extract 6.26

1 C: and all the people ran onto **that plane**. (0.4) Right?

2 A: →   what plane.

3 C: that plane right there. Or this plane. Ya cuz [there]

4 A: [they ran]

5   on to that.

6 A: [mmmmm]

Extract 6.27

1 R: My robot got picked up by **the Toronado**

2   (0.2)

2 A: →   What Toronado.

3 R: A Tornado – it's been round and round

Extract 6.28

1 S: we can have **that army** up there

2 W: Which army.

3 S: that army.

4 W: which army.

5 S: this army ((*points to it*))

In Extracts 6.23 to 6.29 the trouble-source is a referential expression – in Extract 6.23 'the biggie', in Extract 6.24 'those pieces', in Extract 6.25 'it', in Extract 6.26 'that plane', in Extract 6.27 'the tornado' and in Extract 6.28 'that army'. The design of the referring expression in each case conveys that the speaker believes the recipient should be able to use it to identify something in the world. In Extract 6.25 the presupposition is associated with the pronoun 'it' while in the rest it is associated with so-called definite determiners 'the' or 'that'. But in each case the recipient is unable to use the expression to locate some real-world object to which it refers. Interestingly, a range of different formats are used to initiate repair – from a questioning repeat in Extract 6.23, to 'what' in Extract 6.24, and what I have termed 'complex constructions' in Extracts 6.25–6.28. When I searched the 4-year-old data for troubles of this sort I could not find a single clear case.

Rather than explain these distributional patterns in terms of developing 'cognitive capacity' we might seek to understand them in relation to the specific contingencies of interaction for children of different ages. Whereas 4-year-olds use other-initiated repair to maintain and enforce norms and standards of conduct, for 5-year-olds many uses of repair are engendered by complex practices of reference and object transfer. While in both cases, repair is addressed to the progressive realisation of intersubjectivity across turns at talk and sequences of action, this intersubjectivity takes different forms and faces different challenges among 4- and 5-year-old children (on the progressive realisation of intersubjectivity, see Sacks et al. 1974 and Schegloff 1992). I hope it is clear, then, that a purely 'developmental' account that explains differences between these groups in terms of increasing cognitive sophistication risks missing something rather important. Children of different ages have different concerns and must deal with markedly different interactional contingencies – it is hardly surprising that their talk should reflect such differences.

Acknowledgements

Previous versions of this chapter were presented at the ESRC seminar on interactions in childhood, the 106th Annual Meetings of the American Anthropological Association, and the SSHRC-funded workshop on repair. For comments on those occasions I thank Jeffrey Aguinaldo, Nick Enfield, Charles Goodwin, John Heritage, Heather Loyd, Clare MacMartin, Merle Mahon, Doug Maynard, John Rae, Geoff Raymond, Tanya Romaniuk, Federico Rossano, Manny Schegloff, Bill Wells and Tony Wootton. I also thank the volume editors for their careful reading and generous comments on the original manuscript I submitted. Finally, I thank Tanya Stivers – my collaborator in the larger project, part of which I am reporting on here – who has helped me not only to better understand the data used in this chapter but also to become a better analyst in general.

References

Bates, E. (1979) *The emergence of symbols*. New York: Academic Press.
Bloom, L. (1991) *Language development from two to three*. New York: Cambridge University Press.

Brown, P. (1998) Conversational structure and language acquisition: The role of repetition in Tzeltal adult and child speech. *Journal of Linguistic Anthropology*, **8** (2): 197–221.

Drew, P. (1987) Po-faced receipts of teases. *Linguistics*, **25** (1): 219–253.

Forrester, M.A. (2001) The embedding of the self in early interaction. *Infant and Child Development*, **10**, 189–202.

Gallagher, T. (1981) Contingent query sequences within adult-child discourse. *Journal of Child Language*, **8**, 51–62.

Garvey, C. (1977) The contingent query: A dependent act in conversation. In M. Lewis and L. Rosenblum (eds), *Interaction, conversation and the development of language* (pp. 63–93). New York: John Wiley and Sons.

Greenfield, P.M. and Smith J.H. (1976) *The structure of communication in early language development*. New York: Academic Press.

Heritage, J. (1984) *Garfinkel and ethnomethodology*. Cambridge: Polity Press.

Jefferson, G. (1972) Side sequences. In D. Sudnow (ed.), *Studies in social interaction* (pp. 294–338). New York: Free Press.

Jefferson, G. (1979) A technique for inviting laughter and its subsequent acceptance/declination. In G. Psathas (ed.), *Everyday language: Studies in ethnomethodology* (pp. 79–96). New York, NY: Irvington Publishers.

Keenan, E.O. (1974) Conversational competence in children. *Journal of Child Language*, **1** (2): 163–183.

Keenan, E.O. (1976) Again and again: Pragmatics of imitation in child language. *Pragmatics Microfiche*.

Keenan, E.O. (1983) Making it last: Repetition in children's discourse. In E. Ochs and B.B. Schieffelin (eds), *Acquiring conversational competence* (pp. 26–39). Boston: Routledge & Kegan Paul.

McTear, M. (1985) *Children's conversation*. Oxford: Basil Blackwell.

Ninio, A. and Bruner, J.S. (1978) The achievement and antecedents of labeling. *Journal of Child Language*, **5**, 1–15.

Ninio, A. and Snow C.E. (1996) *Pragmatic development*. Boulder, CO: Westview Press.

Ochs, E. (1984) Clarification and culture. In D. Schiffrin (ed.), *Georgetown University Round Table in languages and linguistics* (pp. 325–341). Washington, DC: Georgetown University Press.

Ochs, E. and Schieffelln B.B. (eds) (1979) *Developmental pragmatics*. New York: Academic Press.

Ochs, E. and Schieffelln B.B. (1983) *Acquiring conversational competence*. Boston: Routledge and Kegan Paul.

Sacks, H. (1974) On the analyzability of stories by children. In R. Turner (ed.), *Ethnomethodology: Selected readings* (pp. 216–232). Harmondsworth: Penguin.

Sacks, H., Schegloff, E.A. and Jefferson, G. (1974) A simplest systematics for the organization of turn-taking for conversation. *Language*, **50**, 696–735.

Schegloff, E.A. (1992) Repair after next turn: The last structurally provided for place for the defense of intersubjectivity in conversation. *American Journal of Sociology*, **95** (5), 1295–1345.

Schegloff, E.A., Jefferson, G. and Sacks, H. (1977) The preference for self-correction in the organization of repair in conversation. *Language*, **53**, 361–382.

Sidnell, J. (2006) Repair. In J. Verschueren and J.O. Östman (eds), *Handbook of pragmatics*. Amsterdam: Benjamins.

Tannen, D. (1987) Repetition in conversation: Toward a poetics of talk. *Language*, **63** (3): 574–605.

Tarplee, C. (1996) Working on young children's utterances: Prosodic aspects of repetition during picture labelling. In E. Couper-Kuhlen and M. Selting (eds), *Prosody in conversation* (pp. 406–435). Cambridge: Cambridge University Press.

Tomasello, M. (1999) *The cultural origins of human cognition*. Cambridge, MA: Harvard University Press.

Tomasello, M. (2003) *Constructing a language: A usage-based theory of language acquisition*. Cambridge, MA: Harvard University Press.

Tomasello, M., Conti-Ramsden, G. and Ewert, B. (1990) Young children's conversations with their mothers and fathers: Differences in breakdown and repair. *Journal of Child Language*, **17** (1), 115–130.

Wootton, A. (1997) *Interaction and the development of mind*. Cambridge: Cambridge University Press.

Chapter 7

Children's participation in their primary care consultations

PATRICIA CAHILL

Introduction

Clinicians can be taught skills to promote useful communication in their encounters with patients (Silverman *et al.* 2005; Howells *et al.* 2006). The skills that are taught need to be selected on the basis of clear evidence of their efficacy. However, there is a dearth of such evidence to guide clinicians on the communication techniques that would best promote child involvement in health care consultations. It is likely that to facilitate child participation involves different skills on the part of the clinician to adult-to-adult talk in medical interaction. However, it has not been established exactly that these skills are different or why they are different. This chapter seeks to address the need for data in this area and is based on fine-grained conversation analysis of paediatric encounters as part of a primary care research project in the United Kingdom (UK).

The paediatric consultation comprises usually of at least three people: a health care worker, a child and his or her adult carer. The talk that occurs, unlike ordinary conversation, is institutional, with an orientation towards goals, tasks and professional identity (Drew and Heritage 1992). It is, in fact, doing the work of the consultation, and is likely to be concerned with some health problem the child might have. Sacks *et al.* (1974) discuss the rules of turn-taking in ordinary conversation, including what happens in multi-party talk, which can be applicable to the discussions in these consultations. There are times when three people can be together, but where one is an over-hearer, listening to a two-person conversation. Such a situation might occur when two friends are talking and an interested stranger is listening, but not participating. The stranger is outside the conversation and is not at liberty to join in unless excessively moved to do so. So, although three people are present, the talk is dyadic and not multi-party. This can be analogous with what often happens in paediatric consultations, where dyadic talk occurs between the adult carer and the clinician. The child is outside his own consultation, only occasionally being invited to speak (Tates *et al.* 2001; Cahill *et al.* 2007a). Van Dumen (2004) looked at a large number of paediatric consultations and made the observation that that little triadic talk happened. On most occasions the doctor and the adult spoke in a dyad, and if the child was spoken to there would be brief dyads with the child and one of the adults, but almost no real three-way talk.

The literature on these consultations shows that the child is usually and historically excluded (Strong 1979; Tates *et al.* 2001; Cahill *et al.* 2007a). Korsch *et al.*'s (1968) seminal research into doctor–patient communication was set in a paediatric clinic. The authors stated that, in paediatrics, 'the patient' refers to the patient's parents, although more recent work indicates that children now have a little more say in their medical encounters. Studies set in the UK found that child talk took up 4% to 5.2% of the total discourse space (Wassmer *et al.* 2004; Cahill *et al.* 2007b). Clinician–child talk in the consultations is often social or rapport building, where children might be asked to cooperate with the examination or asked some details of their history. Child concerns are rarely heard and children are unlikely to participate in the later parts of the consultation that concern management plans (Tates *et al.* 2001; Cahill *et al.* 2007a). Tates and her colleagues discuss a series of analyses of videos of primary care paediatric consultations in the Netherlands from the period 1975–1993, which illustrate aspects of how children are involved in the consultations (Tates *et al.* 2000, 2002a, b, c). Doctors spoke in a social and joking way to young children. They did, however, accommodate for age and talked with older children more equally, but parents did not seem to make this accommodation. Doctors also appeared to try to involve the older children initially. However, 90% of consultations ended up with the child having little or no say in the discussion. The doctors appeared to accept the parental role of speaking for the child, aligning themselves with the parents.

Indeed, Stivers (2001), looking at the opening part of paediatric consultations, demonstrated that although doctors and the child's adult carers were oriented towards the child having a right to participate in the interaction and present his or her problem, the adult usually ended up doing so. Child patients themselves complain that when seeing their doctor or nurse, the talk is often more between the adults who are present than with them. They would like more say (Boylan 2004). In addition to children wanting to interact in their health encounters, doing so has shown to be beneficial. This is illustrated by a randomised-controlled trial conducted by Lewis *et al.* (1984), where children aged 8–12 years with asthma were included in 'a self-management programme'. In the intervention group, games were used to teach the children to recognise their symptoms and manage their disease. The asthma in these children significantly improved compared with those in the control group.

Alderson and Montgomery (1996) produced a code of practice for professionals who are consulting with child patients. They advocate that a child in partnership with his adult carer and health worker should be involved in the health decisions that affect him. They presented evidence showing that children over the age of 5 years can be presumed sufficiently competent to share in their own health care choices. They acknowledge that not all children are going to want to or be able to do this, but that all the participants in the child's consultation – including the child – have a right to have their views taken into account. Borland *et al.*'s (1998) qualitative studies with primary school children in Scotland further demonstrated how children in this age group are competent to participate in their health encounters as well as being aware of, and understanding, current health issues. The government and professional bodies now state that it is good practice for health professionals to actively involve children in their medical care (Department of Health 2003; General Medical Council 2007).

The analysis of data that is discussed in this chapter was undertaken with the aim of identifying skills that could be taught to clinicians to promote child involvement in a paediatric consultation. The 'involvement' was loosely defined, but permitted children to talk more in the encounters, and express their views, concerns and preferences if they wished to do so. The data was specifically checked for features of the interaction associated with this involvement, using tools from the methodology of conversation analysis (CA) – a methodology that is increasingly being used in health research (Drew *et al.* 2001). The findings are aimed to be directly applicable to clinicians who may wish to examine their own behaviour in consultations, with a view to introducing factors that might be relevant to their interaction in paediatric consultations.

Method

Details of the methods of the data collection are reported in more detail elsewhere in a paper on the same theme that discusses other aspects of the data analysis (Cahill *et al.* 2007b). Thirty-one consultations between general practitioners (GPs), child patients aged 6–12 years and the children's adult carers were videoed over the period October 2004 to April 2005 in routine surgeries in Suffolk, UK. The GP participants were selected to represent doctors from a diversity of practice types. The final sample included: 13 principal doctors who are partners in their practices; two salaried GPs, the status of these doctors is that of employees for a GP partnership; and one registrar, a qualified doctor who is training to become a GP. Their lengths of service ranged from 30 years to less than one year for the registrar. Children in the correct age groups attending the surgeries in the study were invited to participate. Those who agreed and gave fully informed consent did so. Full ethical approval from the appropriate regulatory authorities was granted prior to commencement of the study. The average age of the child participant was 8.5 years. The videorecordings were transcribed and analysed.

Results

Table 7.1 shows how the participants in the recordings sat in relation to one another. This is further illustrated in Figures 7.1–7.3. The seating and greeting part of the consultation is discussed below, and this is followed by discussion of some extracts of the consultations to demonstrate participant interaction in the encounters studied where there is some child participation. Most of the interaction seen was doctor–adult dyads. The word count and utterances made by the child were counted and found to be 5.2% of all the words and utterances.

The majority of the consultations began with a greeting sequence. This is important since the manner in which the interaction starts sets the scene for the whole consultation. However, it is not seen in some of the recordings where the camera was started after the patient had already entered the room. This happened in consultations where the doctors turned the camera on themselves and also in instances where the doctors collected patients from the waiting room and greeted them there.

Table 7.1 Greeting and seat allocation

Seating	Number of the 31 consultations featuring in this arrangement	Child participation
Child sitting next to the doctor.	16	The children in these consultations had some involvement. They answer questions predominately on rapport building, social talk and history giving. They were not heard to participate in the treatment and planning parts of the consultation.
Adult sitting next to the doctor.	6	In 2 of these consultations the child did not speak at all. In the other consultations the children were seen to answer only a few questions of a social nature or on clarification of the history primarily given to the doctor by the adult.
Adult, doctor and child sitting in a triangular arrangement.	9	The children in these consultations were heard to speak throughout the consultations. This was in the form of social and rapport building talk, exploring history, and expressing views when asked on diagnosis and treatment options.

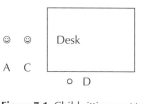

Figure 7.1 Child sitting next to doctor.

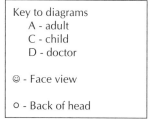

Key to diagrams
  A - adult
  C - child
  D - doctor

☺ - Face view

o - Back of head

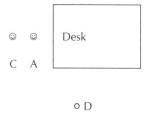

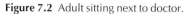

Figure 7.2 Adult sitting next to doctor.

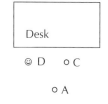

Figure 7.3 Triangular arrangement.

Extract 7.1 illustrates a greeting sequence, as was typically seen in the consultations. Key for the extracts: D = doctor, C = child, A = adult.

Extract 7.1

1 D: hallo: jake
      ((*Doctor sitting in chair looking up at child. Child has been called into room with mother. Doctor waiting for them*))

2 C: ((*Child looks at doctor*))

3 D: hi:↑ have a seat↓
      ((*Doctor gestures to child and mother to sit*))

4 D: ↓you're jake's mum,
      ((*Doctor looking at mother then looking from mother to Jake*))

5 A: I am yes↓ (*laugh*)

6 D: I have seen jake (.) once before
      ((*Doctor looking at computer screen*))

The doctor says 'hallo' to the child in line 1, making this greeting explicit. She does this by looking at the child and using his name when addressing him. Mechanisms of selecting a next speaker in multi-party talk are described in detail elsewhere (Lerner 2003; Sacks *et al.* 1974). No audible answer is forthcoming from the child in response. The doctor rephrases his 'hallo' to 'hi' and directs the child and parent to sit down. Neither the adult nor the child returns the doctor's greeting. The doctor continues to speak, checking on her computer for the last time Jake was seen. The child followed the parent into the consulting room and they sat down in that order, the doctor did not specify where they should sit.

In other consultations when a doctor had greeted the patient, some allocated a seat to the parent and child, as illustrated in the consultation in Extract 7.2. Here the doctor orchestrates the seating, which results in the child sitting next to him.

Extract 7.2

1 D: co:me and take a seat Peter that is your seat there↓
      ((*Doctor points at a seat then touches the seat while looking at the child*))

2 D: hi:↑ mr smith (.) come and take a seat (.) right
      ((*Doctor gestures to the father*))

The doctor uses verbal and non-verbal commands to seat Peter and his father where the doctor chooses. He uses the child's name, points and then touches the seat where Peter is to sit. The preferred response to the doctor's direction is to comply and it would have been unlikely that the parent and child would not sit where they were asked to.

In 16 of the 31 consultations analysed, the child was sitting next to the doctor. This seating arrangement is illustrated in Figure 7.1. In some cases, with the child in this position, the parent would stand. In six of the consultations the adult was closest to the doctor, as illustrated in Figure 7.2. In the remaining nine consultations the doctor sits in front of her desk to place the participants in a triangular set up, as illustrated in Figure 7.3.

As we saw in Extract 7.2 above, the doctor can arrange to have the child sit close to him or her, rather than leaving this to chance. When the child and doctor are in juxtaposition, they do not have to talk across the adult. A small child between the two adults does not pose too much of an obstacle. A child sitting next to the doctor without an adult in-between, in the consultations analysed, was seen to speak more in the consultation than when the child sat farther away from the doctor. This may have been in part because the physical barrier separating doctor and child is absent. However, it may have also been that a doctor who was intent on involving a child might take such measures, while a doctor who was content to conduct the consultation with the adult alone might not feel it necessary. So the arrangement of the physical context can be taken as an index of potential involvement, creating conditions that make interactional engagement more likely. In 12 of the consultation recordings made for this project, the doctors call the patients to come from the waiting room to the consulting room with a buzzer. In these instances the doctor is already in his or her room when the patients come in and in a position to direct all the patients to specified seats. This was the case in the consultation in Extract 7.2. In the consultations where it is the doctors' practice to collect the patients from the waiting room, it could be more difficult to offer the child a seat next to the doctor. For example, in one of these consultations, the child and adult preceded the doctor into the room and the adult selected a seat next to the doctor's desk. Some of the doctors who collect their patients still manage to offer the patients particular seats. In the consultation illustrated in Extract 7.3, the doctor is seen to stand in the doorway, having collected the patients from the waiting room, and directs them to specified seats.

Extract 7.3

1   D: hallo:: there ↑
        ((*Doctor looks at child and points towards chair nearest doctor's chair*))

2   D: have a seat ↓ hallo::

3   (0.3) ((*Child sits down in seat closest to the doctor's chair and the adult sits down in a second seat further away*))

When the doctor, adult and child were seated in the triangular arrangement seen in Figure 7.3, the participants are equal distances apart. When sitting in this arrangement the child spoke more in the consultations from a word count point of view, and the nature of the talk they were involved in was more extensive than was seen in consultations with the other seating arrangements. The children were seen to answer questions not only on social matters and their history, but also in the treatment and planning parts of the consultation. This situation is exemplified in the consultation in Extract 7.4.

Extract 7.4

1   D: I think it is proba::bly worth giving a course of antibiotics yo::u happy with that?
        ((*Doctor looking at the father*))

2   A: (.) yer
        ((*Father looking at the doctor*))

3   D: are yo::u happy to take some antibiotics?
        ((*Doctor looking at the child*))

4   C: (1.0) ye:::rs
        ((*Child looking at the doctor*))

The doctor is sitting in a triangular arrangement with a father and son and a three-way conversation occurs as illustrated in lines 1–4. The doctor offers the child and his father the option of antibiotics. The doctor is able to easily turn his head from the parent to the child and they can all participate in the discussion.

Problem presentation

After the participants have greeted one another and the seating is organised, the reason for the consultation is established and the participants commence exchanging information. Doctors in training in the UK are taught how to consult, so the talk usually follows the fairly universal patterns they have learnt. The consultation is an institutional interaction, and although the talk flows like ordinary conversation it differs in that specific topics need to be covered. The doctor usually starts by establishing the history of the presenting complaint; finding out what the patient's problem is. This part of the consultation in the conversation analysis (CA) literature is usually termed the problem presentation (Heritage and Maynard 2006). Table 7.2 presents the various combinations of turns taken by the doctor, adult and child to establish why the child has come to the doctor. A problem presentation is seen in all the consultations. The doctor can request the information or the adult or child can volunteer it. When the doctor asks for this information she can direct the request specifically to the child or to the adult. Alternatively, she can ask that the problem be presented by the adult

Table 7.2 Patterns of problem presentation in triadic, paediatric consultations

Pattern of problem presentation	Number of the 31 consultations featuring this pattern		
The doctor asks the adult directly for the problem.	7	23%	Adult is in a position to freely express concerns.
The doctor is ambiguous in asking for the problem and the recipient could either be the child or the adult.	6	19%	Adult is in a position to freely express concerns.
The doctor asks the child for the problem presentation but the adult takes the turn without waiting for the child to try answering.	4	13%	Adult is in a position to freely express concerns.
The doctor asks the child to present the problem but the child does not take the turn either passing it to the adult or refusing to take the turn.	9	29%	Adult in a position to freely express concerns.
The doctor asks the child for the problem presentation. The child takes up the turn.	5	16%	Adult needs to compete with the child for floor by self selecting in order to be able to express concerns.

or the child, not showing clearly to whom the question is addressed. The work of Stivers (2001), on paediatric consultations, discusses this issue in detail. In her analysis of data from this problem-presentation part of the consultation, she found that doctors usually selected the child to present the problem – although children only responded in just over half of the cases. She did show, however, that if the children were selected, they were much more likely to present the problem than if they had not been selected.

In the UK doctors are taught to say as little as possible at the beginning of a consultation. Their reticence is to indirectly encourage the patient to speak (Silverman *et al.* 2005). The rationale for this is to prevent the patient's agenda being closed down too quickly, thus allowing a patient-centred consultation to ensue. Many of the doctors seen in these recordings are ambiguous in selecting the adult or the child to present the reason for attendance. The doctors who do overtly select a speaker predominantly invited the child to take the floor first. However, in this study the majority of these children declined the invitation and the adult took the turn. This is similar to that found in settings outside the UK (Stivers 2001, 2007).

Examination of the recordings show that unless the child is actively offered a turn to speak, by being invited to talk by one of the adults at some point in the discussion, he doesn't become involved in the consultation other than minimally, such as by obeying instructions during the examination phase.

Extract 7.5 illustrates an example of a consultation where a doctor takes a very open stance at the beginning, not really specifying whether she is addressing the child or the adult.

Extract 7.5

1   D: hallo there
     ((Doctor looks at child and points towards chair nearest doctor's seat))

2   have a seat ↑hallo
         (0.5)

3   D: oh de::ar ↓
     ((Doctor looking at child's face, child has a sling on. Doctor smiling. Child looking up at doctor))

4   A: he fell over in the school playground (.) on wednesday.

The child is wearing a sling. The doctor has greeted the patient and the adult. When all are seated she says 'oh dear' in line 3. This 'oh dear' has several functions: firstly, it displays empathy for the child's plight regarding the need to wear a sling. It is also a place where the doctor in this type of institutional talk could be expected to inquire why the child has come, so it fills this space. As the doctor has not asked what the problem is, this gives an opportunity for the problem to be presented by either the adult or the child, which in this case is taken up by the adult. It might have been more appropriate for the child to do this from an interactional point of view, as he was sitting closer to the doctor, to whom the information is being related and she is looking at him. The adult, who is the child's grandmother, goes on to explain her concerns and view about the child. When the grandmother has finished, the consultation continues as in Extract 7.6.

Extract 7.6

1   D: Oka:: so::: can you tell me then Paul what happened ?
        ((*Doctor smiling at child, looking away from adult*))
        (0.5)

2   C: u:::m I was playing with my friend and I u::m well he like ( ) fell and<then he fell on
        top of me> and then
        ((*Child eyes looking down, removing his sling and unwinding the bandage around his arm.*
        Doctor's eyes looking down towards his hands))

3   D: ye::r
        ((*Doctor still looking down*))

4   C: then this got on the wrong (0.2) think it bent backwards
        ((*Child leans forward and bends hand backwards*))

5   D: think it was bent u::nder you was it?
        ((*Doctor raises chin and moves head back slightly*))

6   C: yer

The adult has been able to express herself fully at the beginning of the consultation. The child is then explicitly invited to speak by the doctor in line 1. The doctor has clearly designed the question in this line for the child to answer. She has turned her head towards the child away from the adult, gazes at the child and uses his name. The child explains what happened to him in line 2, although he does not do so fluently, leaving, pauses and displaying some word-finding difficulty, creating places his grandmother could have come in but she does not. In line 4 he carries on his account with words and actions. The doctor indicates that she has comprehended what he has said by paraphrasing it back to him in line 5, and the child confirms that she has got this right in line 6 with a 'yer'. The child answers the doctor in response to being asked questions. The doctor carries on talking to the child until, in this consultation, it comes to the diagnosis and explanation, which is then with the adult.

Passing the turn

In 16 of the 31 consultations the doctor turns initially to the child to establish the problem presentation. However, the child does not necessarily take up this opportunity but either passes the responsibility of taking the turn on to the adult, is silent or, as in one case, used the turn to refuse involvement in the consultation. The adults then go on to state the reason for attendance and have the opportunity to express themselves. This is shown in the consultation in Extract 7.7.

Extract 7.7

1 D: °↑right how can I help yo::u Jennifer°
((*Doctor looking directly at Jennifer, child turns gaze away from doctor towards mother*))

2 C: (1.0) (two squeaky like noises)
((*Child holds mother's hand and moves head towards mother and looks down at mother's knees, then holds on to mother's arms*))

3 D: oh dea::r
((*Doctor look away from child and up towards mother*))

4 D: (.)°gos:hhu° (*laughs*)
((*Looks to mother, who then starts to talk*))

5 A: about two:: weeks ago
((*Mother's head lifts up*))

In the example in Extract 7.7, the doctor addresses the child, uses her name and looks directly at her. The mother can see that the doctor is looking at the child. In line 2 the child acknowledges the doctor's question with ill-defined squeaky noises. The child indicates with body language her declination to deliver the information directly. The mother is selected to speak by the doctor and the child, as both of them look at her and she goes on to disclose the reason for the child's attendance herself. The child passes on the responsibility of disclosing the problem presentation to her mother. The doctor's 'oh dear' in line 3 can be interpreted as a reaction to the child's whimper and also fills a potential space created by the girl not answering the question. The mother, when able to take the turn, can speak freely as she is not competing with the child.

The mother goes on to explain the child's problems as she perceives them, telling the doctor that the child has a cough, and her theories on this. After the mother has stopped speaking the doctor turns to the child again and attempts to engage her in the discussion once more. The consultation continues in Extract 7.8.

Extract 7.8

1 D: °↑so what is the main thing that has been upse:::tting yo::u ?°
((*Doctor looks directly at child, bends forward stooping down from her chair, moving slightly closer to the child*))

2 C: (2.0) umm °the cough°
((*Child raises head up still holding on to mother's arm*))

The child has already been asked once what is troubling her, as seen in Extract 7.7 when she delegated her mother to answer the question. It is possible that, when asked initially, the child was not ready to answer. She responds to this question when it is put to her again in Extract 7.8, line 1. Now that her mother has had her say, there is less pressure of someone waiting for a turn, which, as Sacks *et al.*'s (1974) model of turn-taking in conversation explains, is an issue in three-party talk. The mother told the doctor that the main problem is a cough and the child gives the 'right' answer after a short delay and an umm; she also says in line 2 that her main problem is a cough. The consultation continues in Extracts 7.9 and 7.10.

Extract 7.9

1 D: has there been anything else↑
        (.)

2 A: she did say this morning that her ears are starting to hurt and=
        ((*Child looks at mother*))

3 A: = her   [throat is starting]

4 C: [NO: its: really ur::ting]
        ((*Tearful voice, first time clearly and audibly heard, also rubbing right ear*))

In line 1, the doctor asks if there is anything else. The mother answers the doctor's question as the doctor has not been specific regarding to whom she is addressing this question. The immediately prior talk has been a dyad between the mother and the doctor. In line 2 the mother adds briefly that as well as the cough her daughter has had an ear problem. She then quickly, without missing a beat, moves on to talking about the throat. She does not pause after mentioning the ears; there is no downward prosody or any elaboration and she does not emphasise this point. The child comes in here when the word 'ear' has been heard and ratifies this part of the answer. She corrects her mother and states that the ear was really hurting. When making this statement, she directs her gaze more to the mother than to the doctor.

Extract 7.10

1 D: ↑what shall we do first? (.) then sha:ll we have a look at your ears?(.)=
        ((*Doctor points her hand to her ear*))

2 D: =or listen to your chest?
        ((*Doctor moves her hand to her chest while looking directly at child*))

3 A: (1.0) (well [her)] ((almost inaudible))

4 C: [e::n]rs

(Lines of transcription omitted, mother talking about ears and throat)

5 D: actually that ear is ver(hh)y red ((*slight laugh*))

6 A: is, it?

In Extract 7.10 the consultation proceeds to the examination phase. The doctor asks the child if she would prefer to have her chest or ears examined first. The child initially lets her mother start to answer the question for her, but then comes in to state her preference of 'ears' decisively.

The doctor examines the child, and in line 5 of Extract 7.10 states that the ear is very red and she laughs slightly. The mother had said that the problem was a cough. The use of the word 'actually' in line 5 highlights the doctor's orientation to what the child is saying and the disjunction between the child's comment and the mother's assertion. The doctor repeatedly allocates turns to the child throughout the consultation. It is the child's input that leads to a diagnosis of the her problem being the ear rather than the cough. The mother is not prevented in any way from saying what she wants to say and does not interrupt when the child speaks.

In the following example from another consultation the doctor offers the opening request for problem solicitation to the child. The child does not take it and the adult takes the turn, as illustrated in Extract 7.11.

Extract 7.11

1   D: what can I do for you Lisa?
          ((*Doctor looking directly at child*))

2   C: um::
          ((*Child looks towards mother*))

3   A: she had a cold about a month 3 to 4 weeks ago she can't shake (.) she's got
          a cough=
          ((*Looking at doctor*))

4   A: =and it just isn't going
          ((*Eyes glance towards child*))

5   D: ye::h ↓not what you want for your Christmas holidays ↑ is it ˙hhh
          ((*Doctor looking at child*))

6   C: ((*Child shakes her head and looks down*))

7   A: it doesn't seem to be getting any better ( )
          ((*Mother looking at doctor*))

8   D: hhhas anybody else in the family had a cold

9   A: I've had a cold

In the example in Extract 7.11 the doctor asks the child to formulate her reason for attendance in line 1. She makes it clear that this question is meant for the child as she addresses the child explicitly by name. The child makes a sound and indicates that she orients to it being her responsibility to answer this question; however, she looks towards her mother who speaks on her behalf. The mother is able to tell the doctor the reason the child has been brought to the doctor. In line 4 the doctor tries to bring the child into the consultation with a social inquiry, which could be regarded as rhetorical and uses a tag question that invites a 'yes' or a 'no', and therefore facilitating but not obliging the child to speak. She doesn't speak but shakes her head in response. The doctor continues to try to involve the child in the consultation, which continues in Extract 7.12.

Extract 7.12

1   A: it is just the cough I mean her nose and anything her nose isn't running it is just
          the cough she has got now
          ((*Mother looks at doctor and then at child. The child looks up at mother and smiles*))

2   D: hh and is it a kind of cough Lisa (.) that keeps you awake?

3   C: u::m=
          ((*Child smiling and looking forward*))

4   D: = or do you sleep alright with it

5   C: I sleep alright
          ((*Child nodding*))

6   D: okay

(Lines 7, 8 and 9 of transcription omitted, where doctor talks about different kinds of cough)

10   D: do you get gunkey slimy stuff into your mouth

11   C: sometimes

The doctor continues to try to talk to and get information from the child. In line 2 she asks the child a two-part question about the cough and sleep, to which the child responds with an 'um'. The doctor rephrases the question, asking a specific one-part question about the cough and gets the information from the child. Later on the doctor asks the child if she has gunkey stuff in her mouth. Doctors are taught to establish if a cough is dry or productive of sputum; here the doctor is asking the child about this. She uses the words 'gunkey stuff', which is not a medical term, to describe sputum, and this is likely to have been designed for the child with the assumption that it would be easily understood. The child shows that she does indeed understand what the doctor is saying as she is able to respond appropriately. The mother lets the doctor–child dialogue continue and does not step in.

In the two consultations illustrated in Extracts 7.7–7.12 above, the doctor offers an initial turn to the child, but the adult essentially takes it after the child has declined to do so. The adults are able to relay information to the doctor that they may feel is important in a way that does not cause turbulence in the discussion. The consultations proceed smoothly without interruptions from the adult when the doctor is subsequently in discussion with the child.

'Mum has her say'

In most of the 31 consultations the adults had their say almost immediately. However, in five consultations the doctor invites the child to formulate the reason for attendance, which the child accepts, and the child and the doctor go on to converse in a dyad, initially excluding the adult from the talk. In these consultations the longer the doctor–child talk goes on, the more tension is apparent. The adult keeps on self-selecting to speak or actually interrupts doctor–child talk until she is able to express her views.

In the example discussed below, interactional trouble is noted when a doctor engages with a child and excludes the adult. It concerns a 12-year-old girl who has come to the doctor to discuss abdominal pain. The girl is sitting next to the doctor with the adult by her side further away from the doctor. The child and doctor are bent towards each other. As the consultation commences, the recording shows the mother sitting with her shoulders slightly raised and her head to the side and still while the others are talking. Her gaze is fixed on the doctor–child talk. She is physically still and any movement is imperceptible.

Extract 7.13

1   C: ((*laugh*))

2   D: >what can we do for you<
((*Doctor bent forward looking at child and away from the mother*))

3   C.   (0.2) um I keep getting stomach stomach aches
((*Looking at doctor*))

4   D: right

5   C.   (0.1) why (.) or they get pretty painful and they keep getting er (0.1) around lunch time normally they and I have had them for I had them since primary school I think (.) I'm not sure but from year five=
((*Child glances at doctor*))

6   C: =up wards
((*Mother has been looking at child, when child mentions primary school the mother pushes hand to eye and looks up fleetingly. Gaze then fixed on child and doctor, eyes held in one position, in stance of attentive listening*))

7   D: right

8   C: and around lunch time and er (0.3) I don't really know what to::
((*Child looks at doctor and smiles. Mother smiles holding body stiffly as if holding back*))

The greeting exchanges have already occurred in the consultation shown above in Extract 7.13. The doctor and child are sitting down at the desk. The doctor in this instance does not use the child's name but nevertheless explicitly addresses the child by bending towards her and gazing at her. The doctor is clearly not looking at the mother. The child shows by her response that she understands the doctor use of 'you' in line 2 is directed at her. The child presents the problem as abdominal pains. It would be physically and inter-actionally difficult for the mother to come in here as the doctor and child are turned away from her towards each other. The doctor continues to address her questions to the child and they talk for 7 minutes. The mother has not been given the opportunity to speak. She is not invited to join in the discussion by either her daughter or the doctor. The consultation continues in Extract 7.14 where the doctor is exploring the bowel habits of the child.

Extract 7.14 (*Consultation continues from Extract 7.13*)

9   C: any problem with your bo::wels(.) with pooing any (0.1) going more o:ften loo::se being (.) c [onstipated]

10 C: [I hardly] I hardly (.) er I don't go(.) uf as much (.)I don't go as much as other people anyway I don't

11 D: right

12 C: I only go (.) may be twice a day so [mething like that] (.)

13 A: [to the toileth   ] haha you mean
((*Mother moves head and smiles*))

14   D: twice a day I mean that's that's pretty[frequent   ]

15   A: [°harhahar°] ((*Smiles*))

16   A: no that is just [ever]

17   C: [ssh]

18   D: [oh ri]ght=

19   A: so she ((*laughs*))

20   D: ==so that's peeing as well as the poo

21   C: yes

22   D: right

In line 12 the child tells the doctor that she only 'goes' twice a day. To pass stools twice a day would be more frequent than is usual for most people. Mother recognises that this is what the child has implied and comes into the talk to correct any misunderstanding; that this is to pass urine as well as stools, in line 16. There is a preference for self-correction when errors occur in conversation (Schegloff *et al.* 1977). Norrick (1991) argues that this is not necessarily seen when it comes to parents correcting children, as parents step in to correct children's mistakes because they are more experienced and have more knowledge. The mother here corrects what the child is saying to the doctor even though it is possible that the child is asking her not to, with a 'ssh' in line 17. By doing so the mother is able to enter the discussion. It also shows that she is part of the triad and a greater expert on her daughter's problems than the daughter. It demonstrates the mother's intimacy with her daughter, having knowledge about this very personal matter regarding bodily functions even to the point where she can comment on it. The mother starts to move when she is able to make this point. The dyad so far has been very successful with the doctor and child. The mother has been able to have her say, making sure that the doctor understands what the child is saying. The child speaks only once more in line 21. The mother has entered into the talk as a participant. More than 7 minutes into this 10-minute consultation the doctor does not know if the mother has concerns, as these have not been heard. The doctor–mother discussion now ensues. The mother's concerns emerge in Extract 7.15, which is a continuation of the dialogue in Extract 7.14.

Extract 7.15 (*Consultation continues from Extract 7.14*)

23   A: we did wonder if it was tiredness and stress ? or something like that↓

24   D: right

25   A: I (.) have a feeling> it is (0.3) wind ↓=<

26   D: right

27   A: because she does have a (.) p problem that way

28   D: yer

29   A: and I would like that to be considered in the whole thing because she is
          <u>struggling</u> with that issue

In line 25 the mother explains that the child's concern is 'wind' and is thus able to have her say. From this point onwards the consultation is entirely between the doctor and mother, the child being excluded.

Discussion

The doctors in this sample did engage with the children. The extracts shown in this chapter demonstrate this interaction. However, almost 95% of the talk in the consultations recorded was between the adults and the doctors, with the child as a bystander. The children's talk represented just over 5% of the total discourse space, showing that very little of the consultation is child talk, which is in line with what has previously been written about these consultations (Tates *et al.* 2001; Cahill *et al.* 2007a).

As has been reported elsewhere, the clinicians and adults oriented towards the child having the right to present the problem, although the adult usually ends up doing so. (Stivers 2001; Stivers *et al.* 2007). When the child did not take up the opportunity to talk first, these adults were then in a position to express their own views and concerns without having to compete with the child for the floor. After the adult carers had spoken, some children were then heard to participate in the consultation, but usually only when invited to do so explicitly by the doctors. A few went on to express their own thoughts and were able to do so without the adult voice coming in. An example of this is seen in the consultation above regarding the girl with ear pain seen in Extracts 7.7–7.10. She was able to contradict her mother's version of her principal health concern being the cough and to let the doctor know that the worse problem for her was ear pain. In the final example (Extracts 7.13–7.15) a doctor–child dyad is seen. The child in this example was 12 years old. (There can be an issue that when a child reaches the teenage years it is appropriate for some consultations to be held with the child and doctor alone – with the parent only as an observer, or outside the room. However, that issue is beyond the scope of this discussion, which is looking at triadic consultations.) Here initially the doctor talks to the child on a one-to-one basis, treating her as competent to proceed with the consultation. It is well documented that the doctors talk more to older children than to younger ones (Tates *et al.* 2000; Stivers *et al.* 2007). Initially, the mother does not speak, but eventually gets the chance to interpret what the child has said to the doctor and come into the consultation. She has her own concerns and worries about the child. Once she has disturbed the doctor–child talk to recount these concerns, the consultation reverts to an adult–doctor dialogue, the child being excluded. Tates *et al.* (2002c) reported from their examination of data from paediatric consultations that, even in cases where the doctor and parent are supportive of the child's involvement by the end of the consultation, the child would be silent. She also showed that when the parent was non-supportive of child involvement – for example, by asking the doctor a lot of questions – a doctor who may have being trying to engage with the child would shift to an adult–doctor consultation.

Primary care paediatric consultations in the UK at the time when these recordings were made lasted usually less than 10 minutes. The GP volunteers for this study all worked under pressure of time. Adult carers in these paediatric encounters could be expected to have been aware of this. The adults may not always have the luxury of waiting for a doctor–child dialogue to finish. They feel that they may not have time to state their case during the short discussion time and, hence, make it necessary to have a say. The adult carer, usually the parent, has brought the child to the doctor and is also likely to wish to speak in the discussion.

The hypotheses resulting from this analysis is that, if a doctor and child successfully interact together and exclude the adult carer, the adult carer is likely to come into the consultation and disturb the doctor–child talk, with the consequence that the child may have little or no more say. In consultations where the parental views are expressed at an early stage, the child is then in a position to go on to speak unchallenged, without the adult waiting to have her turn. The doctor is are in a position to select the child for questions during the consultation.

Stivers (2001) showed that if the child is selected to present the problem, then that child is 27 times more likely to do so than if not specially selected. It is observed in this current analysis that a child is more likely to speak if invited to do so by the adults. Based on what was seen in this study, clinicians are advised to allow the carers to speak if the carer wishes, and then to actively invite the child to participate throughout the consultation, aiming for all parties having a say.

GPs rooms in the UK are usually set up so that the doctor and patient can sit at a desk at a knee-to-knee angle rather than side by side or directly across from each other (Silverman *et al.* 2005). This arrangement suits one-to-one consultations but in three-way talk it means that the third party can be physically marginalised. The simple measure of sitting in a more triangular arrangement here was associated with episodes of triadic talk – all parties speaking together – and would thus be recommended for doctors to try. This study confirms that to talk to children, doctors should be very explicit in the terms of address they use. It is also suggested that when the parent or the adult carer is able to express his or her concerns during paediatric consultations, the child's contribution should be facilitated.

References

Alderson, P. and Montgomery, J. (1996) *Health care choices, making decisions with children*. London: Institute for public policy research.

Borland, M., Laybourm, A., Hill, M. and Brown, J. (1998) *Middle children*. London: Jessica Kingsley.

Boylan, P. (2004) *Children's voices project: Feedback from children and young people about their experience and expectations of health care*. Commission for Health Improvement, National Health Service England and Wales. Available at: http://www.healthcarecommission.org.uk/NationalFindings/NationalThemeReports/ChildrensWorkDetail/fs/en?CONTENT ID=4010931andchk=4h8wpV

Cahill P. and Papageorgiou, A. (2007a) Triadic communication in the primary care paediatric consultation: A review of the literature. *British Journal of General Practice*, 57, 904–911.

Cahill, P. and Papageorgiou, A. (2007b) A video analysis of communication in paediatric consultations in primary care. *British Journal of General Practice*, 57, 866–871.

Department of Health (2004) *National Service framework for children, young people and maternity services*. Available at: http://www.doh.gov.uk/PolicyAndGuidance/HealthAndSocialCareTopics/ChildrenServicesInformation/fs/en

Drew, P. and Heritage, J. (1992) *Talk at work: Interaction in institutional settings.* Cambridge: Cambridge University Press.

Drew, P., Chatwin, J. and Collins, S. (2001) Conversation analysis: A method for research into interaction between patients and health care professionals. *Health Expectations*, **4**, 58–70.

General Medical Council (2007) *0–18 years: Guidance for all doctors.* London: GMC.

Howells, R., Davies, H. and Silverman, J. (2006) Teaching and learning consultation skills for paediatric practice. *Archives of Disease in Childhood*, **91**, 367–370.

Korsch, B., Gozzi, E. and Francis, V. (1968) Gaps in doctor–patient communication. *Pediatrics*, **42** (5), 855–870.

Lerner, G. (2003) Selecting next speaker: The context-sensitive operation of a context-free organization. *Language in Society*, **32**, 177–201.

Lewis, C., Rachelefsky, G., Lewis, M., De la Sota, A. and Kaplan, M. (1984) A randomized trial of ACT (Asthma Care Training) for kids. *Pediatrics*, **74** (4), 478–486.

Norrick, N. (1991) On the organization of corrective exchanges in conversation. *Journal of Pragmatics*, **16**, 59–83.

Sacks, H., Schegloff, E. and Jefferson, G. (1974) A simplest systematics for the organization of turn-taking for conversation. *Language*, **50** (4), 696–735.

Schegloff, E., Jefferson, G. and Sacks, H. (1977) The preference for self-correction in the organization of repair in conversation. *Language*, **53** (2), 361–382.

Silverman, J., Kurtz, S. and Draper, J. (2005) *Skills for communicating with patients* (2nd edition). Oxford: Radcliff Publishing.

Stivers, T. (2001) Negotiating who presents the problem: Next speaker selection in pediatric encounters. *Journal of Communication*, **51**, 252–283.

Stivers, T. and Majid, A. (2007) Questioning children: Interactional evidence of implicit bias in medical interviews. *Social Psychology Quarterly*, **70** (4), 424–441.

Strong, P. (1979) *The ceremonial order of the clinic.* London: Routledge & Kegan.

Tates, K. and Meeuwesen, L. (2000) Let Mum have her say: Turntaking in doctor-parent-child communication. *Patient Education and Counselling*, **40** (2), 151–162.

Tates, K. and Meeuwesen, L. (2001) Doctor-parent-child communication. A (re)view of the literature. *Social Science and Medicine*, **52** (6), 839–851.

Tates, K., Meeuwesen, L., Bensing, J. and Elbers, E. (2002a) Joking or decision-making? Affective and instrumental behaviour in doctor-parent-child communication. *Psychology and Health*, **17** (3), 281–295.

Tates, K., Meeuwesen, L. and Bensing, J. (2002b) 'I've come about his throat': Roles and identities in doctor-parent-child communication. *Child Care, Health and Development*, **28** (1) 109–116.

Tates, K., Elbers, E., Meeuwesen, L. and Bensing, J. (2002c) Doctor-parent-child relationships : 'a pas de trios'. *Patient Education and Counselling*, **48** (1), 5–14.

Van Dulmen, S. (2004) Pediatrician-parent-child communication: Problems related or not? *Patient Education and Counselling*, **52**, 61–68.

Wassmer, E., Minnaar, G., Abdel Aai, Atkinson, M., Gupta, E., Yuen, S. and Rylance, G. (2004) How do paediatricians communicate with children and parents? *Acta Paediatrica*, **93**, 1501–1506.

Chapter 8

Feelings-talk and therapeutic vision in child–counsellor interaction

IAN HUTCHBY

Introduction

In many areas of their everyday lives, children find themselves managing the contingencies of adult-controlled institutions, including school classrooms (McHoul 1978; Mayall 1994), medical settings (Silverman 1987) and social services such as counselling (Hutchby 2007). These settings involve professionals and other organisational representatives who engage in task-oriented interaction with children. One of the key themes often drawn out in relation to such settings is the way that differing agendas and moral imperatives can inform the participation of adults and children. Of course, such factors are not absent from adult–child interaction in other, more routine settings, such as the home. For example, Wootton's (1997) work on child-requesting clearly shows the child displaying an orientation to understanding as being both public and moral. However, as we will see, institutional forms of talk bring into play distinctive factors associated with the particular activities oriented to, as relevant to a given setting.

There is a two-fold relevance to studying these differences. Firstly, they can reveal how children exercise their situated social competencies (Hutchby and Moran-Ellis 1998) in orienting to those institutional agendas. Secondly, they can illuminate the ways in which professionals, practitioners and policy makers understand (or fail to understand) the social competencies of children.

The interface between children's social competence and the agendas of institutional discourse is nicely illustrated in Silverman *et al.*'s (1998) study of parent–teacher interviews – a space in which children are actively present but at the same time are the objects of discussion between adults. Focusing on cases of silent or non-responsive children in these contexts, they show how silence often follows turns in which adults have proffered advice for future actions (such as 'maybe you can agree to work harder . . .'). The child's silence thus occurs in a particular sequential context – it is, in other words, an identifiable *lack* of speech – but it is treated analytically not as a deficiency on the part of the child but as a display of interactional competence. 'This is because silence (or at least lack of verbal response) allows children to avoid implication in the collaboratively accomplished adult moral universe and thus . . . enables them to resist the way in which an institutional discourse serves to frame and constrain their social competencies'

(Silverman *et al.* 1998: 220). In other words, it is a means of orienting to, and dealing with, the institutional agenda at work in this setting.

Similar themes emerge in my own research on children's talk in counselling sessions following parental separation or divorce (Hutchby 2007). Such sessions are an institutional space that, like all forms of counselling, provide what Silverman (1996) called an 'incitement to speak': in this case, about the 'feelings' generated by the break-up of a family unit. Yet that 'incitement', which forms part of the task-oriented institutional work of child counsellors, is by no means straightforwardly complied with by children. As in most forms of counselling (Peräkylä *et al.* 2008), the willingness of the client (the child) to produce the kind of 'feelings-talk' that counsellors encourage varies widely.

In this chapter I pursue the theme of the elicitation of feelings-talk in relation to a number of central issues. Previous studies (Hutchby 2001, 2002, 2005) have shown how child counsellors are routinely concerned to perform 'translations' of children's talk into therapeutic objects: in other words, to recast what children say in terms that may be amenable to a counselling intervention. The characteristic properties of such translations are: (1) that they refer issues back to the child, especially in terms of their subjective experience, i.e. what they may *think* about given events; (2) that they refer issues to *feelings* the child may have or concerns that they may harbour; and (3) that they refer issues to their *consequences* in terms of child–parent relationships. The institutional work of child counselling therefore involves the counsellor bringing into play events in the child's 'private' or intrapersonal sphere (thoughts, feelings, emotions, experiences) and translating them into the 'public' or interpersonal sphere of talk-in-interaction.

However, as in Silverman *et al.*'s (1998) data, children may choose whether or not to go along with the elicitation of feelings-talk. We thus encounter again the often problematic interface between children's communicative competencies and professional institutional agendas. Using data in which the counsellors ask explicitly about what children 'think' or 'feel' about events or situations, and later, data in which counsellors themselves volunteer their own 'thoughts' on situations, I show how the production of talk about thoughts and feelings (which I collect together under the general heading 'feelings-talk') is both driven and constrained by contrasting discourses and agendas at the heart of child counselling as an institutional discourse.

The data

The data were collected in a British child counselling and family therapy practice where the emphasis was on work with children currently dealing with the prospect of, or consequences of, their parents' separation. The child counsellors in this practice did not deal with children exhibiting severe behavioural problems, who would more likely be referred to clinical psychologists, or at risk of harm, in which case the child would more likely be assigned to social workers. Instead, they tended to deal with children whose parents felt that some sort of help was needed in getting the child to come to terms with the decision they had made to separate. Children were therefore referred for counselling on a voluntary basis; although the volition was more usually that of the parents rather than the child. The overall aim of counselling was to ease the children into acceptance of their parents' separation or divorce, and to encourage them to see that such experiences were not extraordinary, or at least not something for which they should blame themselves.

In all cases in the current data corpus, the policy was that while parents were seen in an initial assessment meeting together with their child, subsequently children were seen by the counsellor on their own for between four and six sessions. At the end, a further meeting was frequently held in which parents, children and counsellors would all be present. Fifteen full sessions were recorded, including sessions conducted by both male and female counsellors. The cases include single children and siblings, both male–male and male–female. In the latter cases, there are recordings of siblings seen by counsellors both together and separately. The age range was from 4 to 12 years.

Informed consent (of both parents and children) was obtained by means of a letter, written in styles that differed according to broad age group categories, which (a) explained some basic facts about the research project, (b) guaranteed that the tape would only be available to the researcher, (c) explained that the child had the right not to agree and, finally, (d) invited them to sign to say that they had read and understood the letter. The process of obtaining the informed consent of parents and children was done prior to the counselling period actually starting, at the initial assessment meeting.

The recordings were carried out with the tape recorder in full view of the participants, the procedure being to place the device (a small battery-operated portable machine) on a table at the side of the room, and situate two small, flat multi-directional microphones in different parts of the room (for example, one near the armchairs where participants would sit, and one near the toy cupboard from which children would choose games, often at the counsellor's invitation) (see Hutchby 2001).

Therapeutic vision

One of the key distinctive features of the current data corpus in comparison to other forms of therapeutic dialogue (e.g. Peräkylä *et al.* 2008) is that children tend to have been brought to the counselling session at the behest of their parents. Therefore, they do not tend to arrive at the session pre-armed with issues, topics, and so on that they wish to 'put on the table'. This means that the work of drawing out therapeutic matters in child counselling can be problematic. While the counsellor may seek to encourage the child to engage in discussion of certain types of topic, the child may seek to avoid that discussion in favour of topics that may be 'easier' to handle. It is important to consider how the situation may appear from both the counsellor's and the child's perspective in order to gain an understanding of the nature of the distinctive discourse practices that result.

Let us look first at counsellors' exercise of what I will call 'therapeutic vision'. Therapeutic vision is a term based on Goodwin's (1994) concept of 'professional vision', which refers to a way of seeing and understanding events according to occupationally relevant norms. It tends to involve three types of practice: (1) 'highlighting' certain features of a perceptual field as opposed to others; (2) 'coding' those features according to given, professionally available knowledge schemas; and (3) producing material representations (such as diagrams, graphs, tables or models) of the salient phenomena. Goodwin (1994) analyses this in the discourse of geologists and in the context of legal argumentation. There are distinct similarities in the professional vision of child counsellors.

The term 'therapeutic' vision is used to foreground the interactional work that is involved in counselling – that is, making the talk-at-hand therapeutic, or relevant for the professional practice of counselling. For example, child counsellors routinely seek to 'highlight' those aspects of children's talk that can be heard to be relevant for family-related or feelings-related matters. The interpretations they produce can be seen as 'coding' events according to specific, counselling-relevant frames or schemas. These frames include what seem to be standard 'positive' messages such as *parents should sort it out*; *it's not the child's fault*; *children often get caught in the middle of parents' fights*; *parents' fights can make children feel angry/sad/guilty*, and so on. Finally, the frames themselves are often represented in literary or graphical form, in the context of manuals for child counselling procedure (e.g. Geldard and Geldard 1997; Sharp and Cowie 1998), or alternatively, storybooks provided within counselling practices themselves for clients – both children and their parents – to view while waiting to see their counsellor.

Therapeutic vision creates a set of competing discourses in child counselling. From the child's perspective, an ambiguous situation results from two major discourse strategies adopted by counsellors. First of all, the talk produced by counsellors tends to place them squarely in the category of 'child' in as much as they are viewed in relation to their *parents*, whose actions have consequences for them *as* children. Extracts 8.1 and 8.2 illustrate this (in all extracts, C represents the counsellor; children are represented by the first letter of the anonymised names I invented for each of them):

Extract 8.1

1	→	C:	Does- do::, (0.2) the fights that mum and dad have, stop
2	→		you doing other things.
3		P:	Yea-a[h.
4		C:	[What kind've things d'they stop you doing.
5			(2.4)
6		P:	Mm-ooh I don't know.

Extract 8.2

1		C:	A::h 'kay so if you did what your da:d (.)
2			a::sked you or suggested, li[ke] go an' play on the=
3		J:	[Yeh]
4	→	C:	=computer, (0.5) would that happen would your mum an' dad
5	→		have an argument about it.
6		J:	Well they- the:y wouldn't me an' my mum would an' me an'
7			my dad would. .hh An' my mum an' dad would tell each
8			other off but they wouldn't argue.
9		C:	A::h. (.) Is that, different do [they-
10	→	J:	[An' my mum would smack
11	→		me an' send me up t' bed.

In Extracts 8.1 and 8.2 children are asked about the consequences upon themselves of actions carried out by their parents. For example, parents' fights may be treated as 'stopping' the child from doing things they may want to do (Extract 8.1); or, slightly more complexly, the child's acquiescence with one parent's wishes may lead to an argument between the two parents, which might ultimately result in the child being smacked and sent to bed (Extract 8.2).

One notable difference between these two examples is in the child's response to the counsellor's questions. In Extract 8.1 there is a lack of engagement with the invitation to think about the consequences of parents' actions (note the pause in line 5 and the non-committal response in line 6). In Extract 8.2, the child readily engages, going so far as to produce her own alternative version of interactional consequences in which she herself is the catalyst for arguments which result in her being sent to bed. These differences in child engagement with counsellor topics are returned to at a later stage in the present chapter.

A second, contrary factor from the child's perspective is that the task-orientation of counsellors within the setting ultimately means that children are routinely invited to speak in ways that are *outside* the normative parameters of 'childhood' as it tends to operate in the context of child–adult interaction. For instance they are frequently invited to speculate on their parents' reasoning, articulate their own feelings and responses to their parents' actions, or even develop proposals for how their parents can improve the situation. Extracts 8.3 and 8.4 illustrate this:

Extract 8.3

```
1  →  C:  Why d'you think, (1.8) mum an' dad said what they said.

2         (0.4)

3      P:  Don't know,

4         (4.1)

5      C:  Cuz it sounds like they were a bit cross.

6         (0.6)

7      P:  Don't know,

8  →  C:  Who d'you think they're cross with.
```

Extract 8.4

```
1  →  C:  Dju think it should stay the sa:me, .h or dju think it

2  →       should be diff'rent tuh how it is now.

3         (1.0)

4      P:  °Diff'rent.°

5      C:  Diff'rent.

6         (1.8)

7  →  C:  So you know it needs to be diff'rent[. . .]But dju know how

8  →       it should be.
```

In Extract 8.3, the child is asked to speculate on his parents' reasons for giving him contradictory messages (in this case, about a cancelled Disneyland trip); while in Extract 8.4, the child is not only asked about whether he thinks life at home should be 'different' but is encouraged to propose a resulting vision of 'how it should be'.

Meanwhile, counsellors are in a similarly ambiguous situation. First of all, their professional ethos and training encourages them to place the child's 'story' at the heart of their work and avoid 'leading' the child or judging their words or actions (Geldard and Geldard 1997). However, this requirement is problematised by the variability in children's willingness to produce the kinds of actions required. This variability itself derives partly from the position that children themselves are placed in – that is, being asked to speak in terms both within and outside the normative parameters of child–adult interaction. Counsellors are thereby placed in the position of having to decide how – or whether – to pursue feelings-talk when children display lack of uptake of such topics.

These competing discourses are mutually intertwined, and they permeate the discourse of child counselling. But more than that, they enable us to account for many of the forms of talk and interactional strategies that the data reveal. The fact that children are both situated as children-within-the-family yet encouraged to speak in ways that are outside the normative bounds for children-in-interaction-with-adults provides the very grounds for their variable willingness to speak in ways that 'communicate' about emotions, feelings and concerns. By the same token, counsellors' orientation to the counselling session as an environment where such 'communication' should ideally take place provides the grounds for their seeking to topicalise emotions, feelings and concerns even where those are not necessarily foregrounded in children's own talk.

In the remainder of this chapter I will examine further some features of the exercise of professional vision by counsellors, and the responses adopted in turn by children. I first illustrate the complex forms of dialogue in which, on the one hand, children are situated by counsellors as competent actors able to account for their own thoughts and feelings; while on the other, children's own means of exercising their communicative competencies – e.g. in resisting such accounts – can result in the counsellor positing accounts of child thoughts or feelings on their behalf. Second, I explore the ways in which counsellors may bring their own thoughts to the fore as a means of framing the interpretive work of the child.

Inviting talk about 'thoughts' and 'feelings'

Let us look at some examples in which counsellors seek to elicit children's personal perspectives on salient events. Child counsellors regularly invite children's thoughts or feelings about things such as the situation at home, having parents living in separate houses, and so on, as we see in Extracts 8.5–8.8:

Extract 8.5

1   C: Amanda what j'think about goin' t'see yuh dad.

Extract 8.6

1   C: Why d'you think they said you couldn't go.

Extract 8.7

1   C: Why d'you think, (0.3) mum an' dad said what they said.

Extract 8.8

1   C: What does it feel like havin' the houses so far apa:rt.

On one level, these invitations index a key aspect of the professional orthodoxy of child counselling: to encourage the child to 'communicate' by placing their own feelings or thoughts about events at the heart of the story. Yet empirical analysis shows that they do not tend to lead to cooperative exchanges in which children go on to produce the requested accounts of thoughts or feelings. This is in stark contrast to work on perspective-display invitations in medical interactions by Maynard (1991), where he found much more cooperative exchanges. The comparison is not straightforward, however, since in Maynard's data the professional invites the perspective of children's parents about the potential causes of their complaints, rather than the children themselves.

As shown in detail in Hutchby (2007), what tends to happen in the child counselling context is that the child *declines* to collaborate in producing a perspective in the slot following such an invitation, leading the counsellor to *pursue* a perspective in a third position slot. What then tends to follow are minimal or downgraded responses from the child, following which the counsellor typically *proffers* a perspective on his own part which the child is invited to take up. The series usually ends by the child refusing this profferance, and the topic is changed.

Extract 8.9 illustrates this pattern. (Note that there are four siblings involved here, and the youngest, Dan, is rather excitable. It is the interaction between C and the elder sister, Amanda (A), in which I am primarily interested.)

Extract 8.9

```
1   →   C:    So what- what d'you think,

2       D:    An' we're ha[vin' this teacher called-

3   →   C:                 [Amanda what j'think about goin' t'see yuh

4             da[d.

5       D:    [We're havin' this [new teacher called ( )

6       C:                       [Yer bein' very >quiet='old it< shh!

7             (.) shush °a minute shush,° ((to D))

8             (0.2)

9   →   A:    I don't mi:nd really.

10            (0.9)

11      (D):  ku[hh ((cough))

12  →   C:       [Mind really.
```

13	(D):	kuh <u>hugh</u>
14		(1.2)
15	D:	Mand[y:,
16 →	C:	[<u>M</u>mm do I sense a bit uv, (.) I'm not so su:re.
17 →		(1.1)
18	D:	([ )
19	C:	[Some good bits (.) an' some <u>not</u> suh good bits.
20 →		(0.8)
21	D:	Ple:ase can I ha-
22 →		(1.6)
23	A:	No jus' the same as P<u>a</u>m really like- [(.) y'get t'miss=
24	D:	[Please c'n I have=
25	A:	=[on some-]
26	D:	[a little] (Man[dy)
27	A:	[.h N<u>o</u>:.
28	C:	[[Yih get t' miss <u>out</u> on bit[s.
29	A:	[[Yih get t'miss out- [Bu- D<u>a</u>n give me back my
30		<u>jui</u>[ce.
31	D:	[([ )
32	C:	[D<u>a</u>:n, (0.3) <u>Da</u>:n,
33	A:	N<u>o</u>::wu[h.
34	P:	[D<u>a</u>n.

((*Talk continues regarding D's purloining of A's drink*))

The counsellor invites A's perspective on the topic of 'goin' t'see yuh dad' in lines 1–4. After a short pause, A's response is brief and non-committal: 'I don't mi:nd really' (line 9). Following this there is a longer pause of almost a second (line 10) before C produces a partial repeat of A's turn (line 12). That partial repeat notably performs a particular operation on the prior turn, recasting it in different terms by shifting the pattern of emphasis. Whereas A placed the emphasis on 'mind' in 'I don't mi:nd really' (line 9), C emphasises 'really' in 'Mind <u>really</u>' (line 12). The effect of this is to transform the perspective from one of mild indifference to one which potentially manifests scepticism or uncertainty about the topic of 'goin' t'see yuh dad'. In other words, C can be understood here to be proffering a version of A's perspective: one which she herself may or may not wish to go along with.

What follows is another silence during which A declines to expand on her viewpoint (line 14); and (leaving out of account for now Dan's interjacent utterances requesting some of Amanda's drink) C subsequently pursues his own perspective on A's feelings about seeing her father. Lines 16 ('Mmm do I sense a bit uv, (.) I'm not so su:re') and 19 ('Some good bits (.) an' some not suh good bits') seek to do this work in the environment of numerous long pauses (lines 14, 17, 20 and 22) during which this alternative perspective receives no uptake from A.

When Amanda does begin to produce the pursued expansion on her perspective (lines 23–25), it is noticeable that she does not explicitly align with C's proffered version emphasising uncertainty, but instead with her sister Pamela's view (expressed in a previous exchange) that seeing their father merely means that they sometimes miss out on other weekend events. C then shifts position in an attempt to topicalise this view (line 28) but the line of talk is disrupted at that point by Amanda directing her attention towards Dan who, following his earlier unsuccessful requests (see lines 21, 24–26, and A's self-interruptive refusal in line 27), has taken Amanda's drink for himself. Others in the room, including the counsellor, now also turn their attention towards Dan's actions, and the perspective-display series is abandoned at that point.

The general pattern that this extract exemplifies (see Hutchby 2007: 59–78) is summarised in Box 8.1.

Although it can often appear as if the counsellor is simply seeking to explore viewpoints with the child in a quasi-conversational exchange, what happens in subsequent turns indicates that there is an institutional agenda at work in which children's perspectives are ideally related to feelings, or to other matters that can be given a counselling relevance. In fact, that agenda is often built into the design of counsellors' perspective-display invitations in the first place, which as noted tend to ask about 'What [X] *feels like*' or 'What the child *thinks about* [Y]' (where [X] and [Y] are matters related to the family situation).

The pattern in Box. 8.1 can be traced to the features of child counselling outlined earlier. The lack of collaboration from the child in producing a perspective and in producing an uptake of the counsellor's proffered perspective can be accounted for, at least in part, by the ambiguous situation facing children – that of being asked to speak both within and outside the normal parameters of 'child' status in interaction with adults. Meanwhile, the impetus for counsellors to produce their own perspective even in the face of non-cooperation from the child derives at least in part from the operation of therapeutic vision – the tendency to highlight and codify just those features of events that are relevant for the professional work of doing therapy.

Box 8. 1 Inviting a child's perspective on events

Turn 1. Counsellor solicits child's perspective
Turn 2. Child produces non-committal response or declines to respond
Turn 3. Counsellor pursues a perspective
Turn 4. Child declines or produces brief/non-committal response
Turn 5. Counsellor produces own perspective
Turn 6. Child declines uptake

'I was just thinking . . .'

Further dimensions of this can be found in a different set of cases: those where child counsellors initiate the topic of what they themselves are, or have been, 'thinking'. Typically, in my data, such interactional moves are initiated in contexts where children are engaged in what I will call 'representational activities': drawing, building, inventing, or developing fictional stories using various materials made available within the counselling room. Such activities are among the kinds of techniques often recommended in the child counselling literature, sometimes under the rubric of 'play therapy'.

In a number of examples, counsellors seek to relate representational activities or fictional events in children's stories to actual situations in their family lives. This tends to be done indirectly, by means of inferentially-based questions and formulations in which alternative, 'real life' interpretations are constructed and, as it were, offered up to the child. In the following examples, the counsellor watches the child for a time, sometimes discussing with them what they are doing, then initiates a turn with a phrase like 'I was just thinking . . .'.

There are at least three different ways in which such 'just thinking' turns are produced, and each has slightly different sequential consequences. Firstly, the counsellor may produce the turn as a freestanding announcement, though one that is in some sense touched-off by the child's activity of drawing, building or writing. As we see in Extract 8.10, such a move may not be built to make any response from the child conditionally relevant. Secondly, the 'just thinking' turn may be produced as a first pair part, as in 'Do you know what I was just thinking?' (Extract 8.11). In such cases, a response from the child (even if only a single word second pair part like 'What?'), is conditionally relevant. Finally, the counsellor's turn may be occasioned by prior talk, often marked as such by a conjunction, as in 'But I was just thinking . . .' (Extract 8.12). Here, the child may elect whether or not to take up the alternative line of talk proposed by that turn.

Extract 8.10 comes from a counselling session with a 6-year-old male child whose parents are separated. The data contains a number of sessions with this child, and in none of them does he get much beyond a very basic level of cooperation with the counsellor. For most of the time, in fact, he exhibits very strong resistance (see Hutchby 2002). In this segment, something has been reported to the counsellor at the start of the session which is quite familiar to those dealing with separated parents and their offspring. One parent (the father) had told the child that he was to go on a trip to Disneyland, Paris. There has then been a dispute between the mother and father over this promise, with the result that the child has now been told (by the mother) he will not be going to Disneyland after all. It turns out, later in the session, that the father has gone anyway, with his girlfriend, and the child knows this.

The counsellor spends some time trying to coax this 6-year old, 'Peter', into talking about how he feels about all this, with little success. Peter then does some drawing. This is when the exchange in Extract 8.10 takes place:

Extract 8.10

1   C: Is that a picture of E̲uroStar.

2   (0.5)

3   P: Yeah.

4   (4.5)

5   C: Cuz I gue̲ss you would've gone on E̲uroStar tuh go to

6   Di̲sneyland wouldn't you.

7   P: Don't know,

8   (.)

9   C: °°Mm°°

10   (4.2)

11 → C: I wz jus' thi̲nkin' if I̲ could've gone tu:h Di̲sneywor:ld

12   an' someone told me I co̲uldn't I mi̲ght feel really cross

13   with them.

14   (1.1)

15   C: .hh Might get really ma̲:d an' cross an' go RRRA̲A̲A̲AAAH!

16   (2.1)

17   C: It would ce̲rtainly make me think it wasn't fai::r,

18   (1.8)

19 → C: I'd be thinkin' (('child' voice)) "it'sh not fa::ir."

20   (4.3)

21   C: "jus' cuz my mum an' dad aren't ge' 'in' on um not

21   allowed to go:tuh Disneyworld."

22   (3.6)

23   It's pre̲tty unfa̲:ir i̲sn' it.

24   (12.5)

25   C: Looks like a r:eally good train that t-train's go̲ing

26   somewhere. (.) Fa̲s:t̲.

Note here that the first two questions, which refer to elements of P's drawing (line 1) and attempt to relate that to the problematic Disneyland issue (line 5), both receive minimal responses showing no uptake of the topic. After a pause (line 10), C then initiates a topic himself (line 11) beginning with the words 'I wz jus' thinkin' . . .'.

This initiates a series of turns that observably seek to foreground an interpretation of the child's hitherto unspoken feelings about the Disneyland trip. That interpretation relies on the kind of therapeutic vision outlined earlier. It highlights feelings of being 'mad' or 'cross' (line 15) and of things being 'unfair' (line 17, line 24). In lines 21–22 it codifies those feelings in terms of the child counselling frame *children often get caught in the middle of parents' fights*.

C thus incrementally produces an account of a suggested emotional state which the child, at each increment, may find himself in a position to identify with; although as we see the child declines uptake of any of the counsellor's proposed 'feelings' as this unfolds (note the pauses in lines 14, 16, 18, 20 and 23). Only in line 23 is an explicit invitation to concur made; although, in line with P's general recalcitrance in this session (see Hutchby 2002), no response is forthcoming, and following a 12.5-second silence C ultimately returns to his previous tactic of topicalising elements of the drawing P is producing (line 25).

In the next example, the 8-year old child 'Jenny' has been engaged for some time in playing with a building game consisting of differently coloured plastic strips and blocks. The counsellor once more has been partly watching, and partly engaging in a conversation with Jenny about what she has earlier described as the 'muddle' that is emerging at home as her parents negotiate their separation. Jenny then announces (line 11) that she has completed the model of the 'muddle' that she has been creating:

Extract 8.11

1	J:	That one was meant- to be on top'v all of them bu:t, .h I
2		put it rou:n:d all of them didn' I.=
3	C:	=So w- sometimes when things go round things they
4		actually, .h end up kind of: .h underneath between an'
5		r:round the sides.
6	J:	Yeah.
7		(5.6)
8	C:	So sometimes it's kinda hard t'know (0.3) where the
9		muddle's gonna be.
10		(0.8)
11	J:	There we are!
12		(0.3)
13	C:	Gre:at.='s a good muddle.
14		(1.2)
15	J:	I think I'll leave it at that.
16		(1.2)

17   J: (I want to.)

18   C: 'S a good muddle.

19   J: (We) can carry it like that.

20   (0.2)

21   →   C: D'you know what I w'z jus' thinkin' 'bout this muddle.

22   J: °hNo.° .h

23   (0.6)

24   C: I w'z thinkin:: (1.4) there's red, in the middle,

25   J: Y:ea:h?

26   C: The smallest one,

27   J: Yea:h,

28   (0.2)

29   J: Me:, ehuh=

30   C: =Jenny!

31   (2.2)

32   C: Who:'s the purple one.

33   (.)

34   J: Mum.

35   (0.4)

36   C: N'who's the green one.

37   J: Dad!

38   C: Ye:ah.

Here, we find a different kind of exchange initiated by the counsellor's 'just thinking' turn in line 21. Following some assessment of the 'good muddle' that J has produced with the coloured strips, C uses a question format to package his proposed thoughts about the muddle: 'D'you know what I w'z jus' thinkin' 'bout this muddle'. This way of formatting the turn makes relevant a next turn response from J (line 22), which in turn acts as a means of topicalising C's 'thoughts'. In that way, it is similar to a common strategy used by children themselves in interaction with adults, where as Sacks (1975) remarks, prefatory questions such as 'You know what Daddy?', which are designed to be followed by the recipient with 'What?', function to provide clear conversational floorspace for the child in a third turn. In Sacks's account, this is intrinsically bound up with the problem of limited rights of access to the floor often encountered by young children in interaction with adults.

Three points are of note in the ensuing sequence. First, the way in which what C is 'thinking' turns out to be a way of linking the representational activity of building a 'muddle' with plastic strips to concrete circumstances in the child's home life. Second, the way that this linkage is achieved incrementally (in a similar sense as the incremental unfolding of the 'imagined emotional state' in Extract 8.10). Third, most significantly, the way that the child herself collaborates in developing the linkage (by contrast with Extract 8.10), to such an extent that it is, in fact, J herself who explicitly verbalises the connections.

C begins, in line 24, simply by picking out one of the colours and observing that it is 'in the middle'. J's next turn takes the form of a continuer, orienting to the 'not yet complete' status of C's utterance. In line 26, C adds another observation, 'the smallest one', which J initially responds to with another continuer. However, after the short pause in line 28, she makes the link between 'in the middle' and 'the smallest one' (two conventional means by which young children are often depicted in family stories) and positions herself as represented by the red strip (line 29, confirmed in the counsellor's latched next turn). From there, J utilises the membership categorisation device 'family' – which children are able to use from a very early age (Sacks 1972) – to position the two colours either side of red as representing 'Mum' and 'Dad'.

Possibly, the counsellor views the connection he is proposing here as too delicate, or too abstract, to be stated baldly. After all, there has been no direct evidence in prior talk that the child herself was anthropomorphising the plastic strips in such an overt way. This may account for the design of his 'just thinking' move such as to have the child state the connection rather than simply have it presented to her. But that design is additionally significant in that it turns the activity of 'concretising' the child's play in terms of family relations into a *joint* one. The joint activity may in turn provide a powerful environment for the counsellor to pursue therapeutically relevant implications of that link.

This in fact is what happens as the session proceeds. In Extract 8.12, taken from slightly later in the same session, we find the counsellor encouraging the child to go further with the linkage between plastic strips and family members. Two particular issues are of note in the light of our concerns in the present chapter. First, the way in which the child is invited to speculate on the future state of family relations, 'when mum an' dad aren't living together' (lines 1–2). This recalls what was said earlier about the complexity of certain forms of talk asked of children in the child counselling session. Second, the way the counsellor again uses a 'just thinking' turn (line 23), but this time to *contrast* with the possible family future that the child has duly produced. This recalls what was said earlier about the complexities of the exercise of therapeutic vision.

Extract 8.12

```
1    C:  How would this muddle be:, (0.5) whe:n, (.) mum an'

2        dad aren't living together.

3        (1.9)

4    C:  What will happen.

5        (1.4)

6    C:  T'your pu[zzle

7    J:            [THIs::::. (0.2) would happen.
```

8		(2.0)
9	C:	Aha: so who's tha[t. Who've you just taken over there.
10	J:	[No no no wait. Wait wait this wouldn't
11		happen, (.) I'll show you what would (happen)
12		(0.8)
13		((BANG))
14		(0.3)
15	J:	(Wait) I haven't finished yet,
16		(2.0)
17	C:	S:so there's, (0.6) Ah ka:y.
18		(3.5)
19	C:	Pulling apart.
20		(0.7)
21	J:	(Yeh they) break hih!
22		(2.1)
23 →	C:	Ah that's your >worry<=.h=But I was jus' thinkin', (0.3)
24		that, maybe this would happen. (.) Instead of them being
25		pulling apart breaking, .hhh (.) I like the way y'did
26		this y'put, .hh that green one over the:re, .h an' that
27		purple one over there cuz they're bo:th .hh having a-
28		(0.3) some ti:me with Jenny, .hh but instead a' pulling
29		they're pushing like this. (0.2) s'they push together.
30	J:	Why::?
31		(0.4)
32	C:	(S'we just move this.) So they're not breaking. But
33		they're both looking a:fter'n, hugging Jenny.

Having been asked to speculate on what may happen once her parents finalise their separation, J complies by moving the coloured plastic strips (lines 7–8). Noteworthy in C's response (line 9) is the continued anthropomorphisation, as he refers to 'who' has been moved 'over there'. J, however, changes her mind in the course of this turn and, as her talk in lines 10–21 demonstrates, produces a different manipulation of the pieces which is ultimately characterised by C as 'Pulling apart' (line 19) and, more strongly, by J, '(Yeh they) break hih!' (line 21).

It is at this point – that is, where a fairly strong imagined future of the family 'breaking' has been introduced by J – that C produces another 'just thinking' turn. This time, he uses the disjunct marker *but* and a stress marker on the first person pronoun ('But I was jus' thinkin'' line 23) to foreground that his own thought is somehow different from that propounded by the child. As we see, he subsequently goes on to produce an alternative possible future in which the two parents, rather than 'breaking', are 'both looking a:fter'n, hugging Jenny' – a far more positive imagined future that the child is invited to consider.

In sum, we see in this section how child counsellors use 'I was just thinking' turns as a means of making connections between children's activities of drawing, building or storytelling and their possible responses to circumstances in everyday home life. Such turns instantiate therapeutic vision by providing interpretive frames by means of which the kinds of events involved in family separation may be understood by children. Such turns function variably, and we have seen at least three different uses. They can either proffer a freestanding 'possible emotional response' presented from the perspective of the counsellor adopting the child's role (Extract 8.10); or invite the child themselves to collaborate in a 'possible interpretation' of their own activities (Extract 8.11); or provide a disjunctive alternative account of a 'possible future' that offers a different (possibly more positive) outlook for the child to consider (Extract 8.12).

In whatever way they function, such interactional moves are closely bound up with the problematic elicitation of feelings-talk with which this chapter has been concerned. I began by describing the ambiguous or contradictory discourses at the heart of child counselling: that children are constructed as competent social agents through being invited to talk about their own feelings regarding the breakdown of their family, while also being invited to move beyond the normative boundaries of adult–child interaction by *accounting for* that breakdown and *speculating about* future scenarios; while counsellors find that children's reluctance to engage in the very talk that their professional ethos promotes often places them in the position of using their own 'thoughts' as a means of encouraging children's engagement with these difficult topics.

We have examined some of the ways in which those factors inform and influence the nature of interaction between children and counsellors. The practices discussed in this chapter are exemplifications of therapeutic vision: the tendency to see and to codify events and accounts of events in terms of the interpretive frames and schemas of child counselling as a professional practice. The variability in children's willingness to go along with these 'concretisations' of counselling frames in relation to their own activities can be accounted for, at least in part, by the ambiguous nature of child counselling discourse and by the relationship between their own social competencies and the institutional agendas of counselling as a professional activity.

Acknowledgements

This chapter is based on research supported by the Economic and Social Research Council. My thanks to the Editors for helpful comments on a previous draft.

References

Geldard, K. and Geldard, D. (1997) *Counselling children: A practical introduction.* London: Sage.

Goodwin, C. (1994) Professional vision. *American Anthropologist,* **96**, 606–633.

Hutchby, I. (2001) The moral status of technology: Being recorded, being heard, and the construction of concerns in child counselling. In I. Hutchby and J. Moran-Ellis (eds), *Children, technology and culture.* London: Routledge.

Hutchby, I. (2002) Resisting the incitement to talk in child counselling: Aspects of the utterance 'I don't know'. *Discourse Studies,* **4**, 147–168.

Hutchby, I. (2005) Active listening: Formulations and the elicitation of feelings-talk in child counselling. *Research on Language and Social Interaction,* **38**, 303–329.

Hutchby, I. (2007) *The discourse of child counselling.* Amsterdam: John Benjamins.

Hutchby, I. and Moran-Ellis, J. (1998) Situating children's social competence. In I. Hutchby and J. Moran-Ellis (eds), *Children and social competence: Arenas of action.* London: Falmer Press.

Mayall, B. (1994) Children in action at home and in school. In B. Mayall (ed.), *Children's childhoods observed and experienced.* London: Falmer Press.

Maynard, D. (1991) Interaction and asymmetry in clinical discourse. *American Journal of Sociology,* **97**, 448–495.

McHoul, A. (1978) The organisation of turns at formal talk in the classroom. *Language in Society,* **19**, 183–213.

Peräkylä, A., Antaki, C., Vehviläinen, S. and Leudar, I. (eds) (2008) *Conversation analysis and psychotherapy.* Cambridge: Cambridge University Press.

Sacks, H. (1972) On the analysability of stories by children. In J. Gumperz and D. Hymes (eds), *Directions in sociolinguistics.* New York: Holt, Rinehart & Winston.

Sacks, H. (1975) Everyone has to lie. In B. Blount and M. Sanchez (eds), *Sociocultural dimensions of language use.* New York: Academic Press.

Sharpe, S. and Cowie, H. (1998) *Counselling and supporting children in distress.* London: Sage.

Silverman, D. (1987) *Communication and medical practice.* London: Sage.

Silverman, D. (1996) *Discourses of counseling.* London: Sage.

Silverman, D., Baker, C. and Keogh, J. (1998) The case of the silent child: Advice-giving and advice-reception in the parent–teacher interview. In I. Hutchby and J. Moran-Ellis (eds), *Children and social competence: Arenas of action.* London: Falmer Press.

Wootton, A.J. (1997) *Interaction and the development of mind.* Cambridge: Cambridge University Press.

Chapter 9

Intersubjectivity and misunderstanding in adult–child learning conversations

CHRIS PIKE

Introduction

Sociocultural studies of adult–child interaction have highlighted the role adults play in children's cognitive development through guiding, or 'scaffolding', their participation in joint activity (Rogoff 1990; Meadows 1996; Gauvain 2001). Numerous studies have shown how adults adjust their assistance in ways contingent upon a child's performance (e.g. Wood *et al.* 1978; Rogoff *et al.* 1984; Pratt *et al.* 1988; Plumert and Nichols-Whitehead 1996), and progressively transfer responsibility for regulating the activity from themselves to the child (e.g. Wertsch *et al.* 1980; Wertsch and Hickman 1987). In this way, adult-teachers are held to create and sustain what Vygotsky (1978) termed a 'zone of proximal development' (ZPD) for the child's ability to carry out a given task. However, much of the research in this area has tended to overemphasise the adult's role in structuring the activity, at the expense of analysing the moment-by-moment dynamics of talk-in-interaction through which the task gets done (Stone 1993; Elbers 2004). As a consequence, others have sought to move beyond dualistic accounts of a ZPD in terms of contingent responding on the part of an adult to a child, and to focus instead on how intersubjectivity, or the *meaning* of what-it-is-to-do a given task, is negotiated and built-up during the course of adult–child interaction.

In an early attempt at reframing the ZPD, Wertsch (1984) proposed that the way an adult and child make sense of their joint activity moves through a series of successively negotiated 'intersubjective situation definitions' of the task they are engaged in (e.g. doing a jigsaw puzzle, solving a maths problem, etc.). In Vygotskyan terms, the 'actual level' (or lower boundary) of the ZPD corresponds to the child's *intra*subjective definition of the task, while the 'potential level' (or upper boundary) corresponds to a working adult–child *inter*subjective definition *through which* the joint activity is accomplished. This definition is different from that of either the child or the adult. According to the model, changes in the child's *intra*subjective situation definition of the activity occur through the appropriation of negotiated changes in the *inter*subjective situation definition, bringing the child's understanding of the activity successively closer to that of the adult (Wertsch 1984; Pontecorvo 1993; Smolka *et al.* 1995). However, to date, very few empirical studies have overtly employed the model (e.g. Henderson 1991; Elbers *et al.* 1992) and have tended to analyse interactions in terms of predetermined categories of speech act, rather than analyse the turn-by-turn process of negotiation directly. As such, even where this analysis is microgenetic (e.g. Elbers *et al.* 1992), the changes tracked are not intrinsic properties of the interaction itself, but rather artefacts of an arbitrarily defined categorisation system imposed from without. The problem with this kind of approach is that it obscures how the adult and child are interactively *generating* their talk and behaviour on a moment-by-moment basis.

More recently, Mercer (2000) has sought to better capture the central importance of intersubjectivity in adult–child learning conversations through replacing the Vygotskyan notion of a ZPD with that of an 'Intermental Development Zone' (IDZ), and the metaphor of scaffolding with the term '*interthinking*'. Like Wertch's model, the IDZ incorporates the idea of language as a means for collective sense-making. However, rather than appeal to abstract theoretical constructs such as situation definitions, it highlights instead the talk-in-interactional processes through which localised 'common knowledge' is created and presupposed across time by specific teachers and learners. As Mercer puts it, the IDZ 'is a continuing event of contextualised joint activity whose quality is dependent on the existing knowledge, capabilities and motivations of both the learner and the teacher . . . this achievement is a joint one, the product of a process of interthinking' (Mercer 2000: 141). The ability to create an effective IDZ is thus a function of a given adult–child dyad, and not the adult alone. The 'scaffolding', as it were, is *jointly* created through talk-in-interaction, not something the adult simply provides for the child. It is a *collaborative* achievement, as evident in the common observation that particular children make more or less progress with particular teachers, arguably reflecting the fact that different pairings of children and teachers are more or less successful at creating an IDZ through their talk-in-interaction.

The talk-in-interactional processes by which interactants create, update and contextualise an IDZ rely fundamentally upon *presupposition*, a key example of which is proplepsis (Stone 1993; Mercer 2000). Prolepsis is a ubiquitous feature of learning conversations and refers to 'a communicative move in which the speaker presupposes some as yet unprovided information' (Stone 1993: 171). In order to make sense of a proleptic utterance (or indeed, any utterance) the listener is forced to make inferences that implicitly recreate the presuppositional basis of the speaker's prior turn. Where this is successful, learning may be said to have occurred. Stone suggests that the effectiveness of prolepsis relies on achieving a balance, or optimal tension, between what is presupposed as intersubjectively known by the speaker, and what is assumed about the context by the listener. 'If too much "common ground" is incorrectly presupposed, the message does not get through. If too little is presupposed, mutual trust might not be maintained' (Stone 1993: 174). There is thus a trade-off between presupposing intersubjectivity for the purpose of maintaining interactional coordination and rapport, and challenging it for the purpose of instruction and learning. This balance in turn relies heavily on the interpersonal relationship between participants and their shared interactional history, both of which are critical in determining the nature of the inferencing involved.

Studies by Clark and associates have shown how conversationalists routinely employ similar techniques to prolepsis in establishing intersubjectivity and updating their 'common ground'. A conspicuous feature of such talk is that utterances dealing with recycled topics, or recurrent patterns of turn-taking, become progressively *abbreviated* over time as more and more aspects of the prior talk become presupposed rather than overtly referred to (Clark and Wilkes-Gibbs 1986; Clark and Brennan 1993; Clark 1996). Abbreviation has been observed in studies of adult–child conversation during joint problem-solving (Wertsch and Hickman 1987; Wertsch 1991), and young children's private speech (Berk 1992). In more general terms, it is an example of *repetition with variation*; the ongoing process by which interactants include modified elements of their own and each others' prior talk in their current talk. Repetition serves both coordinatory and communicative functions in conversation (Norrick 1987; Tannen 1989), and together with anaphoric reference helps build the cohesiveness of the talk (Mercer 2000).

Through studying the dynamics of repetition and variation in conversational structures across the course of a learning conversation, we may understand how the participants develop and refine their orientation to specific features of their ongoing talk, and how these features thereby come to contextualise and presuppose particular understandings of the activity in which they are engaged (Gumperz 1995; Ochs 1996; Wootton 1997; Pike 2000). In so doing, we can study how teachers and learners collaboratively create an IDZ on a moment-by-moment basis. A basic principle of conversation analysis (CA) is that in constructing a next turn at talk, participants *display* an understanding of the prior talk at a multiplicity of levels (both process and content). These displayed understandings are themselves subject to either tacit confirmation or explicit *repair* at any third turn in an ongoing sequence (Schegloff 1993). However, it is important to note here that 'CA's claims about participants' understandings are *not claims about speakers' cognitive states*' (Edwards 1997: 108 emphasis added), but rather about the 'ways in which participants themselves *orient to, display* and *make sense of* one another's cognitive states' (Drew 1995: 77, emphasis added). The emphasis is upon the inferential nature of talk-in-interaction – what counts, and is accountable for, as a *display* of understanding – and the orderly means by which such 'understandings' are collaboratively created and negotiated. CA cannot *in principle* make claims about whether or not learning has 'actually' occurred; it can only ever seek to specify the conditions of talk-in-interaction that participants themselves orient to and treat as evidence for it. The distinction is important because it raises the parallel question of how or in what sense interactants *themselves* can ever 'know' they have achieved shared understanding. How and when do teachers and pupils, or researchers, 'know' that learning is happening?

The main purpose of this chapter is to address this issue by exploring what an analysis of misunderstandings in teacher–pupil discourse can tell us about the nature of intersubjectivity in learning conversations.

The context of the learning conversations

The focus of the following analysis is a series of four learning conversations between a primary school teacher (the author) and Sarah, a 6-year-old, that took place at the child's school over a six-week period as part of a larger study looking at the development of children's estimation skills (Pike and Forrester 1997; Pike 2000). Each session was videotaped and transcribed, and centred around the carrying out of an interactive computer-based task. The four sessions were set within an overarching single-case experimental design in which adult–child sessions alternated with child-alone sessions, following two initial baseline assessments of the child's independent performance at the task. The adult and child had not worked with each other prior to the first session, and hence had no previous interactional history.

A screen-shot of the task as it appeared at the start and end of a session is given in Figures 9.1(a) and 9.1(b).

From a teacher's perspective, the task can be described as an exercise in proportional reasoning. The initial screen displayed 10 'balls' suspended on separate vertical 'strings' of varying lengths, each 'hanging' from a single horizontal line (Figure 9.1(a)). Each ball had a different number, and was fixed to its respective string. The strings could be moved to the left or right by clicking and dragging the corresponding balls with the mouse; each string could only be moved once. The object of the activity was simply to position the strings along the line such that the spaces between the strings reflected the relative magnitude of the numbers on the corresponding balls. For example, given the numbers 0, 24 and 32, one would expect the distance between the 0 string and the 24 string to be three times that between the 24 string and the 32 string. However, the fact that the actual distance between any two numbers depended critically on the values of *all* the other numbers, gave the task an additional strategic dimension. Thus, given the range 0, 5, 10, 16, 32, 50, 68, 72, 95 and 100, it would be strategically better to position the 0, followed by the 100, followed by the 50, etc., than it would be to simply work from left to right along the list. While a different set of numbers was used each week, care was taken to ensure that the spread and/or the ratio properties of each set were kept approximately the same. Hence, the ideal relative spatial positioning for each set remained constant across sessions.

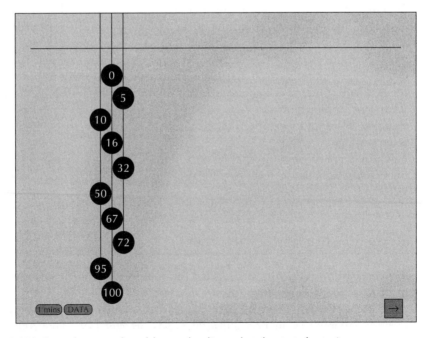

Figure 9.1(a) Example screen shot of the number-line task at the start of a session.

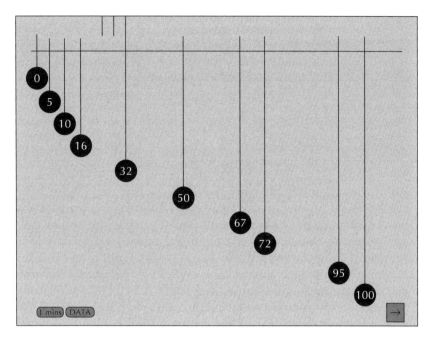

Figure 9.1(b) Example screen shot of the number-line task at the end of a session.

Analysis of the learning conversations

As most institutional discourse is primarily concerned with coordinating goal-directed action, talk-in-interaction in such settings frequently exhibits a context-specific episodic structure, and/or makes use of specialised turn-taking systems (Greenleaf and Freedman 1993; Heritage 1997). Accordingly, initial inspection of the corpus showed much of the turn-taking organisation to adopt the familiar form of a three-part Initiation–Response–Evaluation (IRE) sequence characteristic (and constitutive) of much instructional discourse (Mehan 1979; Cazden 1988; Edwards and Westgate 1994). Furthermore, as with tasks used in previous studies (e.g. Wertsch *et al.* 1980; Henderson 1991; Elbers *et al.* 1992), the number-line task had a fairly predictable episodic structure, comprising a series of more or less discrete 'moves', each requiring a similar action. As such, the trajectory of talk in each adult–child session follows a more or less predictable series of well-demarcated episodes, each concerned with the positioning of a particular number, or group of numbers, on the number-line. In broad terms, this episodic organisation consisted of: (i) positioning the lowest and highest numbers at opposite ends of the line; (ii) positioning the middle number; (iii) positioning the upper group of remaining numbers; and (iv) positioning the lower groups of remaining numbers.

At the same time, close inspection of the corpus shows large stretches of talk within each episode to be organised around the reproduction of a recognisably recurrent *five-part sequential structure*, the organisation of which is summarised in Table 9.1.

By way of example, Extract 9.1 shows the opening exchange of the first session. The sequence comprises two IRE exchanges; the first dealing with the selection of a number to move (1–5), and the second with the rationale for the choice made (5–11).

Table 9.1 Five-part sequential structure recurrent across sessions

IRE	Position	Action
(I)	1st	Initiation and request for number
(R)	2nd	Provision of number
(E/I)	3rd	Evaluation of choice/request for rationale
(R)	4th	Provision of rationale
(E)	5th	Evaluation of rationale and closure

Superimposed on this basic IRE 'scaffolding', as it were, is the locally-specific turn-constructional organisation summarised in Table 9.1. Subsequent analysis shows this turn organisation to be a recurrent feature of much of the ensuing dialogue within and across sessions, and as such it constitutes a spontaneously-produced five-part sequential structure that the teacher and child demonstrably orient to and recycle for the purposes of getting the task done. Considerable evidence for participant orientation to this structure exists throughout the corpus as a whole (Pike 2000), and is amply illustrated in the extracts below; most conspicuously, as we shall see, in the ongoing abbreviation, anticipation and repair of particular turn-positions and turn-constructional units, as the interaction proceeds.

In this and all subsequent extracts, A refers to the adult and C refers to the child. Transcription follows CA conventions, with the exception of all emphases of pitch and/or loudness, which are italicised.

Extract 9.1 *Session 1* {Number set: 0 5 10 16 32 50 67 72 95 100}

1st	1	A:	okay. .. which number shall we move *first*. d'you think ... ...
	2	C:	u:::m:[:::::
1stR	3	A:	[which one would be a good [one to move *first*.]
2nd	4	C:	[one *hundred*..]
3rd	5	A:	*one* hundred. why one hundred. ..
4th	6	C:	because .. u::m::: .. i::f we mo:ve .. th' *biggest* numbe::r, ..
	7	A:	yea::::[::h,
	8	C:	[*the::::re*, .. and then the *sma:llest* number .. the::re.
	9		then we can do:: .. them in the *middle*.
5th	10	A:	alri:ght, sounds like a good id::ea, ..
	11		okay, .. so::: .. you wanna move the hundred *first*.

For present purposes, the following analysis focuses on a misunderstanding that arises in session 3. Having first outlined the nature and local context of the misunderstanding itself, it moves on to consider the possible origins of the difficulty in sessions 1 and 2, and then finally addresses its apparent resolution in session 4.

The nature of the misunderstanding

Extract 9.2 *Session 3* {Number set: 0 3 6 13 30 45 63 66 87 90}

1st	1		okay .. which one .. which one shall we move *first*. then ..
	2		which would be a good one to move first. [this time
2nd	3	C:	[u:::m::, ... the *zero*. hh!
3rd	4	A:	the zero. ... right ..
4th	5	C:	cos there's no numbers *before*. or- .h ..
	6		and um then I *kno:w* .. there's no numbers before. so i can just leave it. ...
	7		the first .. *piece*. ... ((*coughs twice*))
(5th)	8	A:	okay, .. next one, ..

Extract 9.2 shows the unproblematic opening exchange of session 3. In line with previous sessions, one or other of the highest and lowest values in the set – in this instance, zero – is chosen as the first number to move, and the exchange follows the same 5–part structure as that originating in session 1 (Extract 9.1; Table 9.1). Notice, however, that in contrast to the earlier session, Sarah gives the rationale for her choice of number *without* the teacher having explicitly requested it; that is, the 3rd position turn is abbreviated such that the requirement for a rationale is now presupposed, while its request is simultaneously anticipated by the child. A similar abbreviation occurs in the 5th position turn, where the teacher initiates the next exchange without directly closing the current one; a favourable evaluation of the rationale is hence presupposed rather than explicitly given. The opening episode, then, constitutes an apparently clear display of intersubjectivity regarding what-it-is-to-do the task. However, as we can see in Extract 9.3, what happens next calls the status of this intersubjectivity into question.

Extract 9.3 *Session 3* {Number set: 0 3 6 13 30 45 63 66 87 90}

1st	1	A:	okay, .. next one, ..
2nd	2	C:	three. ...
R-2	3	A:	is that the *best* one to move next, ...
4th	4	C:	i *think* so cos its .. the next one after *zero*. ...
	5	A:	hmm::
	6	C:	and we can just .. go *along*. ...
R-4	7	A:	is that the best way to *do* it though. ...
	8		[if you want to get the right *spacing*.]
4th R#1	9	C:	[probably not]
			pause (4.0)

On the basis of previous teacher–child sessions, where the negotiated outcome has been to position the highest and lowest numbers followed by the middle number, *and* the immediately prior child-alone session in which Sarah employed the same strategy without adult facilitation, we might reasonably expect the choice of number here to be '90'. Instead, she chooses '3'. Why is this? The problem arises from the sequential ambiguity of the term 'next' in the context of the number-line task. In its current sequential position, 'next' could potentially mean either adjacency in time (the one to move next) *or* adjacency in space (the one next to zero), and whereas the teacher's attempt at initiating repair clearly presupposes the former (line 3), Sarah's reply presupposes the latter (lines 4–6). Interestingly, neither participant displays any recognition of this as the source of the problem (lines 7–9). Furthermore, notice that Sarah does not actually treat the teacher's turn in line 3 *as* an attempt to initiate repair at all; rather, as her subsequent turn indicates (lines 4–6), she treats it as a straightforward 3rd-position request for a rationale. We should also note that in attempting to initiate repair elliptically, the teacher does not *directly* challenge Sarah's choice of number.

Extract 9.4 shows how the difficulty is resolved.

Extract 9.4 *Session 3* {Number set: 0 3 6 13 30 45 63 66 87 90}

	1	A:	what did you just do:. .. when you did it on your own.
	2		which ones did you move *first*. .. when you did it on your own. ...
	3	C:	lowest *highest* lowest [*highest* lowest] *highest*
	4	A:	[lowest *highest*] ...
	5	C:	[low] *high* low high low high [low high .h heh!]
	6	A:	[yeah.] [.hh hhhhheh! .hh] ..
1st R#1	7		okay. so:: =
	8	C:	= *low* high *low* high *low* high, ..
	9	A:	so if you've moved the zero there first. which would be the
	10		*next* one to move. ...
2nd R#1	11	C:	*ninety*. [:::
3rd R#1	12	A:	[ninety. .. (alright then.) ..
4th R#1	13	C:	highest *one*. ..
5th	14	A:	highest one. ... ...

In an attempt to restore interactional coordination, the teacher appeals to Sarah's recollection of how she did the task in the previous child-alone session. This strategy proves successful, leading to the provision of '90' as the appropriate number, with the resumption and subsequent completion of the five-part sequence. Note that as in the opening exchange of this session (Extract 9.2), Sarah provides a 4th-position rationale for the choice of number (line 13) in the absence of an overt 3rd-part request. However, if we look closely at how repair of the problematic 2nd-position turn is achieved here, we can also note a subtle yet conspicuous difference in its sequential context compared to that of the previous exchange. The difference lies in the way the teacher's initial question (line 2) formulates Sarah's prior independent activity in terms of 'which *ones*' she moved 'first', rather than which 'one' she moved 'next'. The use of the plural together with 'first' presupposes a single strategic move which, together with the subsequent sing-song alternation of 'lowest' and 'highest', effectively disambiguates the meaning of the teacher's subsequent request for the 'next one to move' (line 10). In other words, the problem is resolved *incidentally*, as it were, via a subtle presuppositional change in the formulation of the teacher's 1st-position turn, rather than through addressing the cause of the problem itself. Further evidence for this interpretation, as well as highlighting the fact that neither participant appears to be aware of what is happening, is found in the ensuing exchange (Extract 9.5).

Extract 9.5 *Session 3* {Number set: 0 3 6 13 30 45 63 66 87 90}

1st	1	A:	oka:y. .. *no:w.*
2nd	2	C:	.hh .. (um we::ll) .. i will mo::ve, .. *three*::::.
R-2	3	A:	well. .. just before you *do* that ..
1st R#1	4		.h if you've put the zero *here*. .. and the ninety *there*. .. which of these would be ...
	5		which-which one of *these* would you be able to put ..
	6		in more or less the right place. .. straight away. *pause* (3.0)
2nd R#1	7	C:	u::m *pause* (3.0)
	8	C:	three:. or six:
3rd R#1	9	A:	three or *six*. ... um hmm, ..
1st R#2	10		... h well if you've put the two *end* points down ..
	11		which is the *next* one that you could look for. ..
2nd R#2	12	C:	.h the middle.
3rd/R-2	13	A:	the *middle*. .. alright. .. which one is the middle. ...
4th/2ndR	14	C:	the nearest to *fo:rty* which is forty *fi:ve* ...
3rd R	15	A:	yea::h.. [*omitted insertion sequence dealing with calculation of middle number* ...]
5th	16		okay. .. so you're gonna move forty five.

Having positioned the '0' and '90' at either end of the number-line, from the point of view of accuracy it now makes strategic sense to position '45' half-way between (remember that each number can only be clicked and dragged once). This has in fact been the outcome in both previous adult–child sessions, *and* the immediately prior child-alone session. But what happens? Sarah once again chooses '3' (line 2); moreover, she repeats this choice following the teacher's unsuccessful attempt at initiating repair (lines 4–5). This in itself suggests that, as before, she is not orienting towards the teacher's prior turn *as* an attempt to initiate repair, but simply as a 1st-position request. The fact that she then offers '6' as an alternative, following a transition-relevant stretch and final fall on 'three' in which the teacher does not respond, further suggests that she is still orienting towards the 'next one along' strategy occasioned by the previous exchange (Extract 3). But rather than address this directly, as before the problem is resolved incidentally through a reformulation of the teacher's 1st-position turn (lines 10–11); that is, in describing Sarah's prior action as having 'put the two *end* points down', the teacher's question again presupposes a single strategic move upon which positioning the middle number '45' as the 'next one' becomes contingent. Notice once again the subtle difference in the presuppositional basis of this formulation of Sarah's prior action compared with the previous one in lines 4–5.

To further account for Sarah's apparently anomalous behaviour in session 3, we need to look more closely at the earlier sessions. Can we find any evidence that the ambiguity of 'a next move' lies latent, as it were, in the history of the dyad's talk-in-interaction, and in particular identify the extent to which Sarah's apparent failure to recognise repair initiation, together with her teacher's failure to directly challenge her responses, are conjointly responsible for sustaining this ambiguity?

The origins of interactional difficulty in earlier sessions

Extract 9.6 shows the initial exchange of the episode in session 1 that deals with the selection of the third number to move. Sarah has already positioned the '0' and '100' at either end of the number-line, and so the teacher is now looking for her to select '50' (the middle number) as the next one to move. However, she chooses '5' instead.

Extract 9.6 *Session 1* {Number set: 0 5 10 16 32 50 67 72 95 100}

1st	1	A:	a:lright, which one are we going to move *next*. ...
2nd	2	C:	u:::m:: number *fi:::ve*.
3rd	3	A:	number fi:::ve. ..
(R-2)	4		would that be the *best* one to move next, ..
4th	5	C:	I *think* so 'cos .. u::m::: .. *that* one's the lowest out of a:ll of these. ..
	6		an' tha- .. an' *then* i can put it .. near the ... ze::ro. ...
3rd R/	7	A:	.hh .. oka:::y, .. i::f you *do* that though ..
R-4	8		how- .. how are you going to know how *close* to put it to the ze:ro. ... ...
4th R	9	C:	i'll just *guess::*. .. this time, ..
	10	A:	you'll just *guess*. ri:ght, .. i see,

Clearly, Extract 9.6 displays a similar pattern of interaction to that discussed above; the teacher's attempt to initiate repair in line 4 is treated as a 3rd-position request for a rationale. Furthermore, neither the original choice of number nor the rationale – including the use of 'guessing' – is directly challenged by the teacher. Extract 9.7 shows what happens next.

Extract 9.7 *Session 1* {Number set: 0 5 10 16 32 50 67 72 95 100}

1st R#1	1	A:	oka:y, .. .hhh .. if you *look* at those *numbers.* ... um ..
	2	C:	mmm, =
	3	A:	Sarah though .. is there *one* number there. ..
	4		that you would *know.* .. where to put. ... without having to guess too much. ... ...
2nd R#1	5	C:	*ninety.* five ... over *the::re.* ..
3rd R#1	6	A:	put ninety five over there. .. [uh huh,] ..
	7	C:	[uh huh,]
	8	A:	wh-why why ninety five. ...
4th R#1	9	C:	'cos its the highest number out of all *these* hh!= !
	10	A:	= right. so you're *thinking* ...
	11		the *five* .. would be:: easiest to move 'cos its the nearest to *this* end. ...
	12		and the *ninety* five would be:: .. ea::sy .. to move because its near *that* end.
	13		is that what you mean. ..
	14	C:	((*nods*))
	15	A:	.hh okay, .. what about ... any of the *other* numbers there. ...

The participants now recycle the five-part sequence. But notice that in the context of the prior exchange (Extract 9.6), it is simply presupposed by the teacher's 1st-position turn that the new sequence is attempting to repair the previous one. Yet there is no evidence in the subsequent talk that this is how Sarah orients towards it. In the absence of any overt challenge to her original choice of '5', there is nothing in the talk to suggest that her new choice of '95' is to be construed as an improvement upon it. Indeed, her teacher's attempt to formulate her reasoning with reference to both numbers (lines 10–13) serves to constitute her two choices as independent events. Once again, neither choice is directly challenged. Extract 9.8 shows the ensuing exchange.

Extract 9.8 *Session 1* {Number set: 0 5 10 16 32 50 67 72 95 100}

1st R#2	1	A:	hh okay, .. what about ... any of the *other* numbers there. ...
	2		any of the other *numbers.* ... wh- *pause* (3.0)
	3	A:	what d'you think would be a .. a good next *mo:ve.*
2nd R#2	4	C:	te:n. ..

3rd R-2	5	A:	te:n .. mmhmm, .. what about *fifty*. ... ...
2nd R#3	6	C:	fifty::: ..
R-2/3rdR	7	A:	where would you put *fifty*. ..
4th R#2	8	C:	*i'd* put fifty in the *middle* =
R-4	9	A:	= ri::ght .. how do you *know* that. ..
4th R#3	10	C:	'cos fifty is half of a [hu:ndred .]
5th R#2	11	A:	['cos fifty's] *halfwa::y*. ..
	12		so *that* one might be quite a good one to *mo:ve* mightn't it.=
	13	C:	= mmhmm,
	14	A:	'kay. how about you gi- .. have a go at *that* then.

As before, it is presupposed by the teacher's talk that this cycle is an attempt to repair the previous one. However, Sarah's choice of '10' as 'a good next move' simply continues the alternating pattern of 'next lowest' and 'next highest' established and unchallenged in the prior talk. Hence, when the teacher now asks 'what about fifty . . . where would you put fifty' (lines 5–7) in an attempt to repair the choice of number directly, we have no reason to assume that Sarah orients to it in this way at all. Rather, as before, she may simply treat it as a new event unrelated in any reparatory sense to the preceding talk. There is certainly no evidence here to the contrary. Given this inherent ambiguity, then, we need to question whether – or at least *for whom*, or in what sense – the subsequent display of intersubjective alignment, clearly marked by the teacher's latched and overlapping responses to Sarah's rationale (lines 9 and 11), also constitutes a display of *learning*.

What happens in session 2? Extract 9.9 is concerned with positioning the second number.

Extract 9.9 *Session 2* {Number set: 0 2 4 10 25 40 54 59 78 80}

1st	1	A:	okay, what about the *next* one.
2nd	2	C:	the *next* one wa::s [... sev]enty *eight*. =
R-2	3	A:	[what would be] = we:ll lets *think* about it .. uh shall we ..
	4		just before we *touch* one ... .hh
1st R#1	5	A:	what would be:::: .. what would be anothe::r .. *good* one that you could space,
	6		now that you w- .. you would *know* where it was going to go. ... ...
	7	C:	*if* i knew .. the middle .. i'd do the *middle* [one.] .. like i did last time. =
	8	A:	[.hhh] =w- good *ide::a*
1st R#2	9	A:	okay well h- what could you do *next* ..
	10		so that you would *then* know where the middle was going to be. ...
	11		which one would you move next.

2nd R#3	12	C:	*ze:ro* =
3rd R#3	13	A:	= the zero. ... brilliant ... thats a good *idea* isn't it. ...
4th	14	C:	mmhmm ... ... right on the end again. ...
5th	15	A:	oka:y, .. so *now* which one are we going to move.

Sarah has already (and unproblematically) selected and positioned '80' at one end of the number-line, and so on the basis of her previous performance would now be expected to position '0' at the other end. However, in response to her teacher's request for 'the next one' she chooses '78' instead (the one next to '80'). Once again, rather than challenge her choice directly, the teacher asks for 'another good one' that she would 'know where it was going to go' (lines 5–6). Again, while from the teacher's point of view asking for *another* good one (instead of positively evaluating the current one) pre-supposes a request for an improvement on the previous choice, taken literally it is simply a request for an alternative. In the absence of any evidence that Sarah orients to such turns *as* attempts to initiate repair, then, the relationship between this request and subsequent talk is ambiguous at best. Furthermore, as we have seen in previous examples, the 'next' problem itself remains unacknowledged and unaddressed – latent, as it were – because the interactional difficulty it gives rise to is resolved indirectly via a change in sequential context. Specifically, following Sarah's suggestion of 'doing the middle one' (line 7), the teacher reformulates the problem of what to do next in terms of a strategic contingency between the second and third moves (lines 9–11).

Our analysis of earlier sessions, then, supports and reinforces our original interpretation of how and why the 'next' problem arises in session 3. At the same time, we have also noted that at no point is the nature or cause of the problem itself actually addressed by the participants. Rather, we have seen how in general interactional difficulties are created and resolved *inadvertently* with no apparent awareness of their cause, and how as a consequence important sources of ambiguity and misunderstanding remain unaddressed. With this in mind, let us finish by looking at what happens in session 4.

Resolution of interactional difficulties

Extract 9.10 shows the first three exchanges of session 4, which collectively result in the successful positioning of the lowest, highest and middle numbers.

Extract 9.10 *Session 4* {Number set: 0 9 20 40 62 100,140,145,191 200}

1st	1	A:	h okay. ... alright. ... so if we look at *all* of those
	2		which is=which .. ones are we going to move *first*. ... ...
2nd	3	C:	*zero::*[: !
3rd	4	A:	[the zero. yeah okay. ...
(4th)	5	C:	i *always* [move-
	6	A :	[its like you did on your *own* isn't it = you did that first =

4th	7	C:	=i *always* move the zero first .. [thats why,
3rdR/R-4	8	A:	[mmhmm, .. wh- *why* is that a good idea
4th R	9	C:	because u::m .. *i* can just get it right on the end 'cos there are no numbers *before* it.
5th	10	A:	right. so you know where its gonna go. ..
1st	11		okay good, ... ((*L coughs twice*))
1st R	12	A:	next one, =
2nd/4th	13	C:	=an:::d ((*coughs*)) two *hundred* cos thats the *most.* =
5th	14	A:	=that's the *other* end thats right. ...
1st	15		okay. ...
2nd	16	C:	an:d um *one* hundred, ...

[Omitted insertion sequence dealing with external interruption by sudden loud music emanating from a nearby classroom]

	17	C:	[an]:d a hu:[n:dred.]
3rd	18	A:	[*hundred* .] right. = *thats* a good idea isn't it.
4th	19	C:	'cos thats the middle.
5th	20	A:	'cos thats the *middle* one. .. alright, ...

Clearly, in marked contrast to previous sessions, session 4 shows no signs of any interactional difficulty. Why is this? Significantly, as in the incidental resolution of the 'next' problem in session 3 (Extract 9.4), the teacher's initial question now formulates the impending task in terms of which '*ones*' to move first, rather than which '*one*' (2); that is, it presupposes a single strategic move comprising more than one number. Rather than offer two numbers at once, however, the child's response still offers only one – the 'zero' – which the teacher immediately ratifies (3–4), following which Sarah begins to provide a rationale for the choice in advance of the teacher's request for it (5). The second and third moves are equally unproblematic. The teacher's highly abbreviated first-position requests for the 'next one' (12), and then simply 'okay' (15), elicit the provision of 'two hundred' and 'one hundred' as the highest and middle numbers, respectively. Furthermore, Sarah's use of 'and' at the *beginning* of both her second-position turns (13; 16), together with her unprompted provision of rationales, display a clear orientation towards both the five-part structure *and* the sequential contingency of the three moves concerned. As such, superficially we might conclude (as would presumably the teacher) that Extract 10 constitutes a convincing display of shared understanding with regards to what-it-is-to-do the task. In light of the preceding analysis, however, we may well be more cautious!

Discussion

The above analysis demonstrates how the participants' orientation to completing the five-part sequence of interaction tends to override all other contextualisation cues. There is ample evidence that the child does not orient to the teacher's attempts to initiate repair *as* attempts to initiate repair, but as 3rd-position requests for a rationale, while treating successive exchanges as more or less independent events. At the same time, the teacher treats each resolution of interactional difficulty, and each *local* – and incidental – disambiguation of meaning, as a further display of C's *cumulative* understanding of the task on the presupposition that each successive cycle within an episode is attempting to repair the previous one. As a consequence, the rationale behind C's problematic choices is never directly contested or explored in all four sessions, and the ambiguity of a 'next move' remains unnoticed and unexplored. Given this, we might well ask what if anything has been learned?

Arguably, the indeterminate nature of 'what has been learned' is a direct outcome of the process by which intersubjectivity is negotiated and displayed in conversation. There is a basic tension – or ambiguity – between intersubjectivity as product or precondition, and intersubjectivity as process, that lies at the heart of the notion of 'common ground' (Clark and Wilkes-Gibbs 1986; Clark and Brennan 1993; Smolka *et al.* 1995; Clark 1996). It is a paradox neatly summed up in Rommetveit's often-cited dictum that 'intersubjectivity must in some sense be taken for granted in order to be attained' (Rommetveit 1985: 189). On the one hand, intersubjectivity usefully *replaces* the notion of objectivity with that of 'a reciprocal faith in a shared experiential world' (Rommetveit: 189), yet on the other, objectivity remains the yardstick against which 'degrees', or 'levels of attainment', of intersubjectivity are measured. The sense of intersubjectivity as a *dynamic relationship between interactants* is displaced, through a process of reification, by talk of it in relation to 'actual states' of shared knowledge or experience (Edwards 1997). As such, Clark's notion of a common ground that 'accumulates' is inherently problematic as an explanatory concept. As Edwards (1997) argues, to claim that conversationalists *assume*, or *update*, common ground is of a different order to that of claiming them to actually *have*, and thereby *accumulate*, common ground. While the former is a description of something that participants *do* during talk-in-interaction, the latter is a metaphysical statement about shared experience. Whereas for Clark, 'common ground' is *actual*, what is *presupposed* in conversation is inherently indeterminate and always 'interactionally at issue' (Edwards 1997: 118). It 'accumulates' only in the sense that coordination is maintained over time in the face of ongoing abbreviation. This is inevitable given the impossibility of 'saying' *all* that is presupposed or 'meant' by a given utterance on any particular occasion, as however this presupposition may be formulated, the formulation itself is only intelligible by way of further presupposition.

Elbers (2004) argues that misunderstandings and misattributions of cognitive ability commonly occur in adult–child interactions whenever the 'ground rules' for interpretation and mutual understanding are not shared by the participants. The sharing of such 'ground rules' is essential to effective 'interthinking' and the successful creation of an IDZ (Mercer 2000; Mercer and Littleton 2007). The teacher's avoidance of direct other-repair of the child's problematic 2nd-position turns observed in this chapter is indicative of a common 'ground rule' of pedagogical discourse; namely, the use of other-initiated self-repair as a learning mechanism. As Seedhouse (2001) observes in the context of second-language learning, where teachers and learners do not share this orientation to self-repair the strong dispreference for other-repair is often self-defeating, and while teachers may see other-initiated self-repair as an important part of the learning process, students themselves may often find direct other-repair more helpful. This problem is exacerbated in the current context by the fact that 'ground rules' include not only normative rules governing interactions in particular kinds of institutional settings, but also the implicit local pragmatics of contextualisation operating within any given interaction between specific participants. The analysis presented in this chapter shows just how subtle these 'rules' can be, and how in the main they lie outside the conscious awareness of *both* participants. For example, the teacher's use of *indirect* initiation of repair rather than direct challenge relies predominantly on changes in prosodic emphasis to differentiate such turns from straightforward questions, and yet the child does not attend or orient to such cues as contextualising repair. The teacher, however, is demonstrably unaware of this. Consequently, as successful completion of the 5-part sequence constitutes a display of intersubjectivity with regards to what-it-is-to-do the task, when following a series of supposed cycles of repair it is automatically treated by the teacher as *a display of learning* (as evidenced by his subsequent abbreviation of relevant turn positions). What is also interesting is that the successful positioning of the first three numbers appears to be highly sensitive to the micro-phraseology of the teacher's initial question, and in particular to whether the child's actual or impending action is formulated as a single or composite move. The subtle difference in the presuppositional bases of these two formulations in itself seems sufficient to disambiguate the meaning of a 'next move'. Once again, however, there is no evidence that the participants themselves are aware of this. Clearly, as Elbers (2004) argues, if teachers (and researchers) were able to become more sensitised to the importance of such pragmatic features of talk, they may be less ready to attribute the cause of misunderstandings to cognitive deficits in the child, and be more likely to notice a possible misunderstanding when one arises.

Whereas classical accounts of scaffolding portray the adult as helping the child to unpack the presuppositional basis of the adult's proleptic utterances (Stone 1993), the current analysis highlights the fact that the adult cannot know what is *potentially* presupposed by his/her own utterances beforehand, and that as such the 'unpacking' is necessarily a much more collaborative and indeterminate activity than the standard model would suggest. As noted, however, this is not how participants themselves make sense of what they are doing. Indeed, as shown here, the fact they do not is an important reason why difficulties may arise, persist and/or be resolved inadvertently without either participant being aware of what is happening. It is in the nature of discourse *per se* that participants tend *not* to focus upon the workings of talk-in-interaction, but to act *as if* they are accessing each others' minds directly by means of talk. Language itself provides the categories and means for them to do so, such that people automatically orient to and 'make sense' of their own and each other's actions in terms of thoughts, feelings, intentions, motivations, etc (Edwards 1997). Furthermore, the IRE organisation of instructional conversation is demonstrably aimed at producing displays of 'teaching-learning', and as such presupposes a whole set of developmental assumptions about the pragmatics of learning in interactional contexts, including its facilitation and display. As a consequence, participants in learning conversations are more likely to attribute – or formulate – difficulties in learning as something internal to the child, than to address or explore them as a function of the immediate interactional context in which they arise. However, while participants *in the process* of participation may have little choice but to act 'as if' such realities exist, conversation analysis allows us to study how these realities are built up and presupposed (consciously, or otherwise) across the course of interactions in ways that may in principle inform and facilitate future participatory practice.

Acknowledgements

I am grateful to Ruth Woods and Mike Forrester for their helpful and insightful comments on earlier versions of this chapter.

References

Berk, L.E. (1992) Children's private speech: An overview of theory and the status of research. In R.M. Diaz and L.E. Berk (eds), *Private speech: From social interaction to self-regulation* (pp. 17–53). Hove: Earlbaum.

Cazden, C. (1988) *Classroom discourse: The language of teaching and learning.* Portsmouth, NH: Heinemann.

Clark, H.H. (1996) *Using language.* Cambridge: Cambridge University Press.

Clark, H.H. and Brennan, S.E. (1993) Grounding in communication. In L.B. Resnick, J.M. Levine and S.D. Teasely (eds), *Perspectives on socially shared cognition* (pp. 127–149). Washington, DC: American Psychological Association.

Clark, H.H. and Wilkes-Gibbs, D. (1986) Referring as a collaborative process. *Cognition*, **22**, 1–39.

Drew, P. (1995) Conversation analysis. In J. Smith, R. Harre and L. van Langenhove (eds), *Rethinking methods in psychology* (pp. 64–79). London: Sage.

Edwards, A.D. and Westgate, D.P.G. (1994) *Investigating classroom talk* (2nd edition). London: Falmer Press.

Edwards, D. (1997) *Discourse and cognition.* London: Sage.

Elbers, E. (2004) Conversational asymmetry and the child's perspective in developmental and educational research. *International Journal of Disability, Development and Education*, **51** (2), 201–215.

Elbers, E., Maier, R., Hoekstra, T. and Hoogsteder, M. (1992) Internalisation and adult-child interaction. *Learning and Instruction*, **2**, 101–118.

Gauvain, M. (2001) *The social context of cognitive development.* London: Guilford Press.

Greenleaf, C. and Freedman, S.W. (1993) Linking classroom discourse and classroom content: Following the trail of intellectual work in a writing lesson. *Discourse Processes*, **16**, 465–505.

Gumperz, J.J. (1995) Mutual inferencing in conversation. In I. Markova, C. Graumann and K. Foppa (eds), *Mutualities in dialogue* (pp. 101–123). Cambridge: Cambridge University Press.

Henderson, B. (1991) Describing parent-child interaction during exploration: Situation definitions and negotiations. *Genetic, Social and General Psychological Monographs*, **117**, 79–89.

Heritage, J. (1997) Conversation analysis and institutional talk: Analysing data. In D. Silverman (ed.), *Qualitative research: Theory, method and practice* (pp. 161–182). London: Sage.

Meadows, S. (1996) *Parenting behaviour and children's cognitive development*. Hove: Psychology Press.

Mehan, H. (1979) *Learning lessons*. Cambridge, MA: Harvard University Press.

Mercer, N. (2000) *Words and minds: How we use language to think together*. London: Routledge.

Mercer, N. and Littleton, K. (2007) *Dialogue and the development of children's thinking*. London: Routledge.

Norrick, N. (1987) Functions of repetition in conversation. *Text*, **7** (3), 245–264.

Ochs, E. (1996) Linguistic resources for socialising humanity. In J.J. Gumperz and S.C. Levinson (eds), *Rethinking linguistic relativity* (pp. 407–437). Cambridge: Cambridge University Press.

Pike, C.D. (2000) *The internalisation of adult-child conversation in children's cognitive development: A microgenetic single-case study*. Unpublished PhD thesis, University of Kent.

Pike, C.D. and Forrester, M.A. (1997) The influence of number-sense on children's ability to estimate measures. *Educational Psychology*, **17** (4), 483–500.

Plumert, J.M. and Nichols-Whitehead, P. (1996) Parental scaffolding of young children's spatial communication. *Developmental Psychology*, **32** (3), 523–532.

Pontecorvo, C. (1993) Forms of discourse and shared thinking. *Cognition and Instruction*, **11** (3–4), 189–196.

Pratt, M.W., Kerig, P., Cowan, P.A. and Cowan, C.P. (1988) Mothers and fathers teaching 3-year-olds: Authoritative parenting and adult scaffolding of young children's learning. *Developmental Psychology*, **24** (6), 832–839.

Rogoff, B. (1990) *Apprenticeship in thinking: Cognitive development in social context*. Oxford: Oxford University Press.

Rogoff, B., Ellis, S. and Gardener, W. (1984) Adjustment of adult-child instruction according to child's age and task. *Developmental Psychology*, **20** (2), 193–199.

Rommetveit, R. (1985) Language acquisition as increasing linguistic structuring of experience and symbolic behaviour control. In J.V. Wertsch (ed.), *Culture, communication and cognition: Vygotskyan perspectives* (pp. 183–204). Cambridge: Cambridge University Press.

Schegloff, E.A. (1993) Conversation analysis and socially shared cognition. In L.B. Resnick, J.M. Levine and S.D. Teasely (eds), *Perspectives on socially shared cognition* (pp. 150–171). Washington DC: American Psychological Association.

Seedhouse, P. (2001) The case of the missing no: The relationship between pedagogy and interaction. *Language Learning*, **51** (Suppl. 1), 347–385.

Smolka, A.L.B., De Goes, M.C.R. and Pino, A. (1995) The constitution of the subject: A persistent question. In J.V. Wertsch, P. Del Rio and A. Alvarez (eds), *Sociocultural studies of mind* (pp. 165–186). Cambridge: Cambridge University Press.

Stone, C.A. (1993) What is missing in the metaphor of scaffolding? In E.A. Forman, N. Minick and C.A. Stone (eds), *Contexts for learning: sociocultural dynamics in children's development* (pp. 169–183). Oxford: Oxford University Press.

Tannen, D. (1989) *Talking voices: Repetition, dialogue, and imagery in conversational discourse*. Cambridge: Cambridge University Press.

Vygotsky, L. (1978) *Mind in society: The development of higher psychological processes*. Cambridge, MA: Harvard University Press.

Wertsch, J.V. (1984) The zone of proximal development: Some conceptual issues. In B. Rogoff and J.V. Wertsch (eds), *Children's learning in the zone of proximal development* (pp. 7–18). San Francisco: Jossey-Bass.

Wertsch, J.V. (1991) *Voices of the mind*. Cambridge, MA: Harvard University Press.

Wertsch, J.V. and Hickman, M. (1987) Problem solving in social interaction: A microgenetic analysis. In M. Hickman (ed.), *Social and functional approaches to language and thought* (pp. 251–266). London: Academic Press.

Wertsch, J.V., McNamee, G.D., McLane, J.B. and Budwig, N.A. (1980) The adult–child dyad as a problem-solving system. *Child Development*, 51, 1215–1221.

Wood, D., Wood, H. and Middleton, D. (1978) An experimental evaluation of four face-to-face teaching strategies. *International Journal of Behavioural Development*, 2, 131–147.

Wootton, A. (1997) *Interaction and the development of mind*. Cambridge: Cambridge University Press.

Section 3

Interactions with children who are atypical

Chapter 10

Interactional analysis of scaffolding in a mathematical task in ASD

PENNY STRIBLING and JOHN RAE

Introduction

Adult support of children's engagement with learning has formed an important domain of enquiry within developmental psychology and educational research; some of this research has been conducted under the related terms of 'scaffolding' and the 'Zone of Proximal Development'. As has been noted within the literatures that use these terms, this support is inherently interactional. Nevertheless despite this recognition, such support has not been subjected to fine-grained interactional analysis to reveal precisely what actions it actually consists in, and how these actions are organised with respect to children's actions. In this chapter we present an exploratory analysis that seeks to address these issues by using conversation analysis (CA) to examine how, in a mathematics lesson, a teacher and a learning support assistant help a teenage girl with an autistic spectrum disorder and severe learning disabilities. Our analysis demonstrates how tutors' supportive actions involve fine levels of coordination, both with the student's actions and with each other. This requires a high degree of monitoring of both student *and* co-tutor. We also show that tutors' supportive actions may be delivered in a different modality to the one in which the child is required to respond (e.g. using non-verbal actions in order to support a verbal response). The student's capacity to produce a response in another modality illustrates one way in which she contributed to the activities that are being supported by the tutors. We also explore further contributions that the student brings, such as organising her hands at a relevant point in the interaction to co-construct a display of her skills. Such displays may be initiated by the student, or can be responses to adult initiations. Finally, we discuss how CA can inform our understanding of scaffolding and contribute to our knowledge of how tutors work to develop the intellectual capacities of students with autism and severe learning difficulties.

Scaffolding learning

The work of Lev Vygotsky was pivotal in the development of a sociocultural, constructivist approach in educational psychology (Vygotsky 1978, 1986). Although initially concerned with sensory barriers to learning (e.g. blindness or deafness), Vygotsky's work has profoundly influenced educational provision for all children. His best-known concept is probably the idea of a Zone of Proximal Development (ZPD), where a child's competence can be extended through the support of an adult, or a more able peer. Vygotsky described the ZPD as 'the distance between the actual developmental level as determined through independent problem-solving and the level of potential development as determined through problem-solving under adult guidance or in collaboration with more capable peers' (Vygotsky 1978: 86). This contribution to pedagogy has influenced numerous approaches to the education of both typical and atypical learners throughout the lifespan, including 'situated learning' (e.g. Lave and Wenger 1991), 'instrumental enrichment' (e.g. Feuerstein 1980; Kozulin 2003), the 'Bright Start' programme (e.g. Tzuriel *et al.* 1999) and 'intensive interaction' (Nind 1996). Vygotsky proposed that both our contact with the world, and our learning, are mediated by the use of signs, which may be linguistic, visual or acoustic. The child uses these signs to construct and mediate his or her knowledge of the world, and this mediation can be explicit or implicit (Wertsch 2007). Consequently, much research inspired by Vygotsky's work has focused upon mediation practices and tutor activity involved in the expansion of a child's ZPD. Children's processes in its development have attracted less research attention than tutor activities.

Much Vygotskian-influenced research has been associated with the metaphor of 'scaffolding', which was introduced in the seminal study by Wood *et al.* (1976), describing how learning was fostered by a tutor. The term 'scaffolding' was adopted to describe a procedure whereby an expert adult may support a learner thus extending their competence. Their data consisted of videotaped recordings of young children's engagement with a developmentally challenging block-construction play task. The analysis focused on quantified measures of child performance and adult intervention rather than on the actual learning mechanisms involved, but provided little detail concerning the social interaction through which the adult support actually took place. Although undoubtedly influenced by it, Wood *et al.* (1976) do not actually make an explicit connection to Vygotsky's ZPD; this connection was first made by Cazden (1979).

Subsequent research on scaffolding diversified into a number of domains, the most prominent strand involved the analysis of tutor activities in interactions with their students. Nevertheless, due to their theoretical and practical commitments, such analyses do not pay detailed attention to the unfolding management of these interactions. Although some of these studies provide extracts of transcripts of talk, these tend to be presented for illustrative purposes, the analysis involving the categorisation of events rather than a detailed interactional analysis (Palincsar and Brown 1984). Langer and Applebee (1986) discuss such extracts in terms of discrete classifications of adults' actions, and although they later describe some research which examines the structure of dialogue, this concerns such things as the number of turns, their regulatory character, and the linguistic categories into which they fall.

Stone (1998), reviewing the utility of the scaffolding metaphor in learning disability (LD), identifies four key characteristics of scaffolding. Firstly, learner involvement is elicited by a more knowledgeable individual, although Stone stresses the *bidirectional* nature of scaffolding. Secondly, the tutor monitors and responds to developments in learner knowledge. Although Vygotsky (1987) assumed that collaborative work led to learning ('what the child is able to do in collaboration today he will be able to do independently tomorrow' (p. 211)), the dawn of 'tomorrow' may be much delayed in this population. The acquisition of knowledge may also involve different mechanisms, requiring specifically tailored scaffolding practices. Stone argues for an 'enriched scaffolding' where adult activities are closely calibrated to student competencies. Thirdly, it encompasses a wide range of support activities, including 'verbal regulation of tasks' which he favours as a key scaffolding strategy for students with LD. A fourth feature was the impetus towards learner responsibility for managing their own learning. Despite this, Biemiller and Meichenbaum (1998) report the practice of 'negative scaffolding' in LD classrooms, where there is no progression towards independent learner status or transfer of task responsibility to the learner.

Mascolo (2005) also questions the unitary emphasis on the expert tutor's actions in much prior research, commenting that while the 'concept of scaffolding depicts development as a social process, the metaphor nonetheless directs attention to the actions of the expert' (Mascolo 2005: 186). He proposes a three-part systemic model of *co-active scaffolding*, where individual action emerges from co-action involving all parties (social scaffolding and self-scaffolding); together with physical or psychological objects (ecological scaffolding). This latter category is a useful reminder that scaffolding is not limited to cognitive activities. Unfortunately, Mascolo offers no detailed empirical research to support these categories. Scaffolding can be managed with the support of a whole gamut of interactional resources (e.g. gaze shifts, gestures, body positioning, etc.) and environmental objects; and the analysis of scaffolding practices would benefit from insights into how these resources are organised. Nevertheless, much previous research on scaffolding has focused upon talk. This may be less useful in the case of severely language-compromised students, who may co-manage interaction in quite idiosyncratic ways. The next section will consider the challenges of educating one such group.

Learning in children with autism spectrum disorders

Students with an autism spectrum disorder (ASD) and a severe learning difficulty (SLD) constitute one of the most challenging populations in public education provision. They exhibit a range of developmental delays in spoken and non-spoken language skills, social interactional skills; and a propensity towards restrictive interests, together with repetitive behaviours (APA 1995). The precise manifestation of these core impairments and a range of so-called 'secondary symptoms' (e.g. pica, attention deficits) will vary between individuals.

Other barriers to learning in this population may include sensory (e.g. auditory or visual hypersensitivity; see Ornitz 1985, 1988), cognitive (e.g. 'mindblindness', see Baron-Cohen 1995) and attentional components (e.g. Curcio 1978). Many students with ASD also display receptive language difficulties (Roberts 1989) and a more visual learning style (Grandin 1996), suggesting that Stone's preferred method of 'verbal regulation' may not be the most appropriate for this population.

Formal assessment of these students' learning is notoriously difficult, partly because they are considered to be slow to generalise their learning. Assessment may be further compromised by socio-motivational deficits, reflected in their apparent unwillingness to cooperate (see Koegel and Mentis 1985). Consequently, many tutor activities are designed to assist students in gradually gaining mastery over relevant skills (or their component parts) in the longer term.

Owing to this unusual constellation of developmental delays and learning difficulties, students with autism are typically provided with high levels of staffing and structure to facilitate their access to learning. Vygotsky was concerned with the *quality* rather than the quantity of assistance provided for the learner, and Vygotskian-inspired researchers have attempted to understand the relevance of that assistance to a learner's development (for discussion see Chaiklin 2003). The quality of learning support in autism can be quite different to provision for other school populations, consequently a number of syndrome-specific educational technologies, e.g. Program TEACCH (Schopler and Mesibov 1985), have been developed to provide intensive scaffolding of their learning. These specialist programs are often staffed with additional learning support assistants (LSAs), frequently engaged in one-to-one tuition. There is some empirical support for the efficacy of these practices – e.g. Bellon *et al.*'s story-reading intervention study (1999) – but it is difficult to partial out age-related developmental gains. Nind and Powell (2000) also make the case for a Vygotskian-inspired approach to teaching students with ASD, using 'intensive interaction'; however, this would benefit from more detailed, empirical evaluation of the actual practices involved in delivering this intervention in the classroom.

Collectively, these factors suggest a pressing need to continue research on scaffolding in learning-disabled ASD populations, but they also suggest that some caution is required in relying upon standardised outcome measures to assess its efficacy. An alternative evaluation strategy may include some refocus upon the intersubjective *process* of learning in the ZPD.

This raises the question of how best to research such processes. Although Mascolo's model was not supported by empirical data, he proposed a basis for pursuing this line of enquiry, namely, 'fine-grained analysis of moment by moment activity is needed in order to identify. . . . coactive exchanges' (2005: 189). Such detailed analysis might also illuminate activities that could constitute the category of 'enriched scaffolding' (Stone 1998). Mascolo's agenda would appear to involve a sequential analysis of how parties put actions together. However, if such an analysis only seeks to identify *categories* of action, this could undermine the dynamic focus on the *process* of moment-by-moment activity.

Conversation analysis and the sequential organisation of interaction

Following Wood *et al.*'s (1976) seminal study, the use of video data has continued to be a feature of work on scaffolding, although the focus has generally been on verbal dimensions of the interactions rather than the moment-by-moment organisations of these activities. Recent video-based work involving LD students has been carried out, but has focused upon issues of responsibility and control in teacher–student interaction (Rasku-Puttonen *et al.* 2003) and has examined specific groups of learners.

Conversation analysis (CA) offers a powerful tool for the detailed analysis of how interactions are organised. Unlike other empirical methodologies that involve a micro-analysis, CA is particularly concerned with the sequential organisation of naturally occurring interaction – that is, how one party's actions create a context for subsequent actions. This inductive approach accommodates participants' use of both spoken and non-spoken interactional resources. CA's commitment to an empirically based inductive approach to the resources that the parties themselves use in managing interaction has particular relevance for the analysis of scaffolding. There are two main reasons for this: firstly, it concerns the activities of all parties to an interaction; and, secondly, analyses are not based on assumptions about how interaction should be managed, or indeed which features are important. The latter is prevalent in content analytic studies of video-taped interaction (e.g. Nind 1999).

There is a significant body of work using CA to examine interactions in educational contexts, for example interactions in classrooms (McDermott 1977; McHoul 1978, 1990; Mehan 1979; Heap 1985; Lerner 1995; Macbeth 2004; Markee 2005;). Some of these address specific skills, such as how schoolchildren draw upon teachers' implicit meanings around a mathematical construct (estimation) in their activities (Forrester and Pike 1998). This work has focused on verbal interaction; however, more recent work on learning in other settings has paid detailed attention to non-verbal resources (in particular, objects) in interaction, for example doing school work at home (Goodwin 2007) and learning in operating theatres (Koschmann *et al.* 2007). While much of this work is not motivated by themes drawn from Vygotsky, the connections between CA and Vygotsky have been clearly indicated (Pea 1993; Jacoby and Ochs 1995).

Conversation analysis has also been used to research multi-modal interaction including interactions involving persons with ASDs. Individual case studies (Local and Wootton 1995; Dobbinson *et al.* 1998, 2003; Tarplee and Barrow 1999; Wootton 1999; Stiegler 2007; Stribling *et al.* 2007;) have paid particular attention to non-vocal resources, such as tapping (e.g. Dickerson *et al.* 2007). In the following section we apply CA to a stretch of classroom interaction in which a teacher and a learning support assistant support a severely learning-disabled student, with an autistic spectrum disorder, in the teaching of very early mathematics skills. This type of teaching often involves the use of symbolic objects as a vehicle for communicating meaning, e.g. wooden blocks. An early task in teaching counting skills may be to support the pupil in using these representative objects in this particular context. Given the reported difficulties with inflexibility in this population and substantial language impairment, this might be expected to create difficulty for the student, thus making scaffolding support from the tutors relevant.

Examining the organisation of classroom activities involving a girl with ASD and a SLD

We will examine the organisation of scaffolding processes by applying CA to an every-day interaction that occurred naturally in a classroom and was recorded on videotape. This data is extracted from 16 hours of material whose collection was funded by the UK Economic and Social Research Council. The activities involved direct teaching of National Curriculum content, so they contrast with the playful, student-following style associated with 'Intensive Interaction' approaches (see Nind and Hewett 1988; Nind and Powell 2000). In this data set, a large number of activities were observed that can be characterised as 'scaffolding' – that is, where a student is supported in the accomplishment of a task. Owing to space constraints, we will focus on one stretch of interaction (just 59 seconds long) from a mathematics class. This was selected as representative of a number of action sequences in which the student's co-participation is sought by more than one member of staff.

The interaction involves a 16-year-old girl diagnosed with autism and severe learning difficulties at age 6, whom we will call 'Helen'. She has some limited speech (a large lexicon of mainly single nouns) and attends a non-maintained school in southern England for pupils with complex severe/profound learning disabilities. All students in the small class have their own dedicated Learning Support Assistant (LSA), who usually sits beside them during group instruction by the class teacher. Helen's LSA, whom we will call 'Ginny', has a variety of roles – for example, helping to maintain Helen's engagement with learning materials and her attention to the teacher. The teacher is a maths specialist whom we will call 'Nigel'. In terms of previous research on scaffolding, the present interaction is rather unusual in that it involves one student (Helen) but two expert adult tutors (Nigel and Ginny). The transcripts display not only the participants' talk, but also a number of non-verbal activities which may be salient to the parties' management of the interaction. In making a choice about what to transcribe, we have focused on events that, by virtue of their timing, are apparently relevant for the participants.

The interaction involves working with half a dozen identical small plastic blocks, thus in Vygotskian terms it is explicitly mediated (see Wertsch 2007). During the lesson, staff and students make reference to these blocks using a range of modalities, including talk, gaze and gesture. In this interaction, Nigel arranges the blocks in front of Helen on a rectangular platter. This physical layout constitutes what Mascolo labels as a type of 'positional' scaffolding as it privileges certain locally available activities, making these more interactionally salient. The following gloss of the interaction may help readers to orient themselves with the transcript showed in Appendix 10.1 (note that this introductory gloss is not an analysis). Nigel has put in front of Helen a platter on which five blocks are placed, and announces that he is going to take a block away; however, Helen removes a block and hands it to him. Nigel praises her and then asks how many blocks are left. With Ginny's support, Helen counts the blocks, initially over-counting but getting it right on a second attempt. She is praised by Nigel, who then instructs Helen to take away two blocks, which she subsequently does, again with some support from Ginny. After praising her for this accomplishment, Nigel again asks how many blocks remain. Again, with some support from Ginny, Helen counts the blocks, Nigel praises her and then moves off to attend to another matter.

As with many interactions in educational settings, this interaction involves a number of sequences in which the teacher produces a *sequence initiating action* that requires the student to produce a *responsive action*. Talk has sequential implications for its recipients, and although participants can decline to respond to initiating actions (for example, they might refuse to answer a question) there is a strong implication that they should provide a responsive action that is fitted to the initiating action (e.g. produce an appropriate answer to a question). This sequential organisation is widely exploited by teachers to structure students' progress in educational tasks and, as a resource for organizing students' work, can itself be a form of scaffolding. These sequences, to which the teacher's feedback is commonly added, have sometimes been considered to be three-part sequences (see Ridley *et al.* 2002), although this third action can be considered as a post-sequence expansion (Schegloff 2007).

The interaction examined here consists of four such sequences. There are two *block-removal sequences*, in which blocks are removed from the platter (lines 1–9 and 20–36 in Appendix 10.1), reproduced as Extracts 10.1 and Extract 10.3 respectively below. Each of these is followed by a *block-counting sequence*, in which the remaining blocks are counted (lines 10–19, and lines 37–41 in Appendix 10.1), reproduced as Extracts 10.2 and Extract 10.4. In these extracts, the initiating-actions and their responses are arrowed and numbered (e.g. I1, R1 shows these actions in Extract 10.1; I2 and R2 in Extract 10.2; and so on). In fact, as we will show, the block-removal sequence with which the interaction begins is not actually designed by the teacher and, as such, it is Helen who treats Nigel's announcement that he is going to remove a block as an instruction for her to do so.

In the extracts presented here, each spoken turn (or part of it, if it occupied more than one line) is allocated a line number in series. Concurrent non-spoken activity is arranged around the line of talk, with each non-speaking participant allocated a sub-line for non-talk activity. Unless otherwise indicated, Helen's non-vocal activities are shown *above* the line of talk and other party's non-vocal activities are shown *below* the line of talk. Pauses between talk in these activities are represented by a series of dashes, each representing one-tenth of a second, and if their duration was more than 1 second, the appropriate digit was adopted to mark the boundary between seconds and parts of a second for ease of reading. Therefore, a pause of 1.4 seconds will be represented as '(---------1----)'.

We will now turn to an examination of how these sequences unfold in terms of the implications that are set up for the student, how adult support of the student is organised, and how the student co-participates in the support that she receives. We will first consider the management of scaffolding in the accomplishment of the two *block-removal* sequences starting with the first one, shown in Extract 10.1.

Extract 10.1 'Helen One Block' (Simplified) Block-removal sequence 1

Annotations above lines of talk are Helen's, unless others indicated

1   Nigel: Now: [Helen: (------)   listen

2   (---------1-)

3   Nigel: **I1▶**   I'm going to take awa:y:

4   (-----)

                 [*raises head looks at Nigel*
5   Helen: [Take way take away

                      [*lowers hands reaches left-hand most block*
6   Nigel: **I1▶** One [block

        R1▶   [*arm extended offering block to N*
7   Helen: One block [one block

8   Nigel: [Good girl
                 [*N takes block*
                 ((*there are now four blocks on the table*))

9   Nigel: Excellent well done

Although Nigel announced that *he* was going to take a block away (line 3), Helen undertakes this task herself, offering a plastic block from the board to Nigel (line 7). As she does so, she echoes the last two items of Nigel's talk, 'one block'. Nigel accepts it, praising her efforts (lines 8 and 9). In this sequence then, Helen appears to treat Nigel's announcement as an instruction for her to remove the block. It seems likely that Helen has misunderstood Nigel's announcement; the organisation of Nigel's talk is very similar to an instruction: it is only his 'I'm' at the start that shows that it is an announcement. However rather than indicating that Helen failed to engage with his actions, his praising of her *retrospectively* frames her action as appropriate and correct. Nigel thereby reflexively orients to Helen's understanding and modifies the trajectory of the actions in which he was engaged in order to fit with Helen's actions. In this sequence no support was required in order to elicit a response from Helen, rather supportive work is done after her production of a response to cast that response as an appropriate response. By contrast, in the second block-removal sequence (represented in Extract 10.2), Helen's response comes about through support from the tutors.

Extract 10.2 'Helen One Block' (Simplified) Block-removal sequence 2

```
20   Nigel:        Now. (--------)

                                       [looks at N
21   Nigel: I2▶    can [you:.(--[----)  [take away
     Helen:            [         [(°you°)  [
                      [point at             [grasping
                      [H's abdomen          [gesture

22   Nigel: I2▶    (--[----)    [two blocks
     Helen:            [>take aw[ay<
                      [two fingers

23   Helen:        (Two blocks)

24                 (---------1------)

25   Nigel: I3▶    [Take away (.) two blocks?
                   [lowers two fingers

26                 (---------1---------2---------3

27   Ginny:        °C'n you do it then°°

28   Helen:        (uurh)

29   Ginny:        °yourself°

30   Helen:        (urh)

31   Ginny:        °ready°

     R2▶           Looks at N
                   picks up block 2nd from left and hands to N
                   ┌──────────────────────┐
32                 (---------1---------2----)
```

| 33 | Nigel: | One |

R2▶   *picks up block 3rd from right and hands to N*

| 34 | | (---------1---------2---------3----- |

| 35 | Nigel: | Good Girl |
| | | (((*there are now three blocks on the table*)) |

| 36 | Nigel: | Excellent. Well done? |

This sequence commences with an instruction from Nigel: 'Can you take away two blocks' (lines 21–22) and, subsequently, Helen passes two blocks to Nigel (lines 32 and 34). However, this accomplishment does not immediately follow Nigel's instruction and we will be concerned with the intervening contributions, from Nigel and Ginny, that support Helen. We start by considering Nigel's actions.

Firstly, it is evident that even before he creates an opportunity for Helen to produce a response, Nigel engages in supportive work. In delivering his instruction, Nigel augments the personal pronoun ('you') with a pointing gesture towards Helen and as he says 'take away', he mimes this by slowly producing a grasping gesture (shown in line 21). In contrast to his retrospective framing of Helen's handing him a block in Extract 10.1, this careful delivery of the instruction with accompanying non-verbal actions constitutes a form of *prospective* support. Following Nigel's instruction (lines 21–22), Helen responds by producing talk in which she repeats the final items of his talk 'take away (two blocks)' (lines 22–23) but she does not visibly engage with the task.

After a silence of about 1.5 seconds (line 24) Nigel redelivers this request in a contracted form 'take away two blocks' (line 25). As Schegloff, Jefferson and Sacks (1977) have noted, repair is a multi-faceted activity that can be initiated and carried out using a wide range of resources. Here, in re-doing talk that has proved problematic, Nigel adopts the common strategy of reproducing what he said previously, but in a simplified form. Nevertheless, this does not elicit the required response, in fact, Helen lowers her head, apparently disengaging with, or refusing to carry out, the task. Nigel has thus produced two supportive actions; his sequence-initiating action involved prospective support and, following a lack of an appropriate response, he repaired his instruction. Nevertheless, his attempts do not succeed in eliciting a response from Helen.

Thus far in the interaction, Ginny has been monitoring Helen but has not intervened in her interaction with Nigel. Ginny does not deliver any talk until 3 seconds after Nigel has delivered his reformulated talk (another party in a parallel interaction speaks at this point). Ginny then issues a directive-interrogative – 'can you do it then' (line 27). Helen by this stage is making murmuring sounds and does not respond to the approach. Ginny produces an increment to her just-prior turn by saying 'yourself' (line 29), thus bringing her turn to a second point of completion and thereby providing Helen with a second place to respond. By line 31 Helen still is not engaging with the task she has been invited to perform, and Ginny issues a summons – 'ready'. This apparently elicits the required response from Helen who passes a block to Nigel. He receives it with a prominent 'one' (line 33) thereby acknowledging the block but – by not delivering praise – implying that more is required. Helen picks up and hands another block to Nigel (line 34), and his praise (lines 35–36) closes the sequence.

In this sequence it appears likely that Helen's non-engagement may well be unrelated to her comprehension of the task requirements, or some lack of appreciation of the directive nature of Nigel's talk, because Helen eventually performs the action that was specified by Nigel without any intervening clarification of the task. The intervening talk from Ginny is geared to encouraging Helen to respond rather than to clarifying what it is that is required of her. (During this sequence there are ecological factors that might be influencing Helen – and which Ginny may be taking into account – namely there are some shrieks and cries from other students, and some audible disciplinary talk from another dyad.)

In this sequence then, the two tutors make distinctive contributions. Nigel, the teacher, initiates the sequence, repairs his instruction when no response is forthcoming, acknowledges Helen's compliance with the task, and brings the sequence to a close. Ginny, the LSA, is relatively slow to intervene. Despite Helen's obvious delays in complying with the task Nigel sets for her in Extract 10.2, the LSA limits her participation to encouraging Helen to respond; and she does not respond to Helen's compliance. We will return to a consideration of the LSA's conduct here by contrasting it with her intervention in other segments of the interaction.

In both the block-removal sequences (Extracts 10.1 and 10.2) tutors show ongoing orientation to the student's participation, the *student's* actions influence the design of tutor support in the response phase. In these sequences, Helen does not require a high level of support. However, in the two block-*counting* sequences in which she is instructed to count the remaining number of blocks, higher levels of support are provided. We will begin by considering the organisation of the block-counting sequence that follows the first block-removal sequence, this is shown in Extract 10.3.

Extract 10.3 'Helen One Block'(Simplified) Block-counting sequence 1

```
10   Nigel: I3▶      How many blocks 'ave you left

                                         [touches Ginny's hand
                                         [briefly points
11   Helen:          Got left got left [got lef[t
     Ginny:                             [offers R hand

                                   [points index finger
12   Ginny:          [    ° han[d°              ]

                     [moves and removes L hand]
13   Ginny:          >How many<

                     ((G guides H's hand, counting the blocks, L to R))
                              touching blocks
                     ┌─────────────────────────────────┐
14   Helen: R3▶      °o:ne° (.) two:: three: (four) five °si°

15   Nigel:          [Count slow[ly
     Ginny:          [          [L hand moves in
                     [hand moves back to L handmost block
```

16   Ginny: °(   )°

              ((*G guides H's hand, counting the blocks, L to R*))
                    touching blocks

                ┌─────────────────────┐
17   Helen: **R3▶**   <u>one</u> t<u>wo</u>: th<u>ree</u>: f<u>our</u>: (– [–) four four four
     Ginny: [*releases G's hand*

18   Nigel: Good girl well done

19   (–––––––––1–)
                ┌─────────────────┐
                └─────────────────┘
              N replaces block on the table

The sequence is initiated by Nigel asking 'How many blocks 'ave you left' (line 10). Although this turn is designed to implicate a response from Helen and is thus analysable as a new sequence of activity, it clearly builds on the outcome of the previous block-removal sequence, the phrase 'have you left' referring to how many blocks remain after having just removed some. Helen subsequently produces a correct answer (line 17), having previously produced an incorrect one (line 14). Our focus will be on the supportive actions through which these responses come about.

Helen promptly responds to Nigel's question by repeating a version of the final part of his turn (line 11). As Helen completes her iterations of 'got left', Ginny offers her hand (line 11) and says 'hand' (line 12). Helen very rapidly places her left hand upon Ginny's and briefly forms her index finger into a point (line 11). As Ginny says 'hand', she briefly grasps Helen's hand in both her hands, and offers a reformulation of Nigel's question: 'how many' (line 13). As she says this, Helen again forms her index finger into point. Ginny guides Helen's pointing hand across the blocks and Helen counts them (line 14).

Here then, unlike in Extract 10.2 where Ginny did not co-participate until some time after Nigel had made a second attempt to eliciting a response from Helen, she gets involved much earlier. It is possible that she is treating Helen's repetitions of 'got left' as an indication that Helen is engaged, but requires direction for the sequence to progress, while in Extract 10.2 the issue may have been one of promoting engagement, however more data would be necessary to establish this.

By forming her left index finger into a point, Helen shows that she understands that she is going to be pointing to things with her hand. Ginny withdraws her left hand, and Helen starts counting (line 14) as she does so, Ginny provides support for Helen's participation by guiding her hand across the blocks. This stage has thus come about through Ginny's co-participation, however Helen clearly brings a lot to the support that she is offered: she readily takes Ginny's hand, she prepares her finger for pointing and once her hand is being guided, she counts spontaneously.

As it happens, Helen over-counts the blocks, and Nigel and Ginny both become involved in corrective action. Nigel tells Helen to 'count slowly' (line 15) and Ginny moves Helen's hand back, bringing her left hand in, and augments her support underneath Helen's hand by placing her left hand on top of Helen's (also line 15). This may well provide more controlled guidance of Helen's movements, thus putting Ginny in a better position to stall any potential over-counting; Ginny maintains her hand there during the re-count (line 17). Helen recounts the blocks, with her hand being guided by Ginny, after she says four (the correct number) Ginny releases her hand and Helen repeats the number three times (line 17). Nigel acknowledges the correct answer and praises her (line 18).

As in Extract 10.2, Helen's successful completion of the task comes about through support from both Ginny and Nigel. A particular feature of Ginny's support here is that it involves Helen being physically guided, a further example of this occurs in the second and final block-counting sequence shown in Extract 10.4.

Extract 10.4 'Helen One Block'(Simplified) Block-counting sequence 2

```
37   Nigel: I4▶     [and how many blocks do you have ] left
                    [moves blocks closer together          ]

38   (Helen):      (have left)  (have left)  (have [left)
     Ginny:                                         [offers R hand

39                 (– – – – – – – – [–1  –       [ – –)
     Ginny:                         [            [brings in L hand
     Helen:                         [lowers hand
                                      and points

                   ((G guides H's hand, counting the blocks, L to R))
                     touching blocks
                   ┌───────────────────┐

40   Helen: R4▶    one two three::  ( –[ – )
                                       [looks at N

41   Nigel:        Excellent well done Helen very very well done
```

This sequence again opens by the teacher producing an initiating action (namely Nigel asking a question in line 37) and is again completed by the student producing a responsive action (namely Helen's answer in line 40). While this constitutes a discrete sequence, as with the sequence examined in Extract 10.3, it is built as a development on the just-prior block-removal sequence, as here in addition to a construction relating to the removal of blocks 'how many blocks do you have left' the turn starts with 'and'. As with her response in Extract 10.3, Helen's initial response to Nigel's question involves talk that is echoic of the final items of Nigel's utterance. This talk again displays engagement with Nigel's concerns, but does not constitute the actions that his prior turn implicated. As this talk draws to a close, Ginny offers her hand (which Helen accepts) and the blocks are counted successfully (line 40). On this occasion, there is some evidence that Helen may be counting more confidently, delivering 'three' with item-final prosodic stress. Following this, Ginny withdraws her hand and Nigel moves away to other business.

Thus, in both these sequences (Extracts 10.3 and 10.4), Ginny scaffolds Helen's transition into participating in the counting activity by offering a physical support for one of Helen's hands. In the second sequence, Ginny guides Helen's movements with both hands from the beginning of the count. The design of her action may be a result of her earlier experience, where the initial attempt to scaffolding Helen's activity with less robust hand support, involved an incorrect attempt at the task. Alternatively this design may reflect an attempt to manage Helen's attention given co-occurring noise from other students.

The organisation of adult support

In each of the last three sequences considered (Extracts 10.2–10.4), it is clear that Helen successfully carries out the actions required by her teacher and he follows each of these with words of praise. Moreover, it is evident that Helen's success comes about through support from Ginny or from Nigel. Consider, for example, lines 10–19 in Extract 10.3. Nigel asks Helen how many blocks are on the board (line 10). Helen produces a response to this by echoing the last part of Nigel's talk (line 11). Although this response demonstrates some engagement with Nigel, it does not constitute the actions that Nigel had implicated. Ginny then becomes involved by extending her hand towards Helen (near the end of line 11). In this instance, Helen's counting extended beyond the number of items on the board, and Ginny appears to be preparing for some corrective action. Nigel proposes a recount by saying 'count slowly' (line 15). On the recount, Ginny uses *both* hands to guide Helen, and on this occasion, Helen's number sequence does not move beyond the correct answer (four) (line 17). This sequence thus consists of an *initiating action* produced by the teacher, namely a question that requires the student to count (in line 10) and a subsequent *responsive action* produced by the student (in line 17), which is subsequently accepted as correct by the teacher (line 18). The correct responsive action then, is not produced autonomously by the student but rather comes about through adult support, which is modified in light of the student's over-counting on the first attempt.

The sort of support just considered involves a number of features, concerning (a) *sequential position*: it is in what might be called the response phase, that is, it follows the production of an initiating action and seeks to facilitate the response required by that action; (b) *modality*: it is implemented largely via manual guidance; and (c) *personnel*: it is implemented primarily by the LSA. It can be seen that, in the data examined, supportive actions in this sequential position are associated with the LSA. Indeed, the LSA's participation is restricted to carrying out supportive actions in this sequential position. Conversely the teacher carries out specific kinds of supportive action, namely *prospective* support (delivering an instruction in a specially designed way), *retrospective* support (treating an action as a correct response), and carrying out repair by re-issuing initiating actions. The teacher and LSA thus operate as members of a team, each having distinctive responsibilities. The professional discretion of LSA work in this context has been examined in Stribling *et al.* 2009.

The support that Ginny offers shows three specific features. Firstly, Ginny's guidance is often in a separate modality to the required response (she uses her hand to encourage and support Helen's arm movements), whereas Nigel's initiation actions implicated that a spoken (or perhaps signed) articulation of numbers is required. Secondly, Ginny's guidance highly controls Helen's movement, and provides relatively few degrees of freedom for her student. Nevertheless, although highly controlling of certain aspects of Helen's participation, Ginny leaves it to Helen to make the step from moving her hand over the blocks to actually counting them.

Thirdly, different levels of guidance are offered for two different types of unfolding sequences. In Extract 10.2, Ginny is much slower to intervene than in Extracts 10.3 and 10.4, where she commences her supportive arm actions soon after Nigel completes his sequence-initiating actions. This may be linked to Helen's differing levels of displayed competence. Given that Helen had already produced evidence of competence in the block-removal task in Extract 10.1, silence after Nigel's request in Extract 10.2 suggests that, although there is some problem with Helen responding, the problem is not related to competence. In Extract 10.3 by contrast, Helen's somewhat mitigated echoing of Nigel's talk ('got left') may provide evidence for Ginny that Helen is not yet able to produce the required response, and is in need of her support.

Student co-participation with adult support

Notwithstanding the importance of tutor support, the successful completion of the sequences is clearly not solely due to their actions, but also depends on Helen's contributions. For example, in the sequence where most support is required (Extract 10.3), there are three particular actions in which Helen engages: (a) forming her hand such that her index finger is pointing; (b) responding to an invitation to place her hand on her tutor's hand; and (c) producing echoic talk.

The first of these actions is initiated by Helen, the others are second-part responses to tutor action. Helen's index-finger point is initiated in lines 11 and 13, and maintained during the counting periods. The formulation of the point displays her readiness to engage in the counting activity, and allows her progress across the blocks to be more readily monitored by tutors. She also displays some understanding of the nature of the task in which she is engaged, by pulling her hand away as she reaches 'four' in her second counting sequence (line 19). Wood *et al.* (1976) state that a child's experience of adult scaffolding should leave the child with a better understanding of what is involved in the learning task. While Helen's cognitive processes may be opaque, her actions may suggest some increasing appreciation that she should stop moving through a linear number series when she has pointed towards the last of the blue blocks on display. Indeed, a pervasive feature of the support offered to her is that it presupposes a capacity to understand how the support being introduced relates to the task underway. This is particularly clear in Helen's capacity to enter spontaneously into counting blocks once Ginny takes her hand. Chaiklin (2003) reminds us that Vygotsky's conceptualisation of student learning via 'imitation' requires some understanding by the child of the structural aspects of task requirements. At other times, Helen's responses are fitted to the tutor's initiations and help to co-scaffold her participation in the learning task. For example, when Ginny extends her hand to Helen prior to conducting the counting sequences, Helen responds by placing her hand upon Ginny's (line 11).

One common occasion for tutor scaffolding is when the student shows some difficulty in making progress. When Nigel asks Helen to quantify the remaining blocks on the board (line 10), Ginny does not immediately offer her hand to Helen, but provides an opportunity for Helen to display her current level of competence. In the event, Helen produces talk that appears to be responsive to Nigel's request, yet is not directly addressing his concerns. Helen's response ('got left got left got left') is both echolalic and palilalic in quality. Ginny may infer that Helen will not identify the remaining number of blocks, and deem this an appropriate point to mobilise further scaffolding. Helen's responsiveness to other parties' actions often suggests a high level of commitment to the proceedings, despite being compromised at times, possibly by background noise.

Across the four sequences that comprise the interaction, there are two recurring features that are important for our understanding of scaffolding. Firstly, tutor scaffolding is essentially a reflexive activity and, secondly, scaffolding involves co-participation between students and tutors. As has been noted by Stone (1998) and others, the expert participant adjusts (calibrates) her activities in response to the student's action (e.g. displays of competence or incompetence at the current level of scaffolding). Although the present analysis is limited, we have shown that evidence of student's 'co-authoring' of learning activities in the context of tutor support can be captured in terms of concrete interactional details.

Discussion

Drawing on four sequences within a single interaction, the analysis has shown how there are specific sequential positions where tutors may carry out supportive actions. We have shown how initiating actions, and responses to the student's response to those initiating actions, are associated with the *teacher* and may be used to implement prospective or retrospective support. On the other hand, the *LSA* may take the opportunity to help the sequence to progress by becoming involved in the response phase of the sequence. In the final section of this chapter, we will discuss the implications of this analysis for some aspects of our understanding of scaffolding, and also some of the wider implications for the structuring of learning activities involving students with autism and severe learning difficulties.

Reflexivity in co-participatory scaffolding

Schon's (1983) seminal work on reflexive cognitive process in professional practice highlights the importance of tutor reflexivity in teaching activities. The term 'reflexivity' has a number of different usages in the Social Sciences (for discussion, see Macbeth 2001). Ethnomethodologists use it to refer to the notion that social order is created in talk, rather than existing independently of it. Many researchers adopt the term to describe a process of critical reflection on their own representations of the phenomena under investigation. For psychological practitioners, reflexivity can be a cognitive process of ongoing reflection on their own actions in relation to others in clinical practice. Schon's usage falls into the latter category.

Scaffolding requires a reflexive orientation to the learner's potential for engaging in the developmental tasks, a notion embedded in Stone's (1998) proposal for an enriched scaffolding that is calibrated to the learner's current knowledge. Although CA eschews the modelling of individual cognition, it is deeply concerned with how parties design their actions in light of co-parties' action. Its sequential approach can usefully inform how participants' observable monitoring of others' activities might be reflected in the design of their own subsequent actions.

Other-initiated repair can be conceptualised in terms of a reflexive response to others actions, such as a failure to respond to an initiating action. Both Nigel and Ginny use this as a reflexive response when Helen is not responding to their earlier talk or actions, although there may be differences in the styles that they adopt. Nigel tends to approach this by pursuing the task instructions until Helen appears ready to orient to them. Ginny appears to be more directive, using summons, requests to participate and non-vocal resources. This may reflect their orientation to their different responsibilities in this setting.

In the second counting sequence (Extract 10.4), Helen has her arms across her face and ears as Nigel poses his question and maintains them there. In inviting Helen to co-count the items, Ginny appears to be responsive to Helen's current activity, which may in turn be responsive to the noises of peers. Ginny places her upturned hand in a central position where Helen, despite having her arms across her forehead and head slightly tipped forwards, can visually observe its presence, and the tacit invitation to co-count the items. Helen's actions may elicit a reflexive response in the tutor scaffolding work in other respects. As in other counting events not presented here, Helen marks turn-final items either by repetition, or by using prosodic stress. Ginny appears to be responsive to this, and withdraws the scaffolding hand. Nigel gets up and moves away to another pupil.

Much of the previous discussion has considered the actions of parties in rather discrete terms. Returning to Mascolo's notion of *co-active* scaffolding, an analysis which considers the actions of each party in turn treats the participants as taking up and progressing to different, discrete roles serially, e.g. speaker becomes hearer in the next turn. CA offers a more co-participatory model, and we will argue that the investigation of scaffolding should focus on the organisation of all parties' activities *concurrently*.

From dyadic social scaffolding to co-participatory social scaffolding

In designing their ongoing participation in the learning activities, the LSA and teacher not only require a reflexive orientation to the student's actions, but also to each other. Such co-scaffolding of teaching colleagues' actions may be a common feature in the tuition of these exceptional learners' development, where high pupil staff ratios are common. Analysis of the organisation of scaffolding can thus be usefully extended to incorporate the management and coordination of co-tutors' (or indeed other co-interactants') activities in the current participation framework.

In the episode that we have examined, the respective tutor activities appeared somewhat asymmetric. CA offers useful tools to describe asymmetry in participants' contributions to an interaction (see Drew and Heritage 1992). For example, Ginny generally delivers support in the response phase when Nigel has finished giving instructions. In designing and delivering this support, Ginny must not only observe Helen's actions, but also monitor the teacher's directives and over-arching scaffolding of the learning activity. Throughout its delivery, she must continue to monitor Nigel's actions, and reflect upon the implications for her own scaffolding activities. For example, in Extract 10.3, although Nigel can observe that Ginny may be mobilising for a redoing at line 15, Nigel also issues advice for the management of that redoing – 'count slowly'. This has import not only for Helen, but possibly for Ginny who must coordinate her movement over the blocks with the tempo of Helen's talk.

As with repair styles discussed above, there is some apparent division of labour in the delivery of tutor scaffolding. Nigel manages and often manipulates the physical objects that represent the mathematical problems with which the parties are working. Ginny does not engage directly with the objects. Much of Nigel's contribution to the interaction involves talk. Ginny uses less talk, although this may be about 'doing' a teaching support role, which both minimises any disruption to teacher-led activities and augments the modes of access available to Helen. Thus, both teacher and LSA are working collaboratively in pursuit of Helen's learning. One interesting feature is that Helen, despite the severe social impairment implied in her diagnosis, may recognise that her tutors have distinctive classroom roles.

Helen sometimes displays actions which suggest an ongoing engagement with the classroom proceedings, and the scaffolding work embedded in them. For example, she plays a role in designing the scaffolding of her own learning by forming her forefinger into a point as a counting tool (Extracts 10.3 and 10.4). This follows the placement of her hand on Ginny's prior to commencing counting. It is difficult to judge who may be leading the arm/hand movements from one block to another, but Helen must at least be passively collaborating in the procedure. This co-activity suggests some common motivation and collaborative action design which involves co-monitoring of *all* participants to the interaction.

There are also some occasions within these data when Helen's withdrawal from co-participation also has implications for the design of the parties' actions, e.g. she covers her ears. These actions (often labelled stereotypical behaviour, or attributed to auditory hypersensitivity) may represent significant constraints upon the management and effectiveness of scaffolding. As the progress of learning requires the student's active co-participation, when Helen withdraws, staff have to reconstruct the scaffolding in order to solicit or regain her attention to their actions.

Here, noise emanating from other participants' activities may well be impacting upon the student's willingness or ability to engage with these learning tasks. Some scaffolding work at the environmental level may be helpful in these circumstances, e.g. the provision of acoustically insulated environments. In the absence of these, the tutors appear to display a sensitivity to the impact of the local auditory events on Helen's scaffolding needs, and the scaffold seems to be reformulated in light of the learner's intermittent displays of fluctuating competence, and her current engagement with the learning environment.

The use of non-vocal resources in supporting learning

Helen's propensity to cover her ears may encourage her tutors to design non-spoken actions that are more likely to attract her visual attention. CA's attention to the sequential placement of actions can help us to understand what information is available to the various parties as they design their subsequent contributions to learning encounters.

Much work on scaffolding tacitly assumes that classroom talk is the primary vehicle for eliciting and displaying knowledge, and Stone prioritises 'verbal regulation of tasks' as a scaffolding strategy for students with learning difficulties. However, a key component of the LSA's scaffolding of block-counting used non-vocal resources. It is possible to think of the subsequent counting activity in Extract 10.3 (where a second hand is placed on Helen's during the recount) as a negative scaffolding strategy, decreasing the learner's autonomy (see Biemiller and Meichenbaum 1998). However, fine-grained analysis of the placement of this action appears to be *responsive* to the student's skills as they are displayed, rather than being symptomatic of some retrograde practice in LD classrooms. Curiously, the non-vocal support appears designed to (and succeeds in) student production of talk and the conduct of a different activity (speaking a number sequence). The production of one type of activity in response to actions delivered in another quite different modality in a student with autism and such severe learning needs may surprise some readers who are familiar with the learning challenges that typify this population (e.g. rigid thinking, difficulties with generalising learning, etc.). Thus, consideration of non-vocal activities in analyses of scaffolding activities may be highly relevant where the learner has quite exceptional needs.

Finally, CA's capacity to describe how both spoken and non-spoken resources are managed in the collaborative building of social action may be useful if evaluating some of the many 'interactional' educational intervention, e.g. the 'intensive interaction' programme discussed by Nind and Powell (2000).

Conclusions

While the limits of the database analysed here (just one interaction) preclude the drawing of highly generalisable conclusions, we have nevertheless sought to demonstrate how conversation analysis offers analytic levers that can facilitate exploration of all parties' contributions to scaffolding in pedagogic interaction. It has provided some useful insights into the possibilities for exploring the scaffolding of co-taught lessons – for example, how different types of activity might elicit different levels of support from the LSA.

One focus of analysis has been the student's activities. Although Helen occasionally withdraws from interacting, she frequently displays considerable willingness to engage in learning activities. Her participation may reflect a number of interactional competencies, a matter we have discussed elsewhere (e.g. Dickerson *et al.* 2007; Stribling *et al.* 2007). An incidental finding here is that Helen also manages to perform actions in one modality based on inferences drawn from instructions delivered in another modality, suggesting that she is at least learning to be flexible in mediating between the scaffolding and her own actions, and may have a structure available for the management of imitation in the Vygotskian sense. Whatever insights Helen may be gaining into elementary subtraction procedures, the scaffolding with objects may be facilitating her learning about the management of certain participation frameworks, and thereby enhance her zone of proximal development.

A range of previous work has attempted to refocus upon interactional processes rather than the outcomes of scaffolding. Although previous research has sought to advance a theory of mutuality in scaffolding, studies typically lack a fine-grained analysis of the recipient-sensitive management of learning support, and of the part played by students' orientations to scaffolding activities. As they stand, they tacitly presuppose that adult scaffolding activities are both supportive of student learning, and development in the ZPD. CA offers the possibility of attaining detailed empirical evidence to advance empirically derived knowledge into learning processes.

Acknowledgements

This work arises from an award funded by the ESRC (RES-000-22-0865 – Interactional Competencies in Children with an Autistic Spectrum Disorder); we gratefully acknowledge their support and the support of our colleague Dr Paul Dickerson who was the Principal Investigator on that award. We are also grateful for discussions with numerous colleagues in numerous contexts.

Special thanks to the participants for allowing their conduct to be recorded and studied.

References

American Psychiatric Association (1995) *Diagnostic and statistical manual of mental disorders (4th Edition)*. Washington: American Psychiatric Association.

Baron-Cohen, S. (1995) *Mindblindness: An essay on autism and theory of mind*. Cambridge, MA: MIT Press.

Bellon, M.L., Ogletree, B.T. and Harn, W.E. (2000) Repeated storybook reading as a language intervention for children with autism: A case study on the application of scaffolding. *Focus on Autism and Other Developmental Disabilities*, **15** (1), 52–58.

Biemiller, A. and Meichenbaum, D. (1998) The consequences of negative scaffolding for students who learn slowly – A commentary on C. Addison Stone's 'The metaphor of scaffolding: Its utility for the field of learning disabilities'. *Journal of Learning Disabilities*, **31** (4), 365–369.

Cazden, C.B. (1979) Peekaboo as an instructional model: Discourse development at home and at school. In *Papers and reports on child language development* (No. 17). Palo Alto, CA: Stanford University Department of Linguistics.

Chaiklin S. (2003) The ZPD in Vygotsky's analysis of learning and instruction. In A. Kozulin, B. Gindis, V.S. Ageyev and S.M. Miller (eds), *Vygotsky's educational theory in cultural context* (pp. 39–64). Cambridge: Cambridge University Press.

Curcio, F. (1978) Sensorimotor functioning and communication in mute autistic children. *Journal of Autism and Childhood Schizophrenia*, **8**, 281–292.

Dickerson, P., Stribling, P. and Rae, J. (2007) Tapping into interaction: How children with autistic spectrum disorders design and place tapping in relation to activities in progress. *Gesture*, **7**, 271–303.

Dobbinson, S., Perkins, M.R. and Boucher, J. (1998) Structural patterns in conversations with a woman who has autism. *Journal of Communication Disorders*, **31**, 113–134.

Dobbinson, S., Perkins, M. and Boucher, J. (2003) The interactional significance of formulas in autistic language. *Clinical Linguistics and Phonetics*, **17**, 299–307.

Drew, P. and Heritage, J. (1992) *Talk at work: Interaction in institutional settings*. Cambridge: Cambridge University Press.

Feuerstein R. (1980) *Instrumental enrichment*. Baltimore, MD: University Park Press.

Forrester, M.A. and Pike, C.D. (1998) Learning to estimate in the mathematics classroom: A conversation-analytic approach. *Journal for Research in Mathematics Education*, **29**, 334–356.

Goodwin, C. (1995) Co-constructing meaning in conversations with an aphasic man. *Research on Language and Social Interaction*, **28**, 233–260.

Goodwin, C. (2007) Participation, stance, and affect in the organization of activities. *Discourse and Society*, **18**, 53–73.

Grandin, T. (1996) *Thinking in pictures*. New York: Doubleday.

Heap, J. (1985) Discourse in the production of classroom knowledge: Reading lessons. *Curriculum Inquiry*, **15**, 245–279.

Jacoby, S. and Ochs, E. (1995) Co-construction: An introduction. *Research on Language and Social Interaction*, **28**, 171–183.

Kidwell, M. (2005) Gaze as social control: How very young children differentiate the look from a mere look by their adult caregivers. *Research on Language and Social Interaction*, **38**, 417–449.

Kidwell, M. and Zimmerman, D.H. (2006) Observability in the interactions of very young children. *Communication Monographs*, **73**, 1–28.

Kidwell, M. and Zimmerman, D.H. (2007) Joint attention as action. *Journal of Pragmatics*, **39**, 592–611.

Koegel, R.L. and Mentis, M. (1985) Motivation in childhood autism: can they or won't they? *Journal of Child Psychology and Psychiatry*, **26** (2), 185–191.

Koschmann, T., LeBaron, C., GoodwIn C., Zemel, A. and Dunnington, G. (2007) Formulating the triangle of doom. *Gesture*, 7, 97–118.

Kozulin A. (2003) Psychological tools and mediated learning. In A. Kozulin, B. Gindis, V.S. Ageyev and S.M. Miller (eds), *Vygotsky's educational theory in cultural context*. Cambridge: Cambridge University Press.

Langer, J.A. and Applebee, A.N. (1986) Reading and writing instruction: Toward a theory of teaching and learning. In E. Rothkopf (ed.), *Review of Research in Education*, **13** (pp. 171–194). Washington, DC: American Educational Research Association.

Lave, J. and Wenger, E. (1991) *Situated learning: Legitimate peripheral participation*. Cambridge: Cambridge University Press.

Lerner, G.H. (1995) Turn design and the organization of participation in instructional activities. *Discourse Processes*, **19**, 111–131.

Local, J. and Wootton, A.J. (1995) Interactional and phonetic aspects of immediate echolalia in autism: a case study. *Clinical Linguistics and Phonetics*, **9**, 155–184.

Macbeth, D. (2001) On reflexivity in qualitative research: Two readings, and a third. *Qualitative Inquiry*, 7, 35–68.

Macbeth, D. (2004) The relevance of repair in classroom correction. *Language in Society*, **33**, 703–736.

Markee, N. (2005) The organization of off-task talk in second language classrooms. In K. Richards and P. Seedhouse (eds), *Applying conversation analysis* (pp. 197–213). Basingstoke: Palgrave Macmillan.

Mascolo, M.F. (2005) Change processes in development: The concept of coactive scaffolding. *New Ideas in Psychology*, **23**, 185–196.

McDermott, R.P. (1977) Social relations as contexts for learning in school. *Harvard Educational Review*, **47**, 198–213.

McHoul, A. (1978) The organization of turns at formal talk in the classroom. *Language in Society*, 7, 183–213.

McHoul, A. (1990) The organization of repair in classroom talk. *Language in Society*, **19**, 349–377.

Mehan, H. (1979) *Learning lessons*. Cambridge, MA: Harvard University Press.

Nind, M. (1999) Efficacy of intensive interaction: Developing sociability and communication in people with severe and complex learning difficulties using on approach based on caregiver–infant interaction. *European Journal of Special Needs Education*, **11** (1), 48–66.

Nind, M. and Hewett, D. (1988) Interaction as curriculum. *British Journal of Special Education*, **15**, 55–57.

Nind, M. and Powell, D. (2000) Intensive interaction and autism: Some theoretical concerns. *Children and Society*, **14**, 98–109.

Ornitz, E.M. (1985) Neurophysiology of infantile autism. *Journal of the American Academy of Child Psychiatry*, **24**, 251–262.

Ornitz, E.M. (1988) Autism: A disorder of directed attention. *Brain Dysfunction*, **1**, 309–322.

Palincsar, A.S. and Brown, A.L. (1984) Reciprocal teaching of comprehension-fostering and comprehension-monitoring activities. *Cognition and Instruction*, **1**, 117–175.

Pea, R.D. (1993) Learning scientific concepts through material and social activities: Conversational analysis meets conceptual change. *Educational Psychologist*, **28**, 265–277.

Rasku-Puttonen, H., Eteläpelto, A., Arvaja, M. and Häkkinen, P. (2003) Is successful scaffolding an illusion? Shifting patterns of responsibility and control in teacher-student interaction during a long-term learning project. *Instructional Science*, **31**, 377–393.

Ridley, J., Radford, J. and Mahon, M. (2002) How do teachers manage topic and repair? *Child Language Teaching and Therapy*, **18**, 43–58.

Roberts, J.M.A. (1989) Echolalia and comprehension in autistic children. *Journal of Autism and Developmental Disorders*, **19**, 271–281.

Sacks, H. (1992) *Lectures on conversation: Volumes I and II*. Oxford: Blackwell.

Schegloff, E.A. (2007) *Sequence organization in interaction: A primer in conversation analyis* (Volume 1). Cambridge: Cambridge University Press.

Schegloff, E.A., Jefferson, G. and Sacks, H. (1977) The preference for self-correction in the organization of repair in conversation. *Language*, **53**, 361–382.

Schön, D. (1983) *The reflective practitioner: How professionals think in action*. London: Temple Smith.

Schopler, E. and Mesibov, G.B. (eds) (1985) *Communication problems in autism*. New York: Plenum Press.

Silliman, E.R., Bahr, R., Beasman, J. and Wilkinson, L.C. (2000) Scaffolds for learning to read in an inclusion classroom. *Language, Speech, and Hearing Services in Schools*, **31**, 265–279.

Stiegler, L.N. (2007) Discovering communicative competencies in a non-speaking child with autism. *Language, Speech and Hearing Services in Schools*, **38**, 400–413.

Stone, C.A. (1998) The metaphor of scaffolding: Its utility for the field of learning disabilities. *Journal of Learning Disabilities*, **31**, 344–364.

Streeck, J. (1996) How to do things with things: *Objets trouvés* and symbolization. *Human Studies*, **19**, 365–384.

Stribling, P., Rae, J. and Dickerson, P. (2007) Two forms of spoken repetition in a girl with autism. *International Journal of Language and Communication Disorders*, **42**, 427–444.

Stribling, P., Rae, J. and Dickerson, P. (2009) The facilitation of learning opportunities for a student with an autism spectrum disorder and severe learning difficulties. (Unpublished manuscript).

Tarplee, C. and Barrow, E. (1999) Delayed echoing as an interactional resource: A case study of a 3-year-old child on the autistic spectrum. *Clinical Linguistics and Phonetics*, **13**, 449–482.

Tzuriel, D., Kaniel, S., Kanner, E. and Haywood, H.S. (1999) Effects of the 'Bright-Start' programme in kindergarten on transfer and academic achievement. *Early Childhood Research Quarterly*, **14**, 111–141.

Vygotsky, L.S. (1978) *Mind in society: The development of higher psychological processes*. M. Cole, V. John-Steiner, S. Scribner and E. Souberman (eds). Cambridge, MA: Harvard University Press.

Vygotsky, L. (1986) *Thought and language*. Cambridge, MA: MIT Press.

Wang, X.-L., Bernas, R. and Eberhard, P. (2001) Effects of teachers' verbal and non-verbal scaffolding on everyday classroom performances of students with Down syndrome. *International Journal of Early Years Education*, **9**, 71–80.

Wertsch, J.V. (2007) Mediation. In H. Daniels, M. Cole and J.V. Wertsch (eds), *The Cambridge companion to Vygotsky*. Cambridge: Cambridge University Press.

Wood, D., Bruner, J.S. and Ross, G. (1976) The role of tutoring in problem solving. *Journal of Child Psychology and Psychiatry and Allied Disciplines*, **17**, 89–100.

Wootton, A.J. (1997) *Interaction and the development of mind*. Cambridge: Cambridge University Press.

Wootton, A.J. (1999) An investigation of delayed echoing in a child with autism. *First Language*, **19**, 359–381.

Appendix 10.1 Transcript of a stretch of classroom interaction involving a girl with an autistic spectrum disorder

Extended extract 'Helen One Block' (Simplified)

Annotations above lines of talk are Helen's, unless others indicated. The start of Extracts 10.1–10.4 is shown.

((Extract 10.1, Block-removal sequence 1))

1 Nigel: Now: Helen: (------)   listen

2   (---------1-)

3 Nigel: **I1▶** I'm going to take awa:y:

4   (-----)

              [raises head looks at Nigel
5 Helen: [Take way take away

                 [lowers hands reaches left-hand most block
6 Nigel: **I1▶** One [block

    R1▶   *[arm extended offering block to N*
7 Helen: One block [one block

8 Nigel: [Good girl
               [N takes block
               ((there are now four blocks on the table))

9 Nigel: Excellent well done

((Extract 10.3, Block-counting sequence 1))

```
10  Nigel: I3▶    How many blocks 'ave you left

                              [touches Ginny's hand
                              [briefly points
11  Helen:        Got left got left [got lef[t
    Ginny:                          [offers R hand

                          [points index finger
12  Ginny:        [        ° han[d°            ]

                  [moves and removes L hand]
13  Ginny:        >How many<

                  ((G guides H's hand, counting the blocks, L to R))
                         touching blocks
                  ┌───────────────────────────┐
14  Helen: R3▶    °o:ne° (.) two:: three: (four) five °si°

15  Nigel:        [Count slow[ly
    Ginny:        [          [L hand moves in
                  [hand moves back to L handmost block

16  Ginny:        °(          )°

                  ((G guides H's hand, counting the blocks, L to R))
                         touching blocks
                  ┌───────────────────────────┐
17  Helen: R3▶    one two: three: four: (– [ –) four four four
    Ginny:                              [releases G's hand

18  Nigel:        Good girl well done

19               (––––––––––1–)
                  └───────────────┘
                  N replaces block on the table
```

((Extract 10.2, Block-removal sequence 2))

```
20  Nigel:        Now. (––––––––)

                              [looks at N
21  Nigel: I2▶    can [you:.(––[––––)  [take away
    Helen:            [          [(°you°)  [
                      [point at          [grasping
                      [H's abdomen       [gesture

22  Nigel: I2▶    (––[––––)    [two blocks
    Helen:           [>take aw[ay<
                     [two fingers

23  Helen:        (Two blocks)

24               (–––––––––1––––––)
```

25   Nigel: **I3▶**   [Take away (.) two blocks?
                      [*lowers two fingers*

26   (---------1---------2---------3

27   Ginny: °C'n you do it then°°

28   Helen: (uurh)

29   Ginny: °yours<u>e</u>lf°

30   Helen: (urh)

31   Ginny: °r<u>ea</u>dy°

        R2▶   *Looks at N*
                  picks up block 2nd from left and hands to N

32   ⌐————————————————————⌐
                  (---------1---------2----)

33   Nigel: One

        R2▶   *picks up block 3rd from right and hands to N*

34   ⌐————————————————————————⌐
                  (---------1---------2---------3-----

35   Nigel: Good Girl
                 ((*there are now three blocks on the table*))

36   Nigel: Excellent. Well done?

((Extract 10.4, Block-counting sequence 2))

37   Nigel: **I4▶**   [and how many blocks do you have] left
                      [*moves blocks closer together   *]

38   (Helen):   (have left) (have left) (have [left)
     Ginny: [*offers R hand*

39   (- - - - - - - [–1 –   [– –)
     Ginny: [[*brings in L hand*
     Helen: [*lowers hand*
                                 and points

                 ((*G guides H's hand, counting the blocks, L to R*))
                   touching blocks

                 ⌐—————————————⌐
40   Helen: **R4▶**   one two three:: (–[–)
                                        [*looks at N*

41   Nigel: Excellent well done Helen very very well done

Chapter 11

Multi-modal participation in storybook sharing

JULIE RADFORD and MERLE MAHON

Introduction

The data discussed in this chapter involves the early classroom experiences of children with language learning needs. We include children with specific speech and language difficulties (SSLD) (Dockrell *et al.* 2006). These children are also referred to in the literature as having specific language impairment (SLI). We also include deaf children from hearing families who are being educated in a natural oral environment (using hearing aids or cochlear implants). [The word 'deaf' is used here to refer to children who have permanent, prelingual sensori-neural hearing impairments which are of sufficient severity to lead to problems in communication using spoken language. This use of the term 'deaf' is not to be confused with the term 'Deaf' which is currently used in the UK when referring to the Deaf community and culture whose mode of communication is sign, and for whom British Sign Language (BSL) is their first and home language.]

Our main research interest concerns how such children are provided with opportunities for language learning through discourse with their teacher (a familiar adult), the ways in which they demonstrate uptake of these opportunities and the role of non-verbal resources of gaze and gesture in such discourse. Although sharing a storybook is a frequently used context for language learning with all young children, rarely has the discourse been examined from a multi-modal perspective. In particular, in this chapter we intend to explore how the child's use of speech, gesture and gaze is coordinated with the adult's verbal and non-verbal resources. As we hope to demonstrate through conversation analysis, the nature and timing of manual gestures and gaze have significant implications for the child's interactional competencies.

Storybook sharing

Good oral skills are vitally important during a child's early years because they lay the foundation for emergent literacy skills. Deaf children and children who have SSLD may be particularly disadvantaged and therefore require high quality language learning experiences in the first years of life. For all young children, adult–child storybook sharing is widely acknowledged as a significant site for developing oral language skills. Given that joint attention facilitates language acquisition for most children (Tomasello 2003; see also Tarplee and Wootton, Chapters 1 and 4 in this volume), the reciprocal nature of looking at a picture book offers a valuable shared visual resource (Liboiron and Soto 2006). Studies of typically developing young children in storybook sharing with parents and other adults demonstrate gains in a variety of language parameters: expressive and receptive vocabulary (Soresby and Martlew 1980; Ninio 1983; Senechal 1997) and morpho-syntax (Bradshaw *et al.* 1998).

As far as the classroom is concerned, storybook reading provides a language enrichment activity where the teacher can promote the learning of vocabulary and syntax. When the adult uses techniques, such as expansion of the child's previous turn, or oral prompting of a missing word (cloze procedure), children produce more complex grammar and multi-word combinations (Bradshaw *et al.* 1998). Speech and language therapists also increasingly recognise naturalistic settings, such as storybook sharing, as a key intervention context for children with language delay or impairment (Fey *et al.* 1995). How the adult's language is tailored to the emerging linguistic abilities of the child is crucial for the success of language intervention (Gioia 2001; Kaderavek and Justice 2002).

Within a socio-interactionist perspective on language acquisition (Bruner 1983; Vygotsky 1986), the child's active participation during storybook sharing is crucial. Indeed, where children are active participants, through dialogic reading experience, they make more significant gains in expressive vocabulary than children who receive regular reading episodes (Hargrave and Senechal 2000). Therefore, while a dialogic intervention context has a clear advantage, there are potential risks for children with language learning difficulties. Whereas typically developing children frequently initiate and elaborate topics during storybook reading (Rabidoux and MacDonald 2000), children with SSLD often respond minimally or, at worst, remain passive (Crowe 2000). This is similarly reported for deaf children, in studies where the controlling nature of teacher or parent interaction styles is reported (Wood *et al.*1986; Swanwick and Watson 2007), and this holds whether sign language or spoken language is the mode of communication (Williams 2004; Plessow-Wolfson and Epstein 2005).

A further concern is that the child's active involvement may be reduced if the adult fails to be sensitive and responsive to the child's initiations and current linguistic abilities (Kaderavek and Justice 2002). It is surprising, then, that studies principally concentrate on the adult's strategies, whereas the interactional resources available to the child have been rarely studied in any depth. What is needed is a better understanding of how *children's* contributions are produced, including both verbal and non-verbal resources such as gaze and gesture.

Gesture and gaze

Goodwin and Goodwin (1986) noted that a recipient's gaze towards the speaker is not an accidental alignment, but that within an interactional activity, the alignment of gaze is systematically achieved by the participants. That this is the case for the teacher and child, in the storybook sharing activities in our data, will be demonstrated in the analysis below. In addition, it is a feature of our data that the children co-construct gaze with gesture. By gesture here, we mean manual gestures that are hand movements used to convey information in communicating during periods of mutual attention (Goldin-Meadow 2003; Ozcaliskan and Goldin-Meadow 2005). Integrating such manual gestures with words is part of effective human communication (McNeill 1992) and use of gesture has been shown to be an important and fundamental developmental step in language acquisition (Iverson and Goldin-Meadow 2005; Ozkaliskan and Goldin-Meadow 2005). Volterra *et al.* (2004) suggest that gesture–speech combinations serve to reinforce intended meaning, especially when the child's speech is not fully intelligible. This is particularly relevant for children with SSLD and for deaf children. As children become more competent speakers, gestures are not simply replaced by words, but, as Volterra *et al.* (2004: 22) suggest, 'vocal and gestural modalities are used together'. That this is the case for deaf children was shown in a recent longitudinal study by Klatter-Folmer *et al.* (2006) who noted that for the deaf children, over time, 'mixed (signed and speech) utterances consisting of either simultaneous or alternating language elements are a crucial communication mode'(p. 247). Deaf children's use of gesture has not been studied as much as might be expected, but there is consensus about the crucial role of gesture in their communication (Wedell-Monig and Lumley 1980; Spencer 1993; Goldin-Meadow 2003, 2007). There is even less research into gestures used by children with speech and language difficulties, but here too, the essential nature of the gesture for conveying meaning is reported (Ellis *et al.* 1993; Evans *et al.* 2001; Capone and McGregor 2004; Blake *et al.* 2008). What has not been researched in any detail is the way in which gesture is used interactionally when children and adults talk to each other, in particular, in the talk with children who have language and communication difficulties. In their paper on word search activity between adult interlocutors, Goodwin and Goodwin (1986) revealed how the participants used non-verbal but visible components of each other's turns (gestures, gaze and gaze shifts) in their organisation of this activity. In our sequential analysis set out below, we will demonstrate the interactional work accomplished by our dyads using such turn components.

The conversation analysis (CA) method adopted in this chapter takes the perspective of the participants as opposed to analytical methods which use predetermined categories. In this chapter, with respect to the description of gestures, we include gesture types that have been described by others in the research literature (e.g. Guidetti and Nicoladis 2008) Thus we show examples of *conventional* gestures whose form and meaning are culturally defined (e.g. nodding head for 'yes') and *representational* gestures (aka 'iconic', 'characterising' or 'symbolic' gestures) where the form of the gesture refers to specific referents like objects, actions, persons, events and the meaning of the gesture does not change with different contexts (for example, putting hands together at side of face indicating 'sleep'). The categorisation systems of gesture that have been used in other research with young children (Goldin-Meadow 2003; Gullberg 2008) would have proved inadequate for our data. One complicating issue for the analysis was that our youngsters are older and therefore produce grammatically longer and semantically more complex turns than those studied by Iverson and Goldin-Meadow (2005). In our analysis, we will simply describe the form of manual gestures used by the children and the teachers, while the meaning of a gesture will be found in the response to that gesture by the interlocutor.

Participants

The two deaf children in this study, Frankie and Kevin, have severe to profound hearing losses. Frankie has a cochlear implant in his right ear, and Kevin wears bilateral digital hearing aids. Neither child uses sign language at home, nor are they formally taught sign language at school, but natural gesture is a feature of their communication and of the communication of their teachers. They are being educated in a unit for deaf children within a mainstream primary school, where they are taught by specially trained and experienced teachers of the deaf, as well as being integrated with hearing children for some of their lessons.

The two children with specific speech and language difficulties, Ben and Marcia, are educated in a language resource base attached to a mainstream nursery and infant school. The resource base is staffed by a speech and language therapist and two very experienced teachers who have additional specialist qualifications in the field of teaching children with specific speech and language difficulties. Given the discrepancy with their relatively good non-verbal abilities (e.g. puzzle completion, drawing), Ben and Marcia's language and communication profiles are typical of children with specific language impairment (see Tables 11.1 and 11.2). Note that all the illustrations in this chapter are reconstructed from the original video footage using actors.

Analysis and findings

Role of child's gesture in turn bidding and turn holding

Our argument is that both the timing and the nature of the child's gesture have interactional significance. With respect to timing, this is particularly noticeable in the onset of the gesture, which occurs in overlap with the teacher's verbal turn. The overlap is

Table 11.1 Participant details

Name	Age	Education	*Language and communication profile
Ben	4 years and 4 months	Language resource base	Moderate receptive and expressive language difficulties, including moderate problems with word meaning and naming
Marcia	4 years and 8 months	Language resource base	Severe receptive and expressive language difficulties, including severe problems with word meaning and naming Mild phonological difficulty
Kevin	6 years	Unit for deaf children within a mainstream primary school	Severely delayed speech and language development
Frankie	3 years 10 months	Unit for deaf children within a mainstream primary school	Delayed speech and language development

* Data obtained from child's speech and language therapist and teacher

Table 11.2 Language learning targets and programme

Name	*Language learning targets	*Main intervention strategies
Ben	To improve expressive syntax i.e. subject verb object (SVO) constructions. To maintain topic in conversation	To re-focus his attention To give opportunities for repetition To use structured small group work
Marcia	To increase receptive and expressive vocabulary To increase clarity of speech To relay a simple message	To re-focus her attention To model appropriate syntax and vocabulary To provide regular practice opportunities
Kevin	To improve use and understanding of classroom vocabulary To use spoken vocabulary To label object + action events in class To improve turn-taking	To give K opportunities to practice in individual sessions To model speech To give opportunities to practice in group and individual sessions
Frankie	To improve use and understanding of classroom vocabulary To understand and use 2 word phrases To improve attention	To give F opportunities to practice in individual sessions To model sentences

* Data obtained from child's speech and language therapist and teacher

not treated as being turn-competitive, and the next turn is secured for the child. With respect to the nature of the gesture: if the gesture is sustained either by repeated gestural movements (e.g. miming playing a flute with fingers moving up and down) or by maintaining a gestural movement (e.g. holding a cupped hand behind the ear), the turn is held. Inextricable from gesture is the interactional significance of gaze and that will be discussed at length in a later section.

We will illustrate the above points with examples of data from three child-teacher dyads.

In the case of Marcia (Extract 11.1) the analysis will highlight the timing of her gesture at line 69. The onset of the gesture enables her to bid for a turn at that juncture, despite the fact that the start of her verbal contribution is delayed until the teacher has completed her verbal input.

In order to interpret the data extracts below, in addition to the usual CA transcription conventions, we also use the following notation (Damico and Simmons-Mackie 2002):

Gesture: each gesture is explained in the key presented beneath each extract
Gaze: maintenance and direction of gaze is indicated thus:

T   x book...
M   x book...

Gaze shift is shown by commas, for example when M shifts her gaze from *book* to *T* and back to *book*, thus:

M   x..book...,,,.T,,,book

Extract 11.1 *Marcia (has specific language difficulties, aged 4 years 8 months)*

The shared book is a familiar story called 'Smarty Pants'. At the beginning of line 69 a new page is turned and revealed to both participants.

```
67   T:   What comes next do you remember,

68   M:   Smarty pants

     T:   T  x book...............................................
          M  x book...............................................
69        [     Smarty pants again (.)   [an:d,
          [((T turns page
→    M:                                  [(((ªgesture

          T  x ...M hands...............................................
          M  x..book...,,,.T,,,book...................,,,T,,,book
70   M:   [ fly          a↑wa:::y (.) the ↑pla::ne ]
→         [((ªgesture ᵇgesture ªgesture ::::::::))   ]
              [((T nods:::::: ))                      ]
```

[a] Hands raised at shoulder level, palms down, hands cupped, moved up and down. See Figure 11.1.
[b] Right hand briefly moved to side and then movement continued as in gesture described at ([a]) above.

The teacher (T) receives an answer to her question at line 68 and, although she receives M's response with a repeat at 69 ('smarty pants'), she pursues the topic with a designedly incomplete utterance (DIU) ('an:d') (Gardner 1995; Koshik 2002; Radford 2009). The DIU has features of sound stretching and level intonation (indicated by ',') which suggest an invitation for M to continue with a syntactically and semantically fitted contribution. However, the onset of M's gesture is earlier as it overlaps with the DIU. Furthermore, the gesture precedes M's 'official' verbal take up of the turn at line 70, indicated by her use of words alongside continuation of the gesture. As the onset of M's gesture and verbal contributions are not aligned, our claim is that using the gesture at this point in time secures the turn for M.

The nature of Marcia's gesture at line 70 also warrants detailed attention because it appears to enable her to hold the turn (see Figure 11.1). The gesture is formed with a sustained movement throughout the whole of line 70 in the sense that the hands are in continuous motion while she is speaking. A significant observation, given Marcia's specific language difficulties, is that having secured the turn in this way, she then produces a relatively long verbal turn. The evidence for this turn-holding claim is that T could have taken the turn at the potential verbal transition relevance place (TRP) (the brief pause between 'fly away' and 'the plane') but, instead, chooses to nod in receipt and does not bid for a verbal turn herself until the gesture is completed. Syntactically speaking, Marcia is thus afforded the opportunity to produce not only a verb ('fly away') but also a noun phrase ('the plane').

In our second child–teacher dyad (Extract 11.2), our analysis will show how Frankie bids for the turn (line 64) using gesture, and how by sustaining his gesture he holds the turn in non-competitive overlap with the teacher's next turn (lines 65–66), effectively sharing the turn with T. As was the case for Marcia, the interactional significance of gaze in this example will be fully discussed later.

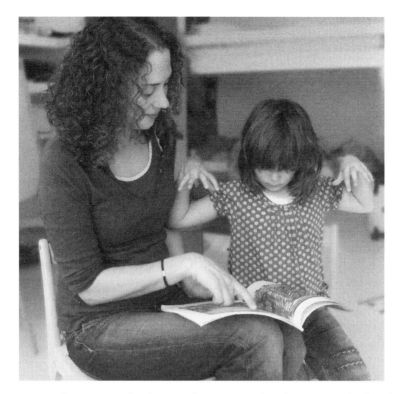

Figure 11.1 Marcia (fly away). Used with parental permission. Photo by Laura Sandwell, with permission.

Extract 11.2 *Frankie 1 (is a prelingually deaf child, aged 3 years 10 months)*

Frankie and his teacher T are looking at photos of a recent school trip and are currently looking down at a picture of the children and other commuters waiting on the station platform.

```
       T x..book...............x
   62  F:  F x..book...............x
           [wait!              ]
           [((ªgesture))       ]

       T x..book...............................................,,,F......x
       F x..book.................,,,T.........................................x
   63  T:  Oh[   wait   ] ok (.)  [everybody's waiting ] that man's waiting]
             [((ªgesture))]       [((points to book))      ]
→  64  F:                         [((ᵇgesture:::::::::::::::::::::::::::::::::::::::=

       T x F.................................................,,,book..............................x
       Fx..T.................................................,,,book..............................x
→  65  T:  [can you hear the train ((makes noise of train))]
           [((ᶜgesture::::::::::::::::::::::::::::::::::::::::::  ]
```

→   66   F: [=ᵇ*gesture*:::] [((smiles))

    67   T: **[ahh you might be right]**

                                            [((*turns page*))]

ᵃ F holds both hands up, palms facing T and moves both hands down slightly.

ᵇ Turns head slightly upwards to fact T, raises cupped hand to hold it around ear, see Figure 11.2.

ᶜ Raises hand to ear holds two fingers up to ear.

Frankie has initiated talk using a gesture and the word 'wait' (line 62). T receipts this by repeating both word and gesture at the start of her turn in line 63, 'oh wait ok (.)'. There is a potential TRP after she says 'ok' (line 63) and Frankie makes a strong gesture, putting his cupped hand to his ear (line 64 and Figure 11.2), thus arguably bidding for the turn. However, T takes the turn, expanding the topic by adding information 'everybody's waiting, that man's waiting'. Frankie sustains his gesture unchanged while she continues her expansion; his sustained gesture overlapping T's expanded turn. T now takes another turn (line 65), overlapping Frankie's sustained gesture, saying 'can you hear the train' and making train noises as well as using a slightly altered (reduced) version of Frankie's gesture (two fingers held up to her ear). Frankie only ends his gesture (line 66) after T has made the train noises. The observation we make here is that because of the timing and nature of F's gesture, the overlap is not competitive, and Frankie and T effectively share the turn.

Another example of a shared turn is found in the data for our third child–teacher dyad (Extract 11.3). Here the sequence is initiated by T who uses a gesture to accompany her verbal turn in line 60.

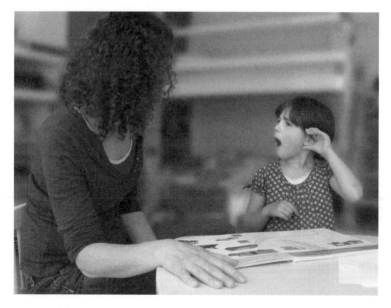

Figure 11.2 Frankie (train listen). Used with parental permission. Photo by Laura Sandwell, with permission.

Extract 11.3   *Kevin (is a prelingually deaf child, aged 6 years)*

T and Kevin are sharing a storybook about a boy going to have a haircut.

```
→  60  T:   [hair                              ]
            [(((points to head briefly, ᵃgesture))]

            T x..K...........................................................
            K x..T...........................................................
→  61  K:   [i: a:::h      ]  (.5)  [u-          i::           ]
            [((ᵇgesture::::::::::::::  ᶜgesture::::::::::::::::::::::::))]
       T:   [((nods))      ]        [                          ]

            T x..,,,K.........................................................
            K x..T...........................................................
→  62  T:   [yeah cut it ]  (.)   [too long                    ]
            [((ᵈgesture))]        [((shakes head, ᵉgesture))]
```

ᵃ T raises cupped hand to touch hair, brings hand down in combing motion.
ᵇ K raises claw handshape to head, see Figure 11.3.
ᶜ K moves open hand, palm down, around head, opening and closing spread fingers, see Figure 11.4.
ᵈ T raises hand to head opening and closing index and middle fingers.
ᵉ T moves hand from top of head down to shoulder.

T has initiated talk in line 60 saying 'hair' and gesturing – raising her hand to her hair and moving it down using a combing motion. In line 61 Kevin mimics a reduced form of T's prior gesture: he raises a claw hand to his head, sustaining the location of the gesture, although he does not perform a combing motion (see Figure 11.3). He simultaneously

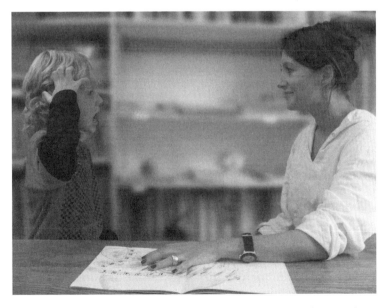

Figure 11.3 Kevin (hair). This image was reconstructed with actors. Used with parental permission. Photo by Laura Sandwell, with permission.

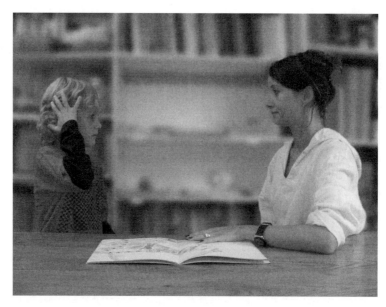

Figure 11.4 Kevin (hair cutting). This image was reconstructed with actors. Used with parental permission. Photo by Laura Sandwell, with permission.

vocalises two vowels. T receipts this gesture with an overlapping nod (line 62), but she does not take the turn at the TRP. Kevin has kept his hand in the location of his gesture in line 61, and he then continues the turn, using a changed gesture in the same location: he adds a further expansion to the topic by moving his hand across his head, opening and closing his fingers in a scissors movement (see Figure 11.4). Arguably, by sustaining his gesture in line 61, K successfully bids for and then holds the turn.

In these three data examples (Extracts 11.1–11.3), we have shown the interactional significance of both the timing and the form of the child's gesture. First, we focused on the onset of the gesture, and how it occurs in non-competitive overlap with the teacher's verbal turn and thus secures the next turn for the child. We also demonstrated how, by sustaining the gesture, a child can secure the turn, thus sharing it during the verbal contributions of the adult.

Role of held gaze in turn holding and turn sharing

Analysis of the previous extracts has shown that adults recognise the child's gesture as a valid way of gaining or holding the turn. However, any account of gesture as an isolated phenomenon is incomplete unless considered as part of a multi-modal turn including gaze and speech. The way in which our children co-construct gesture with gaze will now be examined in more detail. In particular, the direction of the speaker/gesturer's gaze is critically important in turn allocation. One example is where mutual sustained gaze serves to hold the turn for the speaker (Kevin in Extract 11.3). A further example shows, unusually, where the child's held gaze contributes to sharing of the teacher's verbal turn (Frankie in Extract 11.2). Subsequently, we shall demonstrate how the timing of a shift of gaze to the interlocutor, in our data, has interactional significance for turn transition.

Returning, firstly, to the example of Kevin and his teacher quoted above (Extract 11.3), they look at each other consistently throughout the sequence. This held gaze, in combination with Kevin's sustained gesture, enables him to hold the turn and effectively expand the topic (Extract 11.3 line 61).

In the example of Frankie and his teacher as quoted in Extract 11.2, T is looking down at the picture at the start of the talk (line 62) and she continues to look down until the penultimate word of her expansion. Meanwhile, however, Frankie has looked up at her at the onset of his gesture (line 64). He then both sustains his gesture and holds his gaze at her while she continues her expansion. She only looks up at him as she ends her turn. They then gaze at each other during her next turn in line 65. F ends his gesture, smiles and looks back down at the picture only after T has made the train noises. T also then looks down at the picture, and takes the next turn (line 67).

Role of gaze shift in mobilising participation, turn sharing and turn transition

The next example (Extract 11.4) features Ben who illustrates the complex role of gaze shift in mobilising participation, turn sharing and, possibly, in turn transition. More specifically, the timing of both of Ben's gaze shifts in line 23 has interactional significance. In terms of the first gaze shift to the teacher, we argue that it serves to mobilise her active participation in the turn, thus affording her the opportunity to share the floor with the child. A further, perhaps tentative suggestion is that when Ben's gaze is averted away from the adult, and shifted back to the book, that he is relinquishing his turn and signaling a transition point.

Extract 11.4 *Ben (who has specific language difficulties, aged 4 years 4 months)*

Ben and the teacher are reading 'Smarty Pants' together. Since the book has already been shared on many occasions, Ben is familiar with some of the sentences. He is therefore able to anticipate some of the teacher's spoken words while she points to the written words on the page.

```
16   T:   Shall we read it together? (.) [ I am a [ smarty pants rum tum
                                         [ ( ( points to words...............

17   B:                                           [smarty pants rum tum

18   T:   tie (.) here is an (.) [aeroplane (.)

19   B:                          [aeroplane me

20   T:   see::

21   B:   me f[ly

22   T:       [ly
```

```
        T    x book,,,B's hands,,,book...............................
  →     B    x ..hands.............. ,,,T........................,,,book
   23   B:      he's [  doin this            (0.8)         ]
                     [ ( (ᵃgesture::::::::::::::::::::::::::::::::::::) ) ]
        T:                        [ ( ( T nods ) )              ]

   24   T:    yes he i:s.
```

ᵃ Fists together, backs of both hands upward, moved in continuous sideways tilting movement (as if moving a joystick). See Figure 11.5.

Ben's contribution at line 23 does not come out of prior talk related to the printed words. His turn is multi-layered, formed as it is with gaze, spoken and gestural components. Our analysis of the turn will proceed sequentially. B starts producing his fists gesture (suggesting the movement of a joystick) soon after his first spoken word ('he's'). At this juncture, his gaze is directed at his hands and T's gaze suggests that she also can see the gesture. After speaking, B shifts gaze to T and continues looking at her while sustaining his gesture movements (see Figure 11.5). That T has heard him and (probably) seen his gesture is indicated by her nodding several times. Our claim here is that B has triggered her participation through the shift of gaze in her direction. An alternative interpretation of B's gaze shift to T is that it is used simply to check that T has seen the gesture. However, we discounted this explanation because of the sustained nature of B's gaze to T following the shift. Also, whereas B's hands were in her line of sight during his vocalisation, T is looking at the book during most of the time that he produces the gesture.

Ben's second shift of gaze in line 23 is also interesting. While the teacher is nodding B continues to look at her, so he clearly sees her contribution. He then shifts his gaze clearly back to the book. One interpretation is that he is simply orientating to T's gaze, which is already directed there. A further possibility that must be considered is that he is signaling that he is relinquishing the floor. Since the gaze shift coincides with cessation

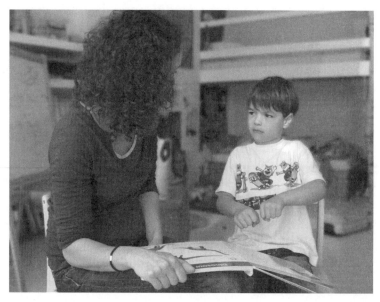

Figure 11.5 Ben (joystick). Used with parental permission. Photo by Laura Sandwell, with permission.

of the gesture is further proof of a transition relevance place. Indeed, T orients to either the gaze shift and/or end of the gesture since she then chooses to take a verbal turn (line 24).

Returning again to Frankie, in the example below (Extract 11.5 which follows on from the earlier Extract 11.2), the timing of his gaze shifts coincides with onset and then cessation of the gesture.

Extract 11.5 *Frankie 2 (is a prelingually deaf child, aged 3 years 10 months)*

T and Frankie are looking at the story of the school trip. In the Extract 11.2, T has acknow-ledged that Frankie's gesture may indicate that, in the picture, the children on the platform can hear the train coming. Having turned the page, she now calls this into question in line 69 as the next picture shows no train approaching. Their gaze is directed down at the book.

```
          T x..book...............................................................x
          F x..book...............................................................x
    69  T:  =can we hear it    [no:::                          (1)
                               [(( points to page, shakes head, ᵃgesture ))

          T x..book..................................,,,FB...................,,,book......
          F,,,T.............................................................,,,book
→   70  F:  [(( ᵇgesture::::::::::::::::::::::::::::::::::::::::::::::::::))]

→   72  T:  [still waiting               (( ᶜgesture ::::::::::))]
            [(( points quickly at book ))       (( makes train noises::::))]
                                                      (( T turns page ))

          T x..book.......................................x
          F x..book............. ..........................x
    73  FB: (( points to book ))

    74  T:  oh: HERE IT COMES (.) HERE IT COMES
```

ᵃ T turns left hand palm upwards.

ᵇ Turns head upwards to face T, raises cupped hand to hold it around ear, see Figure 11.2.

ᶜ Raises hand to ear holds two fingers up to ear.

Frankie and T are gazing down at the book. Frankie takes the turn after the transition point (line 69), shifting his gaze from the book to T and producing his gesture (line 70; and see Figure 11.2). Although she continues to look down at the picture, Frankie's gaze shifts to her, plus his overt head movement and sustained gesture arguably serves both to check that she can see his gesture and also invites her participation. This multi-layered turn is in overlap with T's verbal comment 'still waiting'(line 72), resulting in a shared turn. Frankie sustains his gesture until T shifts her gaze to him, and she then acknowledges his gesture by producing a changed (reduced) version of the gesture, while simultaneously making train noises. Only then does Frankie cease his gesture, drop his gaze, and look back down at the book. T also then shifts her gaze back to the book, turning the page.

We have shown how mutual sustained gaze serves to hold the turn for the speaker (Kevin, Extract 11.3), suggesting that the adult and the child are monitoring each other using gaze. We have also shown how held gaze contributes to turn sharing (Frankie Extracts 11.2 and 11.5) and how the timing of a gaze shift leads to turn transition.

Discussion

One of the key analytical features highlighted in the data is that our children's turns are multi-layered, composed primarily with both verbal and non-verbal behaviours. The rich descriptions of these resources presented in this chapter, by using conversation analysis, have shown how simultaneous use of speech, gaze and gesture achieves important interactional work for the children's participation in turn-bidding and turn-holding. Systematic use of gaze by a child with SSLD is also reported by Radford (2009) but operates differently. Ciara, a child who experiences significant word-finding difficulties, averts her gaze from the adult during solitary searching for words (self-repair). A more comparable finding is that Ciara shifts her gaze towards the adult when she abandons solitary searching in order to mobilise teacher participation in the word search, as was also the case in the adult word search activity reported by Goodwin and Goodwin (1986).

Our analysis now raises an important, yet rarely discussed, question in the study of child language: *'what is a turn in these data?'* While it may be widely acknowledged that a child's turn can be non-verbal (e.g. a nod of the head), rarely (if ever) have the nature and timing of children's manual gestures and gaze alongside speech been examined at a fine level of detail. A challenge for our analysis was to decide whether or not any given behaviour should be attributed as a 'turn' to the adult or the child. For instance, in Extract 4, the verbal silence during Ben's 'turn' at line 23 could have been a TRP. We decided, however, that the nature of the gesture (that it was sustained throughout the silence) held the floor for Ben while the adult nodded in acknowledgement. Indeed co-participation in turns was abundant and permitted turn-sharing between the adult and child when a held or sustained gesture was involved (see also Marcia, Extract 11.1, line 70; Frankie, Extract 11.2 lines 64 to 66 and Kevin, Extract 11.3, line 61).

In the literature on interactions with deaf children there has not been a focus on this level of sequential detail, with turn-taking being categorised in terms of either 'vocal' or 'gestural' (Tait *et al.* 2007). While such quantitative approaches are informative and useful, rich descriptions such as in the above examples provide a level of detail that enhances our understanding and appreciation of deaf children's communicative skills.

This finding leads us to a further, related and interesting question posed by conversation analysts (Goldberg 1990) *'what is interruption and what is overlap?'* So far in our data, overlap of child manual gesture alongside the adult's verbal contribution, is not treated as being interruptive by the participants. Instead, the overlapped gesture is treated as being topically relevant by the adult. Overlap thus proceeds smoothly: it is not treated as a problem that warrants initiation of a side sequence to repair a trouble source. We thus suggest that it is difficult to know who owns the turn which includes verbal and non-verbal components but where other actions from the interlocutor are happening simultaneously, particularly when the simultaneous behaviour is not treated by either party as being interruptive. Hence, we support the idea of a shared turn, which echoes Goodwin and Goodwin's (1986) notion that patterns of co-participation found at certain points during interaction unfold in a systematic way between the interactants.

In our introduction we raised the well-documented issue of joint attention playing an important role in language development in very young children. Clearly there is a great deal of 'joint attention' between the adults and somewhat older children in our data. Yet, having examined gaze at a finer level of detail, we are led to ask: *'What, precisely, is joint attention?'*. Harris and Chasin (2005) studied the active elicitation of visual attention from the deaf child by the hearing mother, suggesting that the 'mapping of the mother's language to the child's focus of attention'is one of the most important factors in determining the deaf child's language development (p. 1122). We have found that our participants' use of gaze is precisely timed, in terms of how it is shared with the other person as well as when and where the gaze shifts. For instance, gaze is aligned in relation to the child's vocalisations (or verbal component of the turn) and to the child's use of gestures. As the timing is very precise, a high level of analytical detail is necessary to provide an ecologically valid description of how joint attention is negotiated, moment-by-moment, between child and adult.

We have discussed some important themes related to the processes of language learning that emerged from our analysis. In future work it will be interesting to investigate whether such non-verbal practices, such as manual gestures and gaze, are employed systematically by typically developing children who do not have language learning needs. It will also be interesting to examine the next turns to uncover how the teacher treats the child's turn, and how her next turn could be the location for launching a language learning opportunity (see also Corrin, Chapter 2 this volume).

Lastly, in addition to giving insight into the way non-verbal resources are used, our conversation analytic approach makes it possible to reveal the interactional competences of both child and adult in book-sharing context. This is especially useful since the language usage of both deaf children and children with SSLD is more often viewed from a deficit-model perspective.

References

Blake, J., Myszczyszyn, D., Jokel, A. and Bebiroglu, N. (2008) Gesture accompanying speech in specifically language-impaired children and their timing with speech. *First Language*, **28**, 237–253.

Bradshaw, M.L., Hoffman, P.R. and Norris, J.A. (1998) Efficacy of expansions and cloze procedures in the development of interpretations by pre-school children exhibiting delayed language development. *Journal of Language Speech and Hearing Services in Schools*, **29**, 85–95.

Bruner, J.S. (1983) *Child's talk: Learning to use language*. Oxford: Oxford University Press.

Capone, N.C. and McGregor, K.K. (2004) Gesture development: A review of clinical and research practices. *Journal of Speech, Language and Hearing Research*, **47**, 173–186.

Crowe, L.K. (2000) Reading behaviours of mothers and their children with language impairment during repeated storybook reading. *Journal of Communication Disorders*, **33**, 503–524.

Damico, J.S. and Simmons-Mackie, N.N. (2002) The base layer and the gaze/gesture layer of transcription. *Clinical Linguistics and Phonetics*, **16** (5), 317–327.

Dockrell, J., Lindsay, G., Letchford, B. and Mackie, C. (2006) Educational provision for children with specific speech and language difficulties: Perspectives of speech and language therapy service managers. *International Journal of Language and Communication Disorders*, **41** (4), 423–440.

Ellis-Weismer, S.E. and Hesketh, L.J. (1993) The influence of prosodic and gestural cues on novel work acquisition by children with specific language impairment. *Journal of Speech and Hearing Research*, **36**, 1013–1025.

Evans, J.A., Alibali, M.W. and McNeil, N.M. (2001) Divergence of verbal expression and embodied knowledge: Evidence from speech and gesture in children with specific language impairment. *Language and Cognitive Processes*, **16**, 309–331.

Fey, M., Catts, H. and Larrivee, L. (1995) Preparing preschoolers for the academic and social challenges of school. In M. Fey, J. Windsor and S. Warren (eds), *Language intervention: Pre-school through the elementary years* (pp. 3–37). Baltimore, MD: Paul Brooks.

Gardner, H. (1995) *Doing talk about speech: A study of speech/language therapists and phonologically disordered children working together.* Unpublished DPhil thesis, University of York.

Gioia, B. (2001) The emergent language and literacy experiences of three deaf pre-schoolers. *International Journal of Disability, Development and Education*, **48**, 411–428.

Goldberg, J.A. (1990) Interrupting the discourse on interruptions: An analysis in terms of relationally neutral, power- and rapport-oriented acts. *Journal of Pragmatics*, **4**, 883–903.

Goldin-Meadow, S. (2003) *The resilience of language: What gesture creation in deaf children can tell us about how all children learn language.* New York: Psychology Press.

Goldin-Meadow, S. (2005) What language creation in the manual modality tells us about the foundations of language. *The Linguistic Review*, **22**, 199–225.

Goodwin, M. and Goodwin, C. (1986) Gesture and coparticipation in the activity of searching for a word. *Semiotica*, **62**, 51–75.

Guidetti, M. and Nicoladis, E. (2008) Introduction to special issue: Gestures and communicative development. *First Language*, **28**, 107–115.

Gullberg, M. (2008) A helping hand? Gestures, L2 learners grammar. In S.G. McCafferty and G. Stam (eds), *Gesture: Second language acquisition and classroom research* (pp. 185–210). London: Routledge.

Harris, M. and Chasin, J. (2005) Visual attention in deaf and hearing infants: The role of auditory cues. *Journal of Child Psychology and Psychiatry*, **46**, 1116–1123.

Hargrave, A. and Senechal, M. (2000) A book reading intervention with children who have limited vocabularies: The benefits of regular reading and dialogic reading. *Early Childhood Research Quarterly*, **15**, 75–90.

Iverson, J.M. and Goldin-Meadow, S. (2005) Gesture paves the way for language development. *Psychological Science*, **16**, 367–371.

Kaderavek, J. and Justice, L. (2002) Shared storybook reading as an intervention context: Practices and potential pitfalls. *American Journal of Speech-Language Pathology*, **11**, 395–406.

Klatter-Folmer, J., van Hout, R., Kolen, E. and Verhoeven, L. (2006) Language development in deaf children's interactions with deaf and hearing adults: A Dutch longitudinal study. *Journal of Deaf Studies and Deaf Education*, 11, 238–251.

Koshik, I. (2002) Designedly incomplete utterances: A pedagogical practice for eliciting knowledge displays in error correction sequences. *Research on Language and Social Interaction*, 35, 277–309.

Liboiron, N. and Soto, G. (2006) Shared storybook reading with a student who uses alternative and augmentative communication: A description of scaffolding practices. *Child Language Teaching and Therapy*, 22, 69–95.

Mahon, M. (2009) Interactions between a deaf child for whom English is an additional language and his specialist teacher in the first year at school: Combining words and gestures. *Clinical Linguistics and Phonetics*, 23, 611–629.

McNeill, D. (1992) *Hand and mind: What gestures reveal about thought.* Chicago, IL: University of Chicago Press.

Ninio, A. (1983) Joint book reading as a multiple vocabulary acquisition device. *Developmental Psychology*, 19, 445–451.

Ozcaliskan, S. and Goldin-Meadow, S. (2005) Gesture is at the cutting edge of early language development. *Cognition*, 96, 101–113.

Plessow-Wolfson, S. and Epstein, F. (2005) The experience of story-reading: Deaf children and hearing mothers' interactions at story-time. *American Annals of the Deaf*, 150 (4), 369–378.

Rabidoux, P. and MacDonald, J. (2000) An interactive taxonomy of mothers and children during storybook interactions. *American Journal of Speech-Language Pathology*, 9, 331–344.

Radford, J. (2009) Practices of other-initiated repair in the classrooms of children with specific speech and language difficulties. *Applied Linguistics*, 23, 598–610.

Radford, J. (in press 2) Word searches: On the use of verbal and non-verbal resources during classroom talk. *Clinical Linguistics and Phonetics*.

Senechal, M. (1997) The differential effect of storybook reading on preschooler's acquisition of expressive and receptive vocabulary. *Journal of Child Language*, 24, 123–138.

Soresby, A.J. and Martlew, M. (1980) Representational demands in mothers' talk to preschool children in two contexts: Picture book reading and a modelling task. *Journal of Child Language*, 18, 373–395.

Spencer, P.E. (1993) Communicative behaviours of infants with hearing loss and their hearing mothers. *Journal of Speech and Hearing Research*, 36, 311–321.

Swanwick, R. and Watson, L. (2007) Parents sharing books with young deaf children in spoken English and in BSL: The common and diverse features of different language settings. *Journal of Deaf Studies and Deaf Education*, 12, 385–405.

Tait, M., Nikolopoulos and Lutman, M.E.T.P. (2007) Age at implantation and development of vocal and auditory preverbal skills in implanted deaf children. *International Journal of Pediatric Otorhinolaryngology*, 71, 603–610.

Tomasello, M. (2003) *Constructing a language: A usage-based theory of language acquisition.* Cambridge, MA: Harvard University Press.

Volterra, V., Caselli, M.C., Capirci, O. and Pizzuto, E. (2004) Gesture and the emergence and development of language. In M. Tomasello and D. Slobin (eds), *Elizabeth Bates: A festschrift. Beyond nature and nurture.* Mahwah, NJ: Lawrence Erlbaum Associates.

Vygotsky, L.S. (1986) *Thought and language.* Cambridge, MA: MIT Press.

Wedell-Monnig, J. and Lumley, J.M. (1980) Child deafness and mother-child inter-action. *Child Development,* 51, 766–774.

Williams, C. (2004) Emergent literacy of deaf children. *Journal of Deaf Studies and Deaf Education,* 9, 354–365.

Wood, D., Wood, H., Griffiths, A. and Howarth, I. (1986) *Teaching and talking with deaf children.* New York: Wiley.

Chapter 12

Child-initiated repair in task interactions

TUULA TYKKYLÄINEN

Introduction

In this chapter I will study and compare playful task interaction of typically developing children and children with specific language impairment (SLI). The focus is on initiating repair after setting the task. The study first looks at examples of playful interaction of typically developing children and their mothers in the home environment, then considers in detail how children with SLI and their speech and language therapists do the same kind of tasks in the environment of speech and language remediation. Studies on children's repair initiators are rare (see McTear 1985a, 1985b) and most studies have focused on the ways adults initiate repair and their consequences in interaction. This chapter will seek to redress the balance. The specific focus of the study is to use conversation analysis to give deeper insight into the sequential organisation of child-initiated repair sequences and to compare the interactions of children with communication difficulties and those with typical language development.

Intersubjectivity, sharing a common understanding of the world (Hutchby and Wooffit 1998), achieved through daily interactions, is a precondition for child's cognitive and language growth. In conversation analytic thinking, intersubjectivity and understanding are intertwined in the sequential process of interaction (Heritage 1984: 225). When intersubjectivity is threatened the participants routinely halt the ongoing sequence and address the problem by initiating repair (Schegloff *et al.* 1977; Sorjonen 1997). Repair can be begun by the speaker of the problematic turn (self) or the recipient of the problematic turn (other). Repair can also be completed by the self or the other. The repair initiation opens a negotiation and invites the other participant to reformulate his or her prior contribution to the task at hand. In the adult–child tasks presented in this data, the repair initiator brings participants to the problem of hearing, attention or minimal understanding (Schegloff *et al.* 1977; Sorjonen 1997) owing to an unclear adult instruction or the child's difficulty with linguistic concepts. A continuum of repair initiation can range from a non-specific request to one that specifies clearly the segment of the prior turn that is particularly problematic. In these interactions, the repair initiation and ensuing talk displays ongoing processing and shifting comprehension of the task in hand.

The children in this chapter attend speech and language therapy because of a specific or suspected language impairment. SLI is a developmental language impairment defined as a significant delay of expressive language and language comprehension in children who have normal hearing and normal cognitive development with no neurological deficits or socio-emotional problems (Stark and Tallal 1981; Bishop 1997; Leonard 1998). The heterogeneity of the SLI population with different subgroups is widely accepted (Rapin 1996; Conti-Ramsden and Botting 1999; Bishop *et al.* 2000), so children with speech and language difficulties vary considerably. Furthermore, language impairment is stabile but with qualitative changes in symptoms over the years (Bishop 1997; Conti-Ramsden and Botting 1999).

Children's language impairments have been approached by research mostly through experimental and group studies. The traditional study design has been a comparison between impaired and typically developing groups of children (Conti-Ramsden and Friel-Patti 1984; Prutting and Kirchner 1987; Bishop and Adams 1989). Case studies with a qualitative approach where children's speech, language and interaction are followed in daily contexts are rare (see, however, McTear 1985a; Conti-Ramsden and Gunn 1986). The findings and the overall picture of the conversation and interaction of language-impaired children vary and are even controversial.

The repair initiators of children with SLI have been approached in several methodologically diverse studies (Brinton and Fujiki 1982; Leonard 1986; Hardgrove *et al.* 1988; Merrison and Merrison 2005; Salmenlinna 2005; Tykkyläinen 2005). The earlier interest has mostly focused on the consequences of the repair initiators or clarification requests the adults have made to the children and how the children clarify their speech (e.g. Brinton *et al.* 1986a, 1986b, 1988). More recently, there have been studies that give qualitative descriptions and analyses of the repair process, how the repair is initiated and the problems are dealt with in interaction (Merrison and Merrison 2005).

The findings on repair initiation in children with SLI vary considerably. According to some researchers, children with SLI initiate repairs more often than typically developing children. According to the others, these children do not initiate repair, or if they do they make unspecific repair initiations. Leonard (1986) found that language-impaired toddlers (2;10–3;6) participated considerably in interaction, and when they had problems with understanding they not only initiated repair but did so more often than the typically developing children. Brinton and Fujiki (1982) studied 5- and 6-year-old SLI and typically developing children in a preschool setting and found that the SLI children initiated repair up to three times less often than the typically developing peers. In the researchers' interpretation of the findings, the SLI group were not as skilful in their grasp of the structure of conversation. Salmenlinna (2005) described a 7-year-old SLI girl who most often initiated repairs that were general in nature and targeted the previous problematic turn as a whole, but also initiated some specific repairs focusing on part of the previous problematic turn. An experimental study by Hardgrove *et al.* (1988) reported that the SLI group expressed their difficulty in understanding both non-verbally and verbally, but in an unspecified manner. The SLI children made general, verbal repair initiations and additionally looked, for example, at the table, whereas the typically developing children looked at their mothers and offered more specific candidate understandings.

An interesting exception among the studies focusing on repair in speech and language therapy is the study of Merrison and Merrison (2005). The study of task interaction combined both quantitative and qualitative methodologies based on conversation and

discourse analysis and examined the repair skills of three groups: children with pragmatic language impairment (PLI), children with specific language impairment (SLI) and
children with typical development. The study has also clinical relevance aiming at developing a tool for assessing and monitoring client's pragmatic skills. According to the
findings, both typical development children and children with SLI tended to initiate
repair through appropriate and relevant questions in order to achieve success in the task
activity. The third group of children, those with pragmatic language impairment, tended
not to initiate repair and the group ended up with a poorer performance in the task.
However, their performance improved after a short intervention.

Participants and task interaction as situated activity

The data of the chapter consist of videotaped task interaction between typically developing children and mothers (8 pairs) doing playful tasks in a home environment (Figure 12.1).
The age range of the typically developing children studied was 4;10–5;1. The home
interactions of typically developing children come from the data corpus of the *Helsinki
Child Cross-Sectional Corpus* 2002–2007. Figures 12.2–12.4 come from the data corpus of speech and language therapy interaction (Tykkyläinen 2005). In the data a speech
and language therapist and a child with SLI (7 pairs) did a routine therapy task together.
The age range of the SLI children was 4;11–6;0. The diagnosis, according to the *Diagnostic and Statistical Manual of Mental Disorders III* (DSM III) was F80.2, which
means that, in addition to problems with expressive speech, the children also had problems with speech understanding. The speech and language therapists participating were
well experienced and had a professional history of 6 to 20 years.

The aims of speech and language therapy are embedded in different activities during
the therapy lessons. Playing games and doing game-like tasks are popular activities
which children enjoy. They are also a popular free-time activity of typically developing
children and parents, and are seen as both amusing and educational. The focus of the
chapter is in interactions in game-like tasks with the aim of practising language reasoning, language comprehension and certain categories of linguistic concepts. The task
activity is an accomplishment of the participants in which talk and non-verbal activity
are interwoven.

The tasks examined in home situations were conducted in the form of hint and guess-
type games (see, for example, Figure 12.1). In the 'hint and guess game' (Figure 12.2) the
child had to pick up, from the cards on the table or floor, the right card according to the
hint or instruction given by the adult. In speech therapy situations, the 'toggle board
game (Figure 12.3) and the 'fish game' (Figure 12.4) were also used. In the 'toggle board
game' the child's task was to choose a toggle and place it according to the given instruction. In the 'fish game' the child moved a fish to the pockets of the board on the table
according to the instructions given by the therapist. The three parts of the prototypical
task sequence were: (1) task setting, (2) child's response and (3) receipting and commenting on the task.

In the interaction to the task, four different paths to its resolution have been found
(Tykkyläinen 2005). The path focused on in this chapter is one where the child displays
his or her difficulty in understanding the speech and language therapist's task-setting
turn (pp. 138–149). Therefore, the next action after the speech and language therapist's

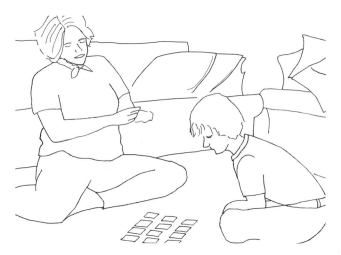

Figure 12.1 A hint and guess game at home between a mother and a typically developing 5-year-old.

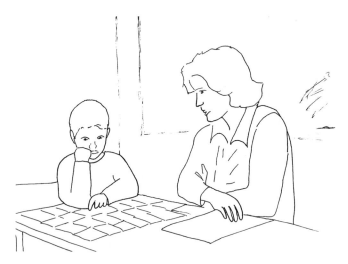

Figure 12.2 Clinical setting: Hint and guess game.

task-setting is not the child's non-verbal target response, but a turn displaying problem in fulfilling the required target. With his or her turn the child addresses something from the task-setting turn which needs more attention (see Schegloff *et al.* 1977). This turn postpones the task resolution and starts the process of repair.

In the following sections I will examine how typically developing children formulated their repair initiations and follow the consequences of the repair initiators. I will then study the children with SLI initiating repair. The data extracts follow typical CA conventions (see Glossary of transcript symbols) with the original Finnish and an English translation placed underneath. An additional diacritic, @word@, with bracketing round an utterance or utterance part, indicates that the bracketed part is pronounced with changed voice quality.

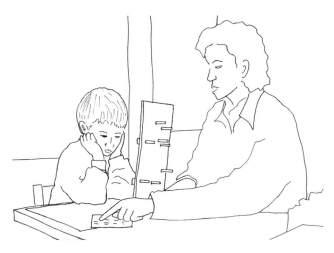

Figure 12.3 Clinical setting: Toggle board game.

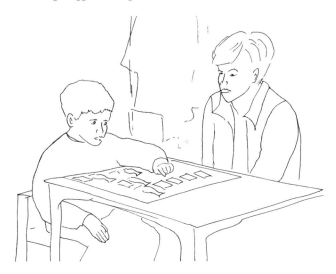

Figure 12.4 Clinical setting: Fish game.

Typically developing 5-year-olds initiating repair in a game-like task

When initiating repair both pragmatic and linguistic knowledge is combined. In the repair-initiating turn the child relates his or her participation to the ongoing activity and selects the appropriate linguistic means for doing it. In the data of eight mother–child pairs playing the hint and guess game at home, repair was rarely initiated. Altogether 70 task sequences were studied. Only four repair initiations emerged, three of which were made by a 5-year-old girl and one by a 5-year-old boy. Three of the repair initiators were questions formulated by using a Finnish question particle –*kO* and one was formulated by simultaneous verbalisation and gaze shift to the mother.

In Extract 12.1 Alina and her mother are sitting on the living room floor and playing the hint and guess game. They have picture cards on the carpet in front of them and the mother is giving Alina a hint about a certain picture.

Extract 12.1 *Hint and guess: Alina and her mother*

1   M: Joo:?
           Yea:h?

2   (1.0)

3   M: minkäs noista voi syödä.
           which one of those can be eaten.

4   (1.9) *Alina looks at the pictures and plays with her toes*

           [PICTURES_____

5   A: [°M-m- ↑m- mm-°(2.9)mm-
           [*Alina plays with her toes, crosses her legs*

6   (1.3) *Alina looks at the pictures*

           MOTHER_____

7   → A: **[puustako,**
           [from a tree,   ]
           [*Alina reaches towards her mother*]

8   (1.6) *Alina looks at her mother*

9   M: [no vaikka puusta,
           [well from a tree though,]
           [*Alina looks at the pictures*]

10   (2.4) *Alina leans on the pictures*

11   M: [minkä voi syödä.]
           [which one can be eaten.]
           [*Alina looks at the pictures*]

12   (1.8)

13   A: [Omenan,]
           [An apple]
           [*points to the picture of an apple*]

14   M: Mmm (.) voikos sen lumiukon syödä,
           Mmm (.) can the snowman be eaten,

15   (2.1)

16   A: En mä tiedä,
           I don't know,

17   (0.5)

18   M: [Ei saa syödä [lun]ta,   ]
           [No you can not eat snow,
           [*Her mother shakes her head, looks at the pictures*]

19   A: [Ei,]
           [No,]

20   A: (1.0) *Alina looks at the pictures and smiles*

21   M: °Joo,°
               °Yeah,°

The hinting, task-setting turn by her mother, *minkäs noista voi syödä / which one of those can be eaten*, opens the task sequence. Alina looks at the picture cards on the carpet for about 1.9 seconds and starts to play with her toes and crosses her legs. At the same time she speaks with a quiet mumbling voice with changing intonation (line 5). Then Alina focuses on looking at the pictures for 1.3 seconds. Then, in line 7, Alina initiates a repair by asking a question *puustako / from a tree* formulated by adding a question particle *–kO* (tree + Q-clitic). While asking the question she turns, shifts her gaze and reaches towards her mother. Alina's question is an interpretation of the previous task-setting turn. With her interpretation she tries to define the number of choices pertaining to a subgroup of edible things from a tree. In line 9 her mother considers Alina's proposed possible definition, *No vaikka puusta / Well from a tree though*, and Alina looks back at the pictures and leans on them. When Alina's answer is still delayed (2.4 seconds) her mother repeats the task-setting turn now formulated as *m̲i̲nkä voi syödä / which one can be eaten*. In line 13 Alina then points at the right picture with her finger and answers *omenan / an apple*. Her mother receives the task-solving turn by the particle *mhm*. Following Alina's correct answer her mother and Alina still puzzle over whether a snowman, one of the pictures remaining in front of them, can be eaten and her mother reminds and advises Alina to avoid it (lines 14–21).

Alina's repair initiation is positioned after a pause in the talk-in-interaction, mumbling voice and another pause (lines 4–6) during which she looks at the cards with both gaze and body orientation aimed at the task cards. When making the repair initiation she changes her body orientation and gazes towards her mother (Figure 12.5). Alina's repair initiation *puustako / from a tree* is formulated as a clarification request to which she seeks her mother's confirmation. With her repair initiation Alina tries to specify her mother's quite generally formulated task. Instead of displaying a problem of hearing

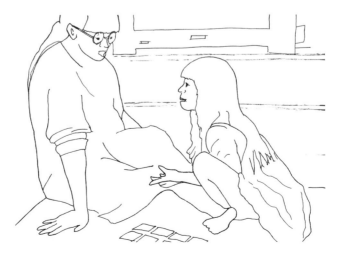

Figure 12.5 Alina initiates a repair.

or understanding a specific part of the task-setting turn, this kind of delayed repair initiation by Alina has a specific function. It demonstrates the process of task-solving and Alina's orientation to the role of task-solver. She displays her cognitive effort in forming a subgroup of candidate solutions in her mind.

Extract 12.2 describes the same phenomenon but now the focus is on giving the correct answer. Alina is eager to give the correct answer and she definitely wants to be sure. In order to do this she asks for clarification on her mother's task-setting and initiates a repair.

Extract 12.2 *Hint and guess – a summer picture*

1		M:	Mikäs niist ois semmonen kesäkuva, (.)
			Which of them is a a summer picture, (.)
2			missä on punainen joka kasvaa.
			where there is red which grows.
3		A:	*Alina looks at the pictures* (5.0)
4		A:	°Mmm,°
5		A:	*Alina looks at the pictures* (8.0)
6	→	**A:**	**Maassako.**
			In the ground.
7		M:	Niin maassa °kasvaa,°
			Yes grows in the °ground°,
8		A:	[Totta.]
			[True.]
			[*Alina points to the right picture*]
9		M:	Mmm? (.) [mikäs se ↑on,]
			Mmm? (.) [what is ↑it,]
10		A:	[(Se on)] kukka. (.) Kukka se oli,
			[(It is)] a flower (.) A flower it was,
11		Ä:	Joo:? (.) hienosti.
			Ye:ah? (.) fine.
12		A:	Se oli kukk:a.
			It was a flower.
13		M:	°Joo,°
			°Yeah,°

Her mother sets the task by hinting at *summer* and something *red which grows*. After leaning on the pictures for 5 seconds Alina takes a turn by using a responding particle *mmm* still leaning on the pictures. By the turn she demonstrates the problem-solving process and keeps it going. After the turn she still continues looking at the pictures for 8 seconds. After looking for a long time, in line 6 she makes a clarification request, *maassako / in the ground*, formulated again with the questioning particle –kO. With her question she delineates the possible candidates for the right answer, to those plants growing near the ground. Alina's repair initiation is followed by her mother's aligning and well-formed turn, *yes grows in the ground* (line 7). Finally, Alina chooses the right picture and underlines her choice by her simultaneous comment, *totta / true.*

To sum up the findings of the two extracts, the repair initiations of typically developing 5-year-olds are rare and tend to have a specific quality. The child here displayed a strong task orientation and motivation to give the correct solution. This was especially audible and visible in the repair initiators and non-verbal body orientation of the child. Alina changed the focus of her gaze and body posture between the task and her mother. The repair initiators formulated did not demonstrate actual, specific problems of hearing and understanding, instead they reflected the ongoing task-solving process of the child. For example, repair initiators addressed the general manner of the mother's task delivery or they were designed to define a possible solution or a group of candidate solutions in the child's mind.

Children with SLI initiating repair

How do the 5-year-old children with SLI initiate repair in a task situation in speech and language therapy? How are the repair initiators designed and formulated in comparison to typical children in a similar context?

The frequency of the phenomenon of a child with SLI initiating repair after the speech and language therapist's task-setting turn was rare, as was the case with typical children in a home context. In the data, there were only 17 sequences in 234 task sequences in which the child initiated a repair. Five of the seven SLI children initiated repairs and two of the children made the majority of the repair initiations. In contrast to the repair initiators of typically developing children, however, the SLI children initiated repair in three ways. They made general repair initiators, specific repair initiators and they offered candidate understandings.

In speech therapy task situations, firstly, there were general repair initiators that marked the whole task-setting turn as problematic ($n = 4$). Secondly, the most often used means for the children to check their understanding and initiate a repair was to formulate a turn that marked part of the task-setting turn in need of clarification ($n = 9$). Thirdly, there were turns where the child interpreted, then offered a candidate solution for the speech and language therapist to confirm or reject. They resemble the turns that Schegloff *et al.* (1977) have called *understanding checks* in adults.

In the cases presented, the turns with which the child initiated a repair and displayed the problem of hearing or understanding were linguistically formulated as questions. Firstly, they were classified as questions by their grammar. In every case except one, there was a question word or a particle that formulated the turn as a question. Secondly, speech prosody and the simultaneous non-verbal action of, for example, gaze switch to the adult, or the use of objects such as offering a toggle as a candidate answer, were also important aspects in identifying the turn as a repair initiator. Thirdly, the character of the speech and language therapist's next turn was crucial in identifying the repair initiators as such, and responding appropriately.

Repair initiators addressing the whole task-setting turn as problematic

In this section, the repair initiators that addressed the whole previous task-setting turn as problematic are analysed. If the repair initiating turns are approached as a continuum, the turns with *mitä / what, huh* are positioned in the other end of the continuum displaying minimal and unspecified understanding of the previous turn (Schegloff *et al.* 1977). Thus the repair initiator is usually interpreted as a sign of a hearing problem or minimal understanding (Schegloff *et al.* 1977; Sorjonen 1997). Extract 12.3 introduces an example of this. The sequence belongs to the toggle board game and the therapist and the boy are just about to begin the game-like task.

Extract 12.3 *Toggle game – black*

1		(1.4)
2	T:	sit sä voit laittaa k<u>aa</u>pin ovet vielä kiinn<u>i</u>, then you can still close the doors of the c<u>a</u>binet,
3		(0.4)
4	C:	JOO (.) [<u>u</u>h (2.1) [joo (0.9) <u>U</u>H (0.7) joo YEAH (.) [<u>u</u>h (2.1) [yeah (0.9) <u>U</u>H (0.7) yeah [*C kicks in the air and moves towards the cabinet*
5		[(.) <u>U</u>h huh [*C kicks the doors of the cabinet shut* [*C turns towards the board, materials and therapist*
6	T:	[.hhh ja etsippäs tuolta (.) Ville musta nappu[lahh [.hhh and look over there(.) Ville for a black togglehh [*T touches the board*
7		(0.4)
8 →	**C:**	**mitä,** **what,**
9		(0.3)
10	T:	missäs [siellä olis musta [nappula where [is there a black [toggle [*T points at the board* [*T points at the toggles*
11		(2.0) *C withdraws his hand, looks at the toggle row*
12	C:	*takes the right toggle* (0.7)
13	T:	j:<u>e</u>p.
14		(0.8)
15	T:	ja laitappa sinne (.) kuvaan missä (0.6) on (0.4) sininen and put there (.) where the picture is (0.6) there is (0.4) a blue one
16		(0.3) hälytysajoneuvo.(0.4) jota ohjaa p<u>o</u>liisi. (0.3) emergency vehicle (0.4) driven by a p<u>o</u>liceman.

The extract begins when the participants are making up the task, taking materials out of the cabinet and moving to the floor. The therapist asks the child to shut the cabinet doors that have been left open (line 2). The child kicks in the air, kicks the cabinet doors shut and turns towards the therapist and the task materials. As soon as the child has turned around, the therapist begins her task-setting turn (line 6) with a directive request *etsippäs tuolta (.) Ville musta nappulahh / and look over there (.) Ville for a black togglehh*. The child has not yet completely focused on the task having just sat by the task materials and the therapist. Consequently, the task-setting turn by the therapist is followed by the child's repair initiator *mitä, / what,* (line 8).

The child's turn *mitä, / what,* in line 8 is an unfocused repair initiator targeting at the therapist's whole task-setting turn. The therapist interprets it as the child not having heard the task-setting turn properly and reformulates the task-setting in line 10. The reformulation is now a concrete question about the position of the black toggle, *missäs siellä olis musta nappula / where is there a black toggle*, question. The turn is formulated multi-modally. The therapist first makes a general waving gesture towards the toggle board, then focuses attention by pointing at the toggle row. By reformulating the task-setting turn the therapist offers the child a new opportunity to make a task-specific response. In line 12 the child chooses the right toggle which the therapist receives with the prosodically emphasised response particle *j:ep / yeah*. This turn closes the task sequence set in line 13.

Repair initiators addressing a specific part of the task-setting turn as problematic

The most typical repair initiators made by the SLI children were questions addressing a specific part of the therapist's task-setting turn. These repair initiators were formulated either by beginning the turn with a *wh*-word or with beginning the turn with the *ai / oh* question particle. The repair initiator in Extract 12.4 begins a long negotiation about the meaning, finally ending in confusion concerning the central concepts of the task. The therapist and a child are playing with cards on the table where the therapist gives the child hints about the cat in the pictures. The child's task is to point out the right picture card (Tykkyläinen 2005, 140–142). The therapist is setting the task and the child is sitting with his hands on his cheeks.

Extract 12.4   *Cat cards – curly moustache*

1		(1.0)
2	T:	@uusinta kissamuotia ovat kiharaiset viikset, (.) mi:nullakin on sellaiset.@
		@the latest cat fashion is a curly moustache, (.) I:: have those too.@
3	C:	*moves on the chair, takes hands away from cheeks, looks at the cards on the table*
		(4.1)
4 →	**C:**	**[mitkä.**
		[which.
5	T:	[(x)

```
6              (0.6)

7      T:     kiharaiset viikset.
              curly moustache.

8              (0.6)

9      C:     tha kirahaiset viik[set
              tha culry   mous [tache

                            [T smoothes her hair
10     T:                   [onks mulla suora vai kihara tukka
                            [is my hair straight or curly
```

The therapist sets the task using a prosodically emphasised voice – she is imitating a cat: @*uusinta kissamuotia ovat kiharaiset viikset, (.) mi:nullakin on sellaiset.*@ / @*the latest cat fashion is a curly moustache, (.) I have those too.*@. After the task-setting there is a long pause (4.1 seconds) in the conversation. The child shifts his posture and also his hands move slightly away from his cheeks (line 3). All the time he is gazing at the cards. The change of posture is followed by the repair initiator *mitkä* / *which*, which is formulated as an overlap of the start of the therapist's turn that is cut off immediately. The linguistic formulation of the child's repair initiator *which* displays a problem in understanding and precisely locates the problem in the words *kiharaiset viikset* / *curly moustache*. Consequently, the therapist repeats the problematic expression '*curly moustache*' (line 7). The therapist's repetition is followed by a pause and after the pause the child formulates a turn with a lexical, morphological error in the word '*curly*' as '*culry*' moustache. With this formulation the problem is located in the concept of *curly*. The therapist is rushing partly with an overlap to explain the unclear concept of curly. A long negotiation on the concept of curly and on the moustache is about to begin.

Another means for the SLI children to formulate a repair initiator pointing at a specific part of the previous task-setting turn was a turn begun with a Finnish particle *ai* (approximately meaning '*oh*' or '*you mean*') which is a questioning particle in Finnish (ISK 2004: 777). In addition to the particle *ai*, the position of the child's turn makes it a questioning repair initiator. In Extract 12.5 the child and the therapist are playing a toggle board game. The task of the child is to first choose the right toggle and then put it in the position according to the therapist's hint.

Extract 12.5   *A toggle board – two blue fish*

```
1              (1.3)

2      T:     ja sitte or:anssi nappulahh
              and then an orange togglehh

3      C:     Ottaa nappulan (2.5)
              Takes the orange toggle (2.5)

4      T:     ja laita siihen miss on kaks sinistä kalaa, (.) ja kolme punasta?
              and put it where there are two blue fish, (.) and three red ones?

5              (2.3)
```

6 → C: **ai kaks sinistä kalaa.**
       you mean two blue fish.

7   T: =mhm?

8   (0.8)

9 → C: **ja kol:me punistah**
       and three red onesh

10   (1.4)

11   T: [(jooh) ((*whispers*))
        [(yeah)
        [*T nods*

12   C: =semmosii
        =like that

The child makes two repair initiators (lines 6 and 9) addressing different parts of the task-setting turn. With these turns he checks the critical substance of the whole task-setting hint. The first repair initiator is formulated by the particle *ai / oh* in the beginning and the other repeats the part of the task-setting turn.

The therapist sets both parts of the task (lines 2 and 4) by beginning the task-setting demand with the particle *and*. *And*-prefaced turns link the new request to the former request and signal moving on to the next part of the whole activity (Heritage and Sorjonen 1994). After the latter *and*-prefaced task-setting turn in line 4, there is first a pause in the interaction and then the repair initiators formulated by the child. With the first repair initiator the child checks the first part of the task-setting turn *ai kaks sinistä kalaa / you mean two blue fish*, and with the second the last part of it *ja kolme punista / and three red ones*. In Finnish, a question beginning with *ai* (Raevaara 1993; Sorjonen 1997; Kurhila 2000; ISK 2004: 777) is a clarification request always looking back to the previous turn.

The therapist confirms the child's turn by immediately responding with the utterance *mhm?*. The intonation of the turn rises towards the end. Such a formulation both receives the child's candidate understanding and moves forward to the continuation of the task. In line 9 the child continues checking his understanding by repeating the last part of the task-setting turn *ja kolme punista / and three red ones*. The word *punista / reds* in the turn is slightly incorrectly articulated. The therapist receives and confirms the last part of the task setting by whispering *yeah* and nodding (line 11). The sequence ends with the child commenting on his performance by a quiet and unclear turn in line 12.

The turns constructed by the particle *ai* and a repetition of a specific part of the turn repeat and check the task setting. They display the child's orientation to the task and the role of the task-solver. At the same time, however, they mark the task understanding as uncertain and display the need for confirmation by the therapist. It may be that the particle *ai* + nominal clause are typical of institutional encounters between an expert and a less knowledgeable person (see also Kurhila 2000, 2003) and also of task situations with a specific focus. In any case, regardless of the continuous checking of understanding by the repair initiations, the ongoing task activity proceeds smoothly.

The child offers the right candidate for the solution

The repair initiators just presented were all aiming backwards, looking back at the task-setting and checking the hearing and understanding of the previous turn. By initiating such repairs the child is checking his or her understanding about the task set *before* solving the actual task. The repair initiators analysed and described next, however, differ from the previous ones. In the following cases the child has proceeded further in the task-solving process. The child has solved the task non-verbally and, in an overlap or immediately after, the child offers his or her candidate understanding to the therapist verbally for confirmation. In Extract 12.6 the child and the therapist are playing the toggle board game. The task is two-fold. Firstly, the therapist decides which of the coloured toggles is to be chosen then hints where to put the toggle on the board. In Extract 12.6 the candidate solution offered by the child in line 5 is the right one.

Extract 12.6 *The toggle board – dark blue*

1	T:	mt (0.6) sitten löytyykö sieltä,
		mt (0.6) then I wonder if there is,
2		(0.8) (*C smacks his lips and hand*)
3		t<u>u</u>m:maa tummaa sinistä (.) ihan tummaa sinistä.
		d<u>a</u>rk dark blue (.) very dark blue.
4 →	**C:**	*C takes a toggle and raises it [over the picture board]*
5 →	**C:**	[tääkö.
		[this+Q-cli.
6 →	T:	°joo°=se menee niille eläimille jotka r<u>ö</u>hkii
		°yeah°=it goes to those animals which gr<u>u</u>nt
7		(0.3) ja joil on k<u>ä</u>rsä ja saparo.
		(0.3) and which have a sn<u>ou</u>t and a t<u>ai</u>l.
8	C:	*Puts the toggle in a hole on the board* (0.7)
9	T:	mitäs ne olikaan=[@röh nröh röhh@]
		what were they= [@röh nröh röhh@]
10	C:	[possuja.]
		[pigs.]

The therapist formulated the task of the toggle-choosing as a question (lines 1–3). The child is very task oriented and looks at the picture board. The child chooses a toggle (line 4), raises it over the board in the front of the therapist's eyes asking *tääkö* / *this+Q-cli* / *this one* (line 5, Figure 12.6). The candidate solution offered by the child is formulated multi-modally combining verbal and non-verbal substance which is typical in game-like activities. The verbal substance consists of a Finnish deictic pronomine *tää* / *this* and a question clitic, particle *–kO*. The non-verbal substance of the candidate solution is constructed by the child's outstretched arm over the picture board towards the therapist. The child is looking at the board not at the toggle. The multi-modal

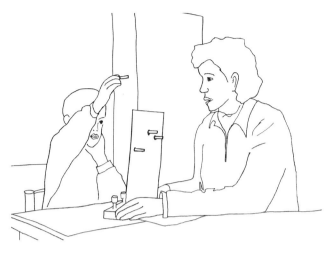

Figure 12.6 The child offers his candidate solution for the therapist to confirm or reject.

candidate task-solution offered seeks for confirmation or rejection of the choice by the therapist. Such action invites correction by the therapist (correction invitation device, Sacks 1992: 380). The therapist receives and confirms the candidate solution with an immediate *joo / yeah* and rushes through to the second part of the task – a request to place the toggle. Despite the side sequence initiated by the child, the main activity proceeds smoothly. The process of repair achieving intersubjectivity between the participants was used minimally and without breaking up the main activity.

The child offers a wrong candidate

A wrong candidate offered for the solution of the task leads to a long negotiation on the interpretation of the task. In a long-lasting repair process the speech and language therapist multi-modally leads the child to the appropriate task solution. Extract 12.7 explicates how the use of the multi-modal resources increases when the sequence and negotiation on meaning proceeds. Besides, the manner of closing the sequence reveals that the intersubjectivity between the participants has been threatened.

The therapist and the child are doing a task where the child moves a paper fish into the pockets of a plastic board according to the instructions of the therapist. The child offers his candidate solution beginning with particle *ai / oh* in line 6.

Extract 12.7 *Fish – another yellow fish*

1   (0.8)

2   T: no sitten (1.0) uita seuraavaksi (.) ↑toinen
            well then (1.0) next swim   (.)↑another

                        [C takes the right fish
3   keltainen kala, (2.3) [ylimmän rivin viimeisen kuvan
             yellow fish, (2.3)   [to the last picture of the uppermost

4		päälle.
		row.
5		(0.6)
6 →	**C:**	**[ai tohon**
		[oh there
		[you mean there
		[*C puts the paper fish in the wrong place*
7		(0.6)
8	T:	mikäs on ylimmän rivin vi̱imeinen kuva.
		which one is the last picture of the uppermost row.
9	C:	*Siirtää kalaa toisen, jälleen väärän kuvan päälle* (2.6)
		Moves the paper fish to another place, the wrong one again (2.6)
10	T:	[tää on se ylin rivi? ja täällä se ihan vika
		[this is the uppermost row? and here the ultimately
		[*T draws her finger along the uppermost line*
11		VII::mei:nen on (.) to̱i.=
		LA::st is (.) that one.=
12	C:	[=kukkaruukku
		[=flower pot
		[*C puts the paper fish in a pocket of the board*
13	T:	kukkamaljakko oli vika viimeinen°
		a flower vase was the very last one°
14		(0.4)
15	T:	hyv̱ä:
		go̱o:d
16		(0.6)

The interactional substance of the therapist's task-setting turn is divided by pausing (lines 2 and 4) and accentuated by emphasising. The turn begins by *no sitten / well then* which moves the participants forward in the task activity. The attention is also focused on something that is ahead with a pause in line 2. Then there is the repeated directive *swim next*. All this interaction substance predicts the critical substance of the tasksolving: the colour of the fish to be chosen (*to̱inen keltainen kala / aṉother yellow fish*) and the position to which the fish should be moved (*ylimmän rivin vi̱imeisen kuvan päälle / to the la̱st picture of the uppermost line*). The child's task-solving action begins during the therapist's turn. The child chooses the right fish simultaneously with the last part of the therapist's prompt that the position of the fish should be moved (line 3). In line 6 the child puts the paper fish on a wrong picture card and asks *ai tohon / oh there / you mean there*. The turn formulated by verbal and non-verbal substance offers a candidate

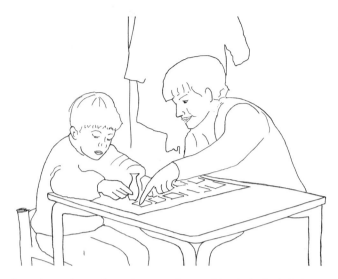

Figure 12.7 The therapist works out the task appropriate position by lexical choices, speech prosody and the therapy material used.

solution which is marked unsure by the question. The child's candidate solution invites the therapist to confirm or reject the choice. Because of the wrong candidate offered the therapist reformulates the position where the paper fish should be moved, this time by a *wh*-question (line 8). The question repeats the original position posed *ylimmän rivin viimeinen kuva* / *the last picture of the uppermost row* (Figure 12.7).

However, in line 9 the child again moves the fish to the wrong position. After the second wrong choice the therapist says what position she is looking for and also utilises the therapy material in her formulation. She divides the description of the targeted position into parts. First she verbalises the right row *tää on se ylin rivi* / *this is the uppermost line* and draws her finger along the right line towards the right picture (Figure 12.7). The utterance used in the beginning of the turn rises at the end indicating a continuation of the turn by the same speaker (see Ogden and Routarinne 2005). The second part of the turn shows the right position by lexical choices, pausing and utilising the therapy material. The right position is formulated by using a word in the child's lexicon *vika viimeinen* / *very last*. The multimodal approach towards the target position is emphasised by stress and prolongation of the word *viimeinen* / *last*. The therapist's moving hand draws attention to the target. After the description of the right position the therapist ends the search by pointing to the right place and saying *that*. The turn formulations described above focus the attention of the child on the task very strongly and invite him to follow and participate in the seeking process. This is also evident in how the child participates after the search is ended. The child names the picture immediately in line 12 *=kukkaruukku* / *=flower pot* simultaneously putting the paper fish to the right pocket of the board. However, the child makes a semantic error calling the picture as a *flower pot* instead of *a flower vase*. In line 13 the therapist makes an embedded correction (see Jefferson 1987) *kukka maljakko oli vika viimeinen°* / *a flower vase was the very last one°*. The task sequence is closed by the therapist's assessment *hyvä* / *goo:d* in line 15.

The verbally and non-verbally distributed candidate solution offered by the child opened a repair sequence and invites the therapist to use the resources available more prominently. As a consequence of the wrong solutions, the therapist emphasised the monitoring of the task, directing and supporting the child's performance towards the right target solution. The therapist worked out the target concept of position multi-modally, utilising different interaction resources. The therapist formulated her hint using special lexical choices designed for the child. She also used marked prosody and the therapy materials at hand. It is also noticeable that the semantic error in the end of the task sequence was followed by a direct but embedded repair. Solving the task, choosing the right paper fish and moving it to the right place, remained the main activity. Additionally, although it was the therapist who actually solved the task, she acted in a way that invited the child to actively participate in solving the task.

Discussion and conclusions

In this chapter I have studied the few child-initiated repair sequences that occurred in a playful task interaction between typically developing 5-year-old children and their mothers at home, and children with SLI with their speech and language therapists during therapy tasks.

To sum up the findings it can be said that the phenomenon of initiating repair was rare in both groups and typically developing children and children with SLI both initiated repair to maintain intersubjectivity to gain success in the task activity. However, the manner in which the repair initiators were formulated, designed and delivered was qualitatively different between the groups.

The repair initiators used by the children with SLI were well suited to the task at hand. Both general and specific repair initiators were made. General repair initiators routinely looked backwards to the speech and language therapist's whole task-setting turn but specific repair initiators checked a specific part of the turn. Besides repair initiators the children with SLI offered candidate understandings for the speech therapist to confirm or reject. Most typically they initiated repair aimed at part of the previous task-setting turn. Initiating a repair was also rare in the task activities of typically developing children. While the repair initiators of the children with SLI pointed to a problem in hearing, attention focusing or understanding, the repair initiators of typically developing children tended to focus more on the task-solving process and a task that had been set on a general level. With their repair initiations the typically developing children defined and specified a possible subgroup of candidate solutions they had to choose from.

The repair initiators were also sensitive to the broader context in which they were used as well as being sequentially shaped by the previous task-setting turn. The repair initiators of the typically developing children revealed the characteristics of unplanned free time activity, where the mothers' task-setting turns were formulated in an unplanned manner and were quite general and even unclear. The typically developing children used the repair process to define the possible group of candidate solutions and sought support for them. The task-setting turns by the speech and language therapists were revealed to be quite long and full of details. The SLI children most typically initiated repair by displaying some part of the therapist's task-setting turn as problematic. But they also formulated repair initiators concerning the whole task-setting turn and offered candidate understandings. By using several types of repair initiators children with SLI demonstrate sensitivity and competence in maintaining intersubjectivity.

The finding of children with SLI using specified repair initiators addressing part of the previous turn is different from the earlier findings of SLI children's repair initiators (e.g. Hardgrove *et al.* 1988; Salmenlinna 2005). The earlier studies mostly describe the repair initiators of SLI children as general and aimed at the whole previous turn. Most of the studies, however, are not very context sensitive and often lack a description of the activity at hand. The game-like tasks studied in this chapter give the child opportunities to check the parts and details of the tasks. The findings of the SLI group of this study are in line with the study of Merrison and Merrison (2005) – both typically developing and children with SLI made appropriate and relevant repair initiators well suited for the task at hand. The finding of an actively problem-solving child also questions the earlier picture of a SLI child as a quite passive interaction partner (e.g. Prutting *et al.* 1978; Panagos *et al.* 1986a; Leiwo 1992). By his or her repair initiation the child points out the problematic part of the task and takes responsibility for solving it. The repair initiations address unclear concepts or difficult linguistic constructions.

Qualitative differences in repair initiations may also have clinical relevance and potential. The findings suggest identifying and analysing the characteristics of repair initiators gives qualitative information, for example, in the diagnostic therapy of a client. The occurrence, quality and distribution of repair initiators may help clinicians, for example, to differentiate between a client with pragmatic language difficulties due to a language impairment, a child with attention difficulties or indeed one with Autistic Spectrum Disorder, where the motivation for intersubjectivity through repair may not be routinely pursued (Gardner 2006).

Initiating a repair in the interactions of children with SLI and speech and language therapists led sometimes to long negotiations with the children's wrong interpretations and candidate solutions and the therapists' reformulations and specifications. In these sequences of meaning negotiation the institutional character of the interaction was both talked and acted into being. The speech and language therapists' use of the multi-modal semiotic resources was prominently present. Using both verbal and non-verbal means and prominent prosody the therapists directed the child towards the target to make task-solving easier for the child. Prompts increased where task-solving was prolonged as it was characteristic of the therapist's manner that they would ensure that the child remained the task-solver.

The problems of understanding have consequences in the child's daily life. An interesting finding of a task interaction was that the SLI children's candidate solutions were formulated in a manner that marked the child's offered solution as unsure and something in need of the confirmation or rejection of the therapist. On the other hand, it says something about the child's orientation to keeping a task flowing, possibly a survival strategy that the child has developed due to his or her difficulty in understanding. If the child confronts recurrent situations in which his or her understanding is unsure, offering a candidate solution is a functional way to handle problematic situations.

It is very important that the SLI child's daily interaction partners are helped to reflect and discuss the moments of daily interaction as part of any speech and language therapy intervention. Interaction partners can become more sensitive to the repair processes the child initiates. Thus, studying repair processes should help to enhance communication in everyday interactions as part of the development of better interventions for children with communication impairments.

References

Bishop, D. (1994) Is specific language impairment a valid diagnostic category? Genetic and psycholinguistic evidence. *Philosophical Transactions of the Royal Society*, B, **346**, 105–111.

Bishop, D. (1997) *Uncommon understanding. Development and disorders of language comprehension in children*. Somerset: Psychology Press.

Bishop, D. and Adams, C. (1989) Conversational characteristics of children with semantic-pragmatic disorder: II. What features lead to judgement of inappropriacy? *British Journal of Disorders and Communication*, **24**, 241–263.

Bishop, D., Chan, J., Adams, C., Hartley, J. and Weir, I. (2000) Conversational responsiveness in specific language impairment: Evidence of disproportionate pragmatic difficulties in a subset of children. *Development and Psychopathology*, **12**, 177–199.

Bishop, D. and Rosenbloom, L. (1987) Classification of childhood language disorders. In W. Yule and M. Rutter (eds), *Language development and disorders. Clinics in developmental medicine* (pp. 101–102). London: MacKeith Press.

Brinton, B. and Fujiki, M. (1982) A comparison of request-response sequences in the discourse of normal and language-disordered children. *Journal of Speech and Hearing Disorders*, **47**, 57–62.

Brinton, B., Fujiki, M., Loeb, D. and Winkler, E. (1986a) Development of conversational repair strategies in response to requests for clarification. *Journal of Speech and Hearing Research*, **29**, 75–81.

Brinton, B., Fujiki, M., Winkler, E. and Loeb, D. (1986b) Responses to request for clarification in normal and linguistically language-impaired children. *Journal of Speech and Hearing Disorders*, **51**, 370–378.

Brinton, B., Fujiki, M. and Sonnenberg, E. (1988) Responses to requests for clarification by linguistically normal and language impaired children in conversation. *Journal of Speech and Hearing Disorders*, **53**, 383–391.

Conti-Ramsden, G. and Botting, N. (1999) Classification of children with specific language impairment: Longitudinal considerations. *Journal of Speech, Language and Hearing Research*, **42**, 1195–1204.

Conti-Ramsden, G. and Friel-Patti, S. (1984) Mother-child dialogues: A comparison of normal and language-impaired children. *Journal of Communication Disorders*, **17**, 19–35.

Conti-Ramsden, G. and Gunn, M. (1986) The development of conversational disability: A case study. *British Journal of Disorders of Communication*, **21**, 339–351.

Crystal, D. (1981) *Clinical linguistics*. Vienna: Springer-Verlag.

Gardner, H. (2006) Training others in the interactional art of therapy for specific needs. *Child Language Teaching and Therapy*, **27** (1), 27–56.

Halonen, M. (2001) Terapeutti elämäkerran tulkitsijana myllyhoidon ryhmäterapiassa [The therapist as an interpreter of biography in the group therapy of Minnesota model]. In J. Ruusuvuori, M. Haakana and L. Raevaara (eds), *Institutionaalinen vuorovaikutus. Keskustelunanalyyttisia tutkimuksia [Institutional interaction. Conversation analytic studies]* (pp. 62–81). Helsinki: Finnish Literature Society.

Halonen, M. (2002) *Kertominen terapian välineenä. Tutkimus vuorovaikutuksesta myllyhoidon ryhmäterapiassa [Telling as a therapeutic tool. A study of interaction in Minnesota model group therapy]*. Helsinki: Finnish Literature Society.

Hardgrove, P., Straka, E. and Medders, E. (1988) Clarification requests of normal and language impaired children. *British Journal of Communication Disorders*, **23**, 51–62.

Heritage, J. and Sorjonen, M.-L. (1994) Constituting and maintaining activities across sequences: *And*–prefacing as a feature of question design. *Language in Society*, **23**, 1–29.

ISK = *Iso Suomen Kielioppi* [*The comprehensive grammar of Finnish*]. Hakulinen, A., Vilkuna, M., Korhonen, R., Koivisto, V., Heinonen, T.-R., Alho, A. Helsinki: Finnish Literature Society.

Jefferson, G. (1987) On exposed and embedded correction in conversation. In G. Button and E. Lee (eds), *Talk and social organization* (pp. 86–100). Clevedon: Multilingual Matters.

Kamhi, A. (1998) Child language. In M. Leahy (ed.), *Disorders of communication. The science of intervention* (pp. 61–95). London: Whurr Publishers.

Kurhila, S. (2000) Milloin natiivi korjaa ei-natiivin kielioppia keskustelussa? [When does a native speaker correct the grammar of a non-native speaker in conversation?] *Virittäjä*, **104** (2), 170–187.

Kurhila, S. (2003) *Co-constructing understanding in second language conversation*. Helsinki: University Press.

Leiwo, M. (1992) Kielitieto ja vuorovaikutus puheterapiassa ja kieltenopetuksessa [Language knowledge and interaction in speech and language therapy and language teaching]. *Finlance: A Finnish Journal of Applied Linguistics*, XI, 56–73.

Leonard, L. (1986) Conversational replies of children with specific language impairment. *Journal of Speech and Hearing Research*, **29**, 114–119.

Leonard, L. (1998) *Children with specific language impairment*. Cambridge, MA: MIT Press.

McTear, M. (1985a) Pragmatic disorders: A case study of conversational disability. *British Journal of Disorders of Communication*, **20**, 29–142.

McTear, M. (1985b) *Children's conversation*. Oxford: Basil Blackwell.

Merrison, S. and Merrison, A. (2005) Repair in speech and language therapy interaction: Investigating pragmatic language impairment of children. *Child Language Teaching and Therapy*, **21**, 191–211.

Ogden, R. and Routarinne, S. (2005) The communicative functions of final rises in Finnish intonation. *Phonetica*, **62**, 160–175.

Panagos, J., Bobkoff, S. and Scott, C. (1986a) Discourse analysis of language intervention. *Child Language Teaching and Therapy*, **2**, 211–229.

Panagos, J., Katz, K., Kovarsky, D. and Prelock, P. (1986b) The nonverbal component of clinical lessons. *Child Language Teaching and Therapy*, **2**, 278–296.

Prutting, C. and Kirchner, D. (1987) A clinical appraisal of the pragmatic aspects of language. *Journal of Speech and Hearing Disorders*, **52**, 105–119.

Prutting, C., Bagshaw, N., Goldstein, H., Juskowiz, S. and Umen, I. (1978) Clinician-child-discourse: Some preliminary questions. *Journal of Speech and Hearing Disorders*, **43**, 123–149.

Raevaara, L. (1993) *Kysyminen toimintana. Kysymys-vastaus vieruspareista arkikeskustelussa* [*Questioning as action. On question-answer adjacency pairs in everyday talk*]. Licentiate thesis. Helsinki: University of Helsinki.

Rapin, I. (1996) Developmental language disorders: A clinical update. *Journal of Child Psychology and Psychiatry*, 37, 643–656.

Rapin, I. and Allen, D. (1983) Developmental language disorders: Nosological considerations. In Ursula Kirk (ed.), *Neuropsychology of language, reading and spelling* (pp. 155–183). New York: Academic Press.

Rapin, I. and Allen, D. (1987) Developmental dysphasia and autism in preschool children: Characteristics and subtypes. *First international symposium. Specific speech and language disorders in children* (pp. 20–35). University of Reading.

Sacks, H. (1992) In G. Jefferson (ed.), *Lectures on conversation*, Vol. 1. Oxford: Blackwell.

Sacks, H., Schegloff, E. and Jefferson, G. (1974) A simplest systematics for organization of turn-taking in conversation. *Language*, 50 (4), 696–735.

Salmenlinna, I. (2005) Korjauskäytänteet puheterapiakeskustelussa seitsemänvuotiaalla lapsella, jolla on kielen kehityksen erityisvaikeus [Conversational repair of a seven-year-old language-impaired child in speech and language therapy]. *Puhe ja kieli*, 25 (2), 87–101.

Schegloff, E., Jefferson, G. and Sacks, H. (1977) The preference for self-correction in the organization of repair in conversation. *Language*, 53, 361–382.

Simmons-Mackie, N., Damico, J. and Damico, H. (1999) A qualitative study of feedback in aphasia treatment. *American Journal of Speech-Language Pathology*, 8, 218–230.

Sinclair, J. and Coulthard, R. (1975) *Towards an analysis of discourse. The English used by teachers and pupils*. Oxford: Oxford University Press.

Sorjonen, M.-L. (1997) Korjausjäsennys [Repair order]. In L. Tainio (ed.), *Keskustelunanalyysin perusteet* [*Foundations of conversation analysis*] (pp. 111–137). Tampere: Vastapaino.

Sorjonen, M.-L. (1999) Dialogipartikkelien tehtävistä [On the use of response words]. *Virittäjä*, 103, 170–194.

Stark, R. and Tallal, P. (1981) Perceptual and motor deficits in language impaired children. In R. Keith (ed.), *Central auditory and language disorders in children* (pp. 121–144). San Diego, CA: College Hill Press.

Tainio, L. (ed.) (1997) *Keskustelunanalyysin perusteet* [*Foundations of conversation analysis*]. Tampere: Vastapaino.

Tykkyläinen, T. (2005) *Puheterapeutti ja lapsi puheterapiatehtävää tekemässä – ohjailevan toiminnan tarkastelua* [*Speech and language therapist and a child performing a language therapy task – analysing interaction in directive sequences*]. Dissertation in logopedics. Publications of Department of Speech Sciences at the University of Helsinki 50. Helsinki: University of Helsinki. http://ethesis.helsinki.fi/julkaisut/kay/fonet/vk/tykkylainen/

Chapter 13

Communication aid use in children's conversation: Time, timing and speaker transfer

MICHAEL CLARKE and RAY WILKINSON

Background

It is a recognised, and oriented to, feature of conversation that talk can be continuous or discontinuous (Sacks *et al.* 1974). Talk may be described as continuous when, for example, speaker transition occurs with minimal gap or overlap between speakers, and discontinuous when, for instance, one speaker stops talking at a place of speaker transfer and does not restart, and no new speaker starts. The immediate progression of turns at places of speaker transition is one facet of the more pervasive features of talk's progressivity (Schegloff 1979, 2007; Lerner 1996), which, in brief, concerns the ways in which successive elements of talk – be they words in an utterance, or turns transferring between speakers for example – are designed and displayed as contiguous. In Schegloff's words: 'it appeared to me that this is a specification, for "sequences", of a more general preference for "progressivity", that is for "next parts" of structured units (e.g. turns, turn construction units like sentences, stories, etc.) to come next' (Schegloff 1979: 268). Interference with talk's progressivity is noticeable and accountable, and the ways in which participants manage such disruption is contingent, in part at least, on the local sequential context of its emergence. For example, delays in an allocated speaker's taking-up of a next turn is one practice in the realisation of dispreferred next turns, that is where a lack of take-up, and the positioning of a delay at speaker transition, may foreshadow the allocated next speaker's non-alignment with the prior turn (e.g. declining an invitation) (Atkinson and Drew 1979; Levinson 1983; Sacks 1987; Schegloff 2007).

For people with communication disability, problems in talk related to features of progressivity may be especially exposed and pervasive. This appears particularly evident in conversations involving people with little or no functional speech and who utilise communication aids (e.g. Sweidel 1991; Beukelman and Mirenda 1992; Robillard 1994; Higginbotham and Wilkins 1999; Clarke, 2005). A proportion of children with significant and ongoing difficulties producing intelligible speech may be provided with augmentative and alternative communication (AAC) systems including for example, voice output communication aids (VOCAs) (e.g. Clarke *et al.* 2001). While important efforts have gone into developing communication aid technologies, and concerns for the ways in which people with disability interact with the communication technology itself, a central (and seemingly under-represented) matter for researchers (and interventionists) in the field concerns how participants manage the constraints on, and possibilities for, face-to-face interactions provided by VOCA technology in everyday talk.

Perhaps the most commonly observed feature of VOCA use in conversation is that VOCA-mediated contributions are significantly slower in their production than spoken contributions, such that progressivity of episodes of talk involving VOCA use is regularly disrupted. Distinct and recurring patterns of conversational organisation observed in such talk are deemed to emerge largely as a consequence of natural speakers' adaptations to the 'alternative metrics' that these conversations, and communication aid use particularly, engender (e.g. Light *et al.* 1985a, b, c; Sweidel 1991; Beukelman and Mirenda 1992; Robillard 1994; Von Tetzchner and Martinsen 1996; Higginbotham and Wilkins 1999). For instance, interaction between adults and children using communication aids has broadly been characterised as asymmetric whereby speaking adults produce a higher frequency of contributions, and a markedly high proportion of turns designed as 'yes/no' questions, than would be expected in interaction between adults and speaking children. Thus children's contributions may be seen to be 'limited' to responses, commonly designed as confirmation or rejection / denial of adults' prior turns signalled through kinesic modalities such as head nods and shakes, with VOCAs and non-technology-based communication aids being used relatively infrequently (e.g. Light 1985a, b, c; Von Tetzchner and Martinsen 1996; Pennington and McConachie 1999, see also Mehan 1979; Goodwin 1995; Tarplee 1996; Mahon 2003 for examples of similar conversational practices observed in adults' and children's talk, including where one participant may possess limited communication resources). Light and colleagues (1985a) propose that adults may work to structure their adult–child interactions in the ways outlined here so that non-speaking children's contributions may be delivered without significant delay and the interaction may adopt a "rhythmic turn passing structure" (Light *et al.* 1985a: 82) considered more typical of interaction between adults and naturally speaking children. More generally, literature in the field suggests that naturally speaking participants may tend not to orient to the different organisation of time and timing within which conversations using communication aids operate.

Very similar patterns of interaction are observed in children's peer interactions in which one child has little or no functional speech and has been provided with a communication aid (Clarke and Kirton 2003). Notably in children's peer talk naturally speaking children have been seen to use specific practices to allocate the placement, and aspects of the content, of their non-speaking co-participants' VOCA-mediated turns (Clarke 2005). Most commonly it seems, VOCA-mediated contributions occur as second parts in adjacency pair-based sequences which are commonly designed as question – answer – response sequences. In such instances natural speakers' first pair parts implicate VOCA use in the immediately next turn where non-speaking children cannot provide meaningful second pair turns using kinesic modalities, such as through sign or iconic gesture (Clarke and Wilkinson 2007). First pair parts designed as questions also project the relevance of VOCA turns coming next functioning as answers and being concerned with particular types of content (Heritage 1984). A second most common sequential location for the realisation of VOCA-mediated turns is following 'meta-interactional' prompts for VOCA use next (Wilkinson and Clarke 2007). Meta-interactional prompts share the design features of first pair parts constructed as questions in that they invite VOCA use in the immediately next turn, and often to conduct a particular class of action (e.g. 'now you ask me a question about football', Extract 13.2). They also provide a 'meta-interactional' function by proposing how the immediately next sequence of turns may be organised. Such sequences of turns are commonly developed as: Prompt – VOCA turn – response. Where for example natural speakers' prompt VOCA users in the production of questions, such prompts regularly initiate sequences of turns which take the form of: prompt – VOCA users' question – natural speakers' answer – VOCA users' response (plus follow-up). Although overwhelmingly, VOCA-mediated turns come about 'in response' to the natural speakers' prior turns, VOCA-mediated turns may also be brought about outside the relevance constraints of a prior turn, although they are relatively rare in these data, and their occurrence is related to the emergence of gaps (i.e. delays between turns) (Sacks *et al.* 1974) in the children's talk (see Clarke 2005). Positioning VOCA use 'in response' to prior turns has been shown to provide structural frameworks for speaking children to understand VOCA – mediated contributions that may be limited in grammatical form, and delayed in both onset and production, and for aided speakers' in being understood (Clarke and Wilkinson 2007; 2008). Like adult–child interactions, it is possible that delays related to VOCA use may also affect how these children's conversations are organised, where for example complex relationships can evolve between VOCA users' physical capabilities, the operational demands of VOCA use, and the normative practices of (children's) conversational interaction (Higginbotham, Mathy-Laikko and Yoder 1988; Higginbotham and Wilkins 1999; Hutchby 2001, see also Pennington and McConachie 2001a,b). Notably however, not all delays related to VOCA use are the same, or are oriented to in the same ways by children (Clarke and Wilkinson 2006), and in adult–child interaction, communication aid use in interaction has been described as not slow in a regular sense, but is characterised by fluctuating 'rhythm' (Light *et al.* 1985a).

The analysis presented here aims to begin to examine in detail something of the nature of delays intrinsic to VOCA use, and the ways in which children orient to disrupted progressivity. As far as we are aware, progressivity has not been systematically investigated in children's peer talk. However, it is notable that the delays in progressivity presented here are massively significant compared with conversation between natural speakers. As the distribution of delays related to VOCA use in conversation is diverse, this analysis limits its scope to an examination of the emergence of delays at places of speaker transition where VOCAs are utilised. Thus the analysis seeks to build on and contribute to broader questions concerning the ways in which normative practices of conversation shape VOCA use, and how VOCA use shapes conversational practices. The study draws on principles and findings from conversation analysis to examine speaker transfer in three sets of video recordings of peer dyads in which one participant has little or no functional speech and has been provided with a VOCA. Thus the analysis is founded on the principle that it is the participants themselves that display that, and how, they orient to delayed progressivity as a feature of this talk. The recordings were taken in the children's schools, and the analysis presented derives from a period of time when each dyad was not in the company of an adult, and had not been provided with guidance or instruction as to how they should spend their time. Firstly, the analysis examines speaker transfer where VOCA-mediated turns are generated in response to natural speakers' prior turns, and, secondly, features of speaker transition in initiated VOCA-mediated turns – that is, turns not generated in repose to prior turns.

In addition to standard CA notation, the transcripts presented in this chapter use brackets to demarcate salient features of the children's interaction that occur simultaneously, including, for example, vocalisations, body movement and physical orientation, as in:

⌈((*looking at VOCA*))⌉.

| ((*looking at T*)) |

⌊   (3.0)   ⌋.

Where non-speaking children produce vocalisations, an orthographic approximation of the sound is provided. The following notation is also used to represent aspects of VOCA use:

talk	bold and italicised text indicates synthesised speech generated by a voice output communication aid.
*	an asterisk represents a 'bleep' generated by a VOCA.
((*switching*))	the term switching represents activation of switches in operation of the VOCA.

Analysis and findings

Pre-beginnings of VOCA-mediated turns

The transition between the end of speaking participants' turns and the beginning of VOCA-users' next turns are distinct from turn transition in typical spoken interaction in particular ways related primarily to the marked delay in the onset of the 'spoken' element (i.e. synthesised speech) of VOCA users' contributions. An example of such a delay is illustrated in Extract 13.1, taken from a conversation between two boys: Jamal and Colin. Jamal (aged 7;11) has physical disability affecting all four limbs. He is unable to generate speech and has been provided with a VOCA. He activates the device via an infrared light source mounted on a headband. By gazing at the VOCA interface he is able to direct an infrared beam to light sensitive cells on the interface (the device presents Jamal with a fixed overlay of 128 cells). By allowing the light source to settle on a cell he can activate it and the device produces an audible bleep (marked by an asterisk (*) in the transcript). Jamal can generate single letters, words and pre-stored phrases by activating assorted cells in specific predetermined sequences. Colin (aged 7;05) is a non-disabled classmate of Jamal. The boys are sitting side-by-side in a room outside the classroom in their school.

From the start of their conversation they have been posing each other known-answer-questions (Schelgoff 2007) in a game of football-related test questions. A significant delay emerges between the completion of Colin's question and the start of Jamal's answer. In Extract 13.1 Colin's orientation of gaze and body position display how he orients to the delay as a relevant feature of the talk.

Extract 13.1 *Jamal and Colin*

→   1   C: ⌈how many times have Brazil⌉ ⌈won the world cup

　　2　　　　│ ((*looking ahead and to right*)) │ │((*looks at VOCA*

→   3   J: │((*head tilted and turned towards C*))

→   4   J: ⌈((*orients to VOCA*)) ⌉ * ⌈((*oriented to VOCA*))⌉ * ***of course***

　　5   C: │((*looking at VOCA*))│ │ ((*looking at VOCA*)) │

　　6　　　　⌊　　(3.0)　　⌋ ⌊　　(1.6)　　⌋

　　7   J: ⌈((*oriented to VOCA*))⌉ * ⌈((*oriented to VOCA*))⌉ * ***four*** ⌈((*looks at C*))⌉

　　8   C: │((*looking at VOCA*)) │ │ ((*looking at VOCA*)) │　　　⌊((*looks at J*)) ⌋

　　9　　　　⌊　　(0.8)　　⌋ ⌊　　(1.0)　　⌋

　10   C: ⌈ye:　　　　　　⌈:eah

　11　　　　⌊((*punches the air*))⌋⌊((*looks at VOCA*))

　12   C: ⌈　　　　spot on　　　　⌉

　13　　　　│((*leaning back looking at VOCA*)) │

　14   J: │　　　　　hur　　　　│

　15　　　　⌊　((*turns head left and down*)) 　⌋

The point at which the spoken element of Jamal's response '*of course*' (line 4) is generated as synthesised speech by the VOCA, comes 4.6 seconds following the completion of Colin's question. The delay of 4.6 seconds is significantly greater than would be expected in conversation between speaking participants, and is in stark contrast to a possible standard maximum silence of approximately 1 second (Jefferson 1989). It has been noted that following a question, an answer is due immediately next (Sacks *et al.* 1974; Heritage 1984). Therefore, the moment that Colin's question is complete, the expectation for who should rightfully speak next shifts unambiguously to Jamal, and thus any delay may be seen to be attributable to Jamal. On completion of Colin's question Jamal is seen to turn his head towards the VOCA and gaze at the interface, directing his infrared pointer towards the device. Cells on the VOCA interface light up as they detect the infrared light source, and after 3.0 seconds Jamal's sustained orientation to the device brings about two bleeps separated by 1.6 seconds, as a cell sequence is triggered and the speech device is activated. Although a spoken next turn is delayed the transition space is occupied or filled with Jamal's visible activity in VOCA operation, and audible VOCA bleeps, in his possible preparation of a next turn and possibly an answer. A particular class of *intra-turn* silence termed 'no-trouble' silence (Lerner 1996) has been reported within activities such as shared list writing. In this context a silence may evolve as participants wait for the writing of the list to catch up with the spoken construction of the list. In this instance, the silence is caused by the activity of constructing a written list and is 'filled' by the writing. It is possible also to speculate that similar 'no trouble' delays may emerge in, for example, children's shared computer work. However, it is the occurrence of such delay in these children's everyday mundane talk that is notable and distinct from natural speakers' conversation. In the conversation between Colin and Jamal, Colin cannot be unequivocally certain of the purpose of Jamal's actions although the ambiguity is mitigated somewhat by the relevance for an answer next cast by the prior turn. As it turns out, Jamal is producing an answer and a known fact, although arguably in this instance the class of turn signalled by '*of course*' is ambiguous. It can be seen retrospectively that Jamal's VOCA-directed activity serves to project the onset of VOCA speech. Schegloff (1996) describes elements of the beginnings of turns 'which project the onset of talk, or the beginning of a (next) TCU [turn construction unit] or a turn, but are not yet proper recognisable beginnings' (Schegloff 1996: 92). Examples of such pre-beginnings include orienting head and gaze direction towards a potential addressee, emphasised in-breath and throat clearing. Jamal's VOCA-oriented activity here is analysable as a class of pre-beginning – a signal that the next turn is literally 'in the works' (Schegloff 2007: 70).

One germane issue for Colin here concerns how he might handle a delay of unknown period in speaker transition. Colin displays how he orients to the work of turn-preparation the delay embodies through his gaze-behaviour and shifting physical alignment at, and around, speaker transition. Colin is seen to shift his gaze towards the VOCA in advance of his own turn-completion (lines 1 and 2), and at a time that Jamal is looking at him (see also Wilkinson *et al.*, in press). Colin's gaze-shift to the VOCA appears indicative of his anticipation of the locus of Jamal's gaze in VOCA use, and suggests a collaborative orientation to the VOCA as the 'animator' (Goffman 1981; see also Wilkinson *et al.*, in press) of the expected response. Significantly, by waiting in silence while gazing at the VOCA interface, Colin treats the delay in speaker transition and VOCA generated bleeps as noticeably relevant features of turn-transition within the context that an answer is due next. Such practices in gaze and body alignment differ from common practices observed in 'natural' speakers' talk, whereby an expectation exists for the speaker to secure the gaze of the intended recipient(s) at the start of a turn (Goodwin 1980, 1981; Higginbotham and Wilkins 1999). Notably also, relevance constraints projected by the prior question allow for the VOCA-oriented activity initiated in this slot to be seen *as* a preparation of an answer.

Two further examples of similarly occurring pre-beginnings are presented in Extracts 13.2 and 13.3. Extract 13.2 is again taken from the conversation between Jamal and Colin. In this instance Jamal's VOCA-mediated turn comes about following Colin's 'meta-interactional' prompt for VOCA use, 'wu (.) now you ask <u>me</u> a question about football' (line 1). Colin's prompt initiates a question–answer–response sequence, on this occasion with Jamal taking the role of questioner. A delay of 9.4 seconds emerges between the end of Colin's prompt and the start of the VOCA turn and, as observed in Extract 13.1, this transition space is occupied, in part, by Jamal's VOCA-oriented activity and the generation of VOCA bleeps signalling its use. In this instance Colin orients his gaze to the VOCA interface somewhat later than observed above, here turning his gaze to the device as the main locus of the boys' shared attention just after the first pre-beginning bleep is generated.

Extract 13.2 *Jamal and Colin*

```
→   1   C:   ⌈wu (.) now you ⌈ask me a      ⌉question about football⌉
    2        |                 ⌊((points at J))⌋                     |
    3        ⌊          ((J and C looking at each other))            ⌋
→   4   J:   ⌈       ((turns and looks at VOCA))       ⌉ * ⌈((oriented to VOCA))⌉ *
    5   C:   |((looks down at his hand on J's w'chair tray))|   |((looks at VOCA))  |
    6        ⌊              (2.2)                       ⌋  ⌊       (0.9)          ⌋
→   7   J:   ⌈((oriented to VOCA))⌉ * ⌈((oriented to VOCA))⌉ * **how**
    8   C:   |((looking at VOCA))  |   |((looking at VOCA)) |
    9        ⌊       (4.2)         ⌋  ⌊         (2.1)       ⌋
```

Extract 13.3 is taken from a conversation between Martin and David. Like Jamal, Martin (aged 10;8) has a severe physical disability affecting all four limbs. He has profoundly limited functional speech and has been provided with a VOCA of similar operational design to Jamal's. Unlike Jamal, Martin accesses his VOCA through switches mounted in a headrest. Using his head, he can control the activation of sequences of cells to generate speech. David (aged 10;6) is a close friend of Martin. He has a very mild speech dysarthria but is normally fully intelligible. The boys are in a room in school but outside the classroom, and sitting side-by-side. This extract is taken from the very start of their recorded conversation. In the moments before the extract an adult has left the room and David has been prompting Martin to use his VOCA to 'start' the conversation, saying 'go on you start' and using his hand to orient Martin's head onto his headrest and thus into the proximity of his VOCA switches.

Extract 13.3 *Martin and David*

```
    1   D:   °go on°
→   2   M:   ⌈((orients to VOCA and starts switching))        ⌉*
    3   D:   |((looks at VOCA, then to M, then into room))|
    4        ⌊                  (6.5)                         ⌋
→   5   M:   ⌈   ((switching))    ⌉ * ⌈    ((switching))    ⌉*
    6   D:   |((looking at VOCA))|   |((looking at VOCA))|
    7        ⌊       (5.9)       ⌋  ⌊       (9.7)        ⌋
→   8   M:   ⌈((turns and looks at David))⌉ **D**⌈**a p h n e** =
    9        ⌊            (0.3)            ⌋  ⌊((starts to smile))
   10   D:   = ((looks at M))
```

At line 1, David's turn 'go on' functions as a command for Martin to use his VOCA. Immediately following David's command Martin orients to the VOCA, and is seen to utilise the device by triggering his head-switches, leading to VOCA generated bleeps after

6.5 seconds. On completion of his turn at line 1, David looks at the VOCA interface, then to Martin and then into the body of the room in which they sit. Like Colin in Extract 13.2, David orients to the VOCA interface just after the first VOCA-generated bleep of the pre-beginning, and he maintains his gaze here throughout the remainder of the pre-beginning. After 22.4 seconds, Martin generates the name 'Daphne'. Here again a very significant pre-beginning delay is evident which is occupied by Martin's VOCA-directed activity. David's explicit location of Martin as the next speaker, his bodily support of Martin's head in relation to the VOCA head-switches, and his waiting in silence during Martin's preparation to speak all display features of his collaborative orientation to the embodied and sequential consequences of VOCA use at speaker transfer. (It is notable here that Martin orients away from his VOCA in the moments before the word is produced. It transpires that this action is used to signal the end of the pre-beginning. More generally this movement can be used to signal the completion of a VOCA-mediated contribution – see Clarke 2005.)

The location of extended pre-beginnings of VOCA-mediated contributions at places of speaker transfer is a common and recurring feature of these children's interaction. The implicit or explicit positioning of VOCA turns following questions or prompts provides for the emergence of significant delay at speaker transfer which is not treated as a source of trouble. However, it is also a feature of these children's talk that pre-beginnings of VOCA-mediated turns are vulnerable to co-occurring talk by a co-participant. By co-occurring talk we mean here talk that occurs concurrently with pre-beginnings. The next section will explicate this practice in these children's interaction.

Natural speakers' (pre-emptive) talk co-occurring with pre-beginnings

This section explores another way in which the issue of delayed progressivity at speaker transition may be seen to be an oriented-to feature of these children's talk. While speaking children may wait in silence during VOCA-turn pre-beginnings, it is evident also that pre-beginnings are vulnerable to speaking participants' co-occurring talk. Such talk is hearable as designed to promote the progressivity of speaker transition by providing for the possibility that the VOCA-user may next produce a less VOCA-work-intensive turn than implicated by the speaker's prior turn. Here we illustrate this feature as it is seen to occur in pre-beginnings developed in response to speaking participants' prior turns. The next example (Extract 13.4) provides a representative illustration of the natural speaker's talk co-occurring with pre-beginning activity.

Extract 13.4 *Jamal and Colin*

```
→   1   C:   tell me your best song
→   2   J:   ⌈((orients to VOCA))⌉*
    3   C:   |   ((looking at J))   |
    4        ⌊      (2.1)          ⌋
    5   J:   ⌈((oriented to VOCA))⌉*
    6   C:   |   ((looking at J))   |
    7        ⌊      (2.9)          ⌋
```

```
→    8   C:  ⌈    is      it    ⌉ ⌈Asha
     9   J:  ⌊((oriented to VOCA))⌋ ⌊*
→   10   J:  ⌈((oriented to VOCA))⌉ * Asha you make me wanna
    11   C:  |    ((looking at J))    |
    12       ⌊        (2.4)          ⌋
```

Here Colin is seen to re-model his initial command, and request for information, 'tell me your best song' (line 1) by providing a candidate response 'is it Asha' (line 8) 5 seconds into the pre-beginning of Jamal's response. Having issued his command, Colin has no obvious way of determining when the pre-beginning of Jamal's turn will end and the turn itself begin (or indeed, as noted above, whether the VOCA-directed activity is aimed at producing an answer). Proffering this candidate implicates acceptance or rejection as a possible, minimally relevant next-turn action. Such a turn could be produced as a single word 'yes' or 'no', communicated through the VOCA, or non-vocally, for example, with a nod or shake of the head – this latter option providing a more economical and immediate modality of response. In this data it is also possible that a 'no' response may initiate a guessing sequence for the intended answer. It transpires that Jamal generates a pre-stored whole phrase next, presumably the title of his favourite song *'Asha you make me wanna'* (line 10), and an answer to Colin's initial question (see also, Harris 1982; Hjelmquist and Sandberg Dalghren 1996).

Extract 13.5 provides a further example of the natural speaker speaking after the VOCA user has initiated pre-beginning activities, again with the apparent intent of promoting progressivity in speaker transition. Like Extract 13.4 the speaker's talk co-occurring with the VOCA pre-beginning makes a different type of answer relevant next. On this occasion, however, the aided speaker goes on to answer the new question.

Extract 13.5 is taken from a conversation between two young people named here as Tina and Lucy. Tina (aged 14;10) has severe physical disability and experiences profoundly restricted movement. She is unable to produce intelligible speech and has been provided with a VOCA of the same design as Jamal's. Like Martin she accesses her device using head-switches mounted in a headrest, although her access method differs from Martin's as her device is configured to operate a switch-scanning procedure. Briefly, upon activation, the device automatically scans through each row of cells on the interface. When the scanning routine has reached a row in which a desired cell is located, Tina can initiate scanning of cells in that particular row by triggering her head-switch. Hitting her head-switch again at the moment at which the specific targeted cell in that row is highlighted activates that individual cell. Like Jamal and Martin, Tina can produce letters, words and phrases by triggering sequences of cells. On each occasion that the VOCA scanning procedure highlights a row or individual cell it produces a bleep, and if no further selection is made the scanning procedure will pass through an array of rows, or individual cells in a row, three times before stopping. Consequently once activated, the VOCA generates frequent and persistent bleeps as it passes through its scanning cycle. The presence of bleeps generated by the automatic scanning procedure is represented by as asterisk (*) in the left margin of the transcript, and within the body of the transcript where the bleeps are deemed to be of particular relevance. Lucy (14;4) is Tina's classmate. She has a physical disability that affects her lower limbs and she uses a wheelchair. Her speech is only marginally affected by her physical disability, and does not present a significant challenge to her speech intelligibility. In this conversation the girls are sitting alone and opposite each other in a teaching/therapy room outside their main classroom.

Extract 13.5 *Tina and Lucy*

```
→    1      L:  ⌈what do you do normally in swimming⌉
     2      T:  ⌊          ((looking at VOCA))          ⌋
→    3   *  T:  ⌈(((sits motionless, then hits switch and bleep heard immediately)))⌉ *
     4   *  L:  |                        ((looking at T))                        |
     5   *      ⌊                            (0.5)                            ⌋
     6   *  T:  ⌈(((looking at VOCA then hits switch and generates a bleep)))⌉ *
     7   *  L:  |                        ((looking at T))                        |
     8   *      ⌊                            (1.7)                            ⌋
     9   *  T:  ⌈* ((looking at VOCA))
→   10   *  L:  ⌊who normally takes ya
→   11   *  T:  ⌈          ((oriented to VOCA, switching))          ⌉ m
    12   *  L:  |((variously looking at T and into the room or down))|
    13   *      ⌊                    (26.0)                    ⌋
```

At line 3 Tina is seen to respond to Lucy's question by engaging in seeming pre-beginning activity of a VOCA-mediated contribution. After 2.2 seconds Lucy recasts her question 'what do you do normally in swimming' (line 1) by asking 'who normally takes ya' (line 10). The new turn implicates a next response from a more restricted category of possible answers by making relevant the generation of a name from a group of people that 'normally' take Tina swimming, rather than an account of swimming as initially implicated. The generation of a name rather than an account of swimming activities is also analysable as being a more economical whole next turn to produce. After 26.0 seconds in which Lucy waits in silence Tina responds to the immediately prior question by generating a single letter '*m*', which Lucy subsequently treats as the first letter of the name Margaret (Clarke 2005).

In these extracts, pre-beginnings are exposed as vulnerable to natural speakers co-occurring talk. The natural speakers' co-occurring talk here alters the 'respondability' of the next due turn by making relevant next turns of potentially reduced production demands. Such talk pre-empts the forthcoming turn, and displays the natural speakers' active engagement in, and sensitivity to, analysis of progressivity at speaker transfer. VOCA users may variously take-up the possibilities provided by speakers' co-occurring talk. Where they do this it is possible that they may be required to restart, or redirect the design of the (start of the) turn in preparation. That is, the recasting may introduce additional (less visible) VOCA-use demands, although the overall 'cost' of production of the complete turn may be reduced (e.g. Extract 13.5).

Natural speakers' (pre-emptive) talk co-occurring with pre-beginnings of initiated VOCA turns

Although most typically, VOCA-mediated contributions come about as responses to speaking participants' prior turns, children may utilise VOCAs outside these specific sequential positions. Here we will refer to such turns as initiated VOCA turns, that is VOCA-mediated turns produced not as responses to prior turns. In this data, pre-beginnings of initiated VOCA-mediated turns are particularly exposed to the co-occurrence of speaking children's talk. Speaking children's talk here can instigate two or three part exchanges whereby confirmation of the status of VOCA-oriented activity as a possible pre-beginning is sought. These short sequences embedded within possible pre-beginnings can be seen to be in the service of the forthcoming VOCA-mediated contribution and the organisation of (unproblematic) sequences of turns more generally. However, such talk may leave the VOCA-turn itself as vulnerable to abandonment.

Extract 13.6 from Tina and Lucy's conversation provides an example of natural speaker's talk co-occurring with the pre-beginning of an initiated VOCA-mediated turn. In this extract the VOCA-mediated turn is successfully started. The first point of significance for this discussion concerns Tina's orientation to her VOCA and activation of her head switch (line 5) within a brief gap following the completion of a prior exchange (lines 1–3).

Extract 13.6 *Tina and Lucy*

```
        1    L:   did ⌈you wanna come back to school⌉
        2             ⌊          ((raises arms))          ⌋
        3    T:   ((nods, head falling forward with chin down to chest))
        4    L:   ((looks away))
→       5    T:   ⌈((lifts head up looking at VOCA, hits switch twice))⌉*⌈((oriented to VOCA, switching))⌉
        6    L:   |          ((looking away))          | |     ((looks at T))     |
        7         ⌊              (3.0)              ⌋
→       8    L:   ya g⌈un⌉na say something =
        9          ⌊*⌋
       10    T:   ⌈              *              ⌉
       11         ⌊((small head movement forward and back))⌋
       12    T:   ⌈((looking at VOCA, hits switch))⌉*
       13         ⌊          (0.8)          ⌋
→      14    L:   ya gonna⌈say⌉↑something
       15            ⌊*⌋
→      16    T:   ((nods looking at VOCA))
```

→   17   L: ⌈yes⌉

      18   ⌊ * ⌋ * *

→   19   *   T: ⌈((switching))⌉ **g** ⌈((switching))⌉

      20   *   ⌊   (29.7)   ⌋ ⌊   (2.2)   ⌋

Following the generation of a VOCA bleep (line 5) Lucy, who has been looking away, directs her gaze to Tina. Lucy is seen to treat Tina's VOCA-directed activity and the production of a bleep as a possible pre-beginning saying, 'ya gunna say something' (line 8). Lucy's question has a meta-interactional function, working as an explicit inspection of the status of the organisation of the talk. Lucy appears to treat Tina's subsequent actions as not a response to her inquiry, and she re-issues her question, which on this occasion initiates a three-part exchange whereby Tina nods and Lucy provides a public treatment of Tina's actions as a response (lines 14–17). Subsequently, Lucy waits in silence and after 29.7 seconds Tina's VOCA-mediated turn begins with the letter 'g'. As seen in Extracts 13.4 and 13.5, it is evident that pre-beginnings are vulnerable to natural speakers' co-occurring talk. In Extracts 13.4 and 13.5 however the VOCA-oriented activity is seemingly treated as a pre-beginning, in part at least, because of the relevance for VOCA-oriented activity cast by the speakers' prior turn. Here, where the VOCA-oriented activity is initiated outside such relevance constraints, the speaking participant seeks to introduce a relevance framework in order to determine the potential implications of the VOCA-user's actions (e.g. that the bleeps are functioning as pre-beginnings and are not, for example, occurring randomly or as a continuation of a prior project). Tina's VOCA-oriented activity taking place after the three-part clarification exchange (line 19) operates within a sequential environment made explicitly relevant for that activity. That is, the pre-beginning is essentially resumed at this point, and Lucy waits a full 29.7 seconds before hearing the first letter of Tina's turn.

In Extract 13.7 the exchange between lines 1–6 is hearable as potentially complete when Tina initiates switch activation (line 7). The possible emergence of a pre-beginning is seen to become an explicitly oriented-to feature of the talk with Lucy saying, 'you're telling something to me' (line 16), instigating a three-part exchange whereby Tina nods in response (line 18) and Lucy provides an overt treatment of her understanding of Tina's nod and consequently Tina's VOCA-oriented actions as a pre-beginning (line 19). Lucy then waits in silence as Tina works with her VOCA in apparent turn preparation. However in this instance, Tina's VOCA-mediated turn is not begun.

Extract 13.7 *Tina and Lucy*

      1   L: don't know

      2   T: ((*small head shake*))

      3   T: ⌈((*raises eyebrows, lifts head looking at VOCA*))⌉

      4   L: | ((*looking forward*)) |

      5   ⌊   (2.0)   ⌋

      6   L: °right.°

```
→   7    T:  ⌈((head hits switch and holds switch down))⌉
    8        ⌊              (1.2)                        ⌋
→   9    T:  ((releases switch))  * ⌈((looking at VOCA))⌉ * ⌈((looking at VOCA))⌉ *
    10   L:                        | ((looking ahead)) | | ((looking ahead)) |
    11                             ⌊      (0.8)        ⌋ ⌊      (1.0)        ⌋
→   12   T:  ⌈((looking at VOCA))⌉*
    13   L:  |   ((looks at T))   |
    14       ⌊       (1.0)        ⌋
    15   T:  ⌈          ((looking at VOCA))              ⌉ ⌈*
→   16   L:  |((raises finger and then closes it into a fist))| ⌊you're telling something to me
    17       ⌊                   (1.2)                     ⌋
→   18   *  T:  ((nods, head dropping forward and down))
→   19   *  L:  ⌈yeh
    20   *  T:  ⌊((raises head up to look at VOCA, switching)) ⌈((switching))⌉
    21   *                                                     ⌊   (23.0)    ⌋
→   22   *  L:  did you have a good weekend ⌈              as well              ⌉
    23   *  T:                              ⌊((head drops forward, looking at VOCA))⌋
    24   *  T:  ((head drops further forward, looking at VOCA))
→   25   *  L:  yeh
    26   *  T:  ((slight forward nod bringing head further down, raises head, looks at VOCA))
→   27   *  L:  ⌈what did you do over the weekend⌉
    28   *  T:  ⌊         ((switching))           ⌋
    29   *  T:  ⌈((looking at VOCA))⌉
    30   *  L:  |  ((looking at T))  |
    31   *       ⌊      (3.0)        ⌋
→   32   *  L:  ⌈shall I um: (1.0) say some words and you stop me⌉
→   33   *  T:  ⌊              ((switching))                     ⌋((nods head))
→   34   *  L:  ok
```

Twenty-three seconds after Lucy establishes the status of the talk as a pre-beginning she initiates a second three-part exchange asking, 'did you have a good weekend as well' (line 22). By asking a question here Lucy appears to disregard the publicly endorsed status of the talk as being a period of preparation for Tina's turn to begin. Notably, however, Lucy's turn is delicately designed in respect to the sequential context. By completing the turn with 'as well' Lucy's talk is hearable as cognisant of the pre-beginning in progress; 'as well' perhaps intended to be taken as signalling that Tina might respond to this question as well as pursuing the start of her own turn. Tina may provide a relevant answer to this question through a nod or shake of the head as a 'yes' or 'no', without irretrievably diverting herself from the work of turn-beginning preparation, although this action may delay the onset of the turn. As noted in Extract 13.5, speech co-occurring with VOCA users' pre-beginnings may introduce a potential ambiguity for how the natural speaker should treat the start of the VOCA-mediated turn. Following Lucy's question here (line 22) it is unknown whether Tina will develop her turn-beginning in relation to her weekend or something else.

Lucy then talks again, posing another question, this time asking, 'what did you do over the weekend' (line 27). This second question is one that makes relevant a VOCA-mediated answer, and therefore contravenes most explicitly the current arrangement for how the talk is being organised by introducing a new relevance framework within which she might seek to understand Tina's turn, and in relation to which Tina may now build the start of her turn. Tina does not obviously respond to this action but remains looking at her VOCA (line 29). After 3.0 seconds Lucy speaks again for the third time and asks yet another question, this time proposing, 'shall I um: (1.0) say some words and you stop me' (line 32). This proposes an explicit strategy with which the girls can develop the talk by introducing the possibility of engaging in a type of guessing sequence (Goodwin 1995) concerned with weekend activities. This also provides a possibility to delete the explicitly negotiated understanding that Tina will produce a turn. Tina is observed to endorse this course of action by nodding (line 33), abandoning her initial independent initiation of a VOCA-mediated turn (see also, Harris 1982; Hjelmquist and Dahlgren Sandberg 1996).

For these initiated VOCA-mediated turns, pre-beginnings can become a site for the realisation of adjacency-pair-based sequences geared specifically to identifying the status of the talk towards possible turn beginning, and therefore expectations for the talk's progressivity at these places. While this may lead to the start of a VOCA-mediated turn (seen here in Extracts 13.5 and 13.6), such talk may be used to negotiate an exit from that explicitly identified course of action (seen here in Extract 13.7, lines 32–34), or can otherwise lead to the abandonment of a VOCA turn (see Clarke 2005).

Summary and discussion

For people with physical disability who have little or no functional speech, and who have been provided with communication aids, delays inherent in communication aid use in conversation may lead participants in talk to manage their conversation in ways that are untypical of conversation between natural speakers. Using conversation analysis as an analytical approach, this chapter has presented an examination of recurring organisational features of speaker transfer related to VOCA use in children's peer conversation. The evidence has been drawn from episodes of interaction in three child–child dyads. VOCA use in these children's conversations is most commonly positioned in response to speaking participants' prior questions or prompts. Although far less common, VOCAs are also seen to be used to initiate turns. Distinct practices in speaker transfer have been observed, in particular how pre-beginnings (Schegloff 1996) which are occupied by VOCA-users' activity of turn preparation, emerge as a manifest feature of VOCA use, and the particular ways in which both children may orient to these distinct sequential locations.

For pre-beginnings developed in response to natural speakers' prior turns, it has been shown that naturally speaking children may treat delays in speaker transition as noticeably relevant, evidenced for example by their physical orientation and sustained gaze towards the VOCA interface during pre-beginnings, and waiting in silence in apparent anticipation of VOCA speech as the 'animator' (Goffman 1981) of their co-participants' turn (Extracts 13.1–13.3). It is evident also, however, that VOCA-mediated turn pre-beginnings are vulnerable to natural speakers' co-occurring talk, both in the sequential context that a VOCA-mediated turn is due next (Extracts 13.4 and 13.5), and for initiated VOCA turns (Extracts 13.6 and 13.7). Where this is seen to occur in pre-beginnings of VOCA-mediated responses, it appears that such co-occurring talk is motivated and designed to enhance the progressivity of speaker transition by potentially reducing the production demands of the next due VOCA-mediated speech. Non-speaking children may variously take up possibilities for (the start of) next turns made relevant by their co-participants' talk co-occurring within pre-beginnings. It would seem therefore that such natural speakers' talk co-occurring with pre-beginnings may introduce a potential uncertainty as to which of the prior turns the forthcoming VOCA-mediated contribution will relate.

The realisation of initiated VOCA-mediated turns in these children's talk has been seen to give rise to other distinctive practices happening in tandem with pre-beginnings. Firstly, it is notable that where VOCA-mediated activity is initiated outside a second turn slot, speaking children may seek to establish explicitly the possibility that such actions are pre-beginnings (Extracts 13.6 and 13.7). Speaking children's co-occurring talk here is intentionally sequence initiating by making relevant a response in addition to, and concurrent with, VOCA-turn preparation. Note, for example, in Extract 13.6, Lucy's pursuit of a response from Tina during her VOCA-directed activity. Pre-beginnings in these sequential positions represent a site where seemingly distinctive displays of multi-modality are evident, that is, where VOCA-directed activity in preparation for turn beginning, and head gestures in response to natural speakers' co-occurring talk, are used independently and concurrently (see also Wilkinson *et al.*, in press).

Within the context of interaction between adults and children using communication aids, it has been proposed that adult practices in organising interaction primarily through question–answer sequences, where children's answers are provided non-vocally, may be a consequence of adults' drive to emulate the 'metric' of turn exchange between natural speakers. One outcome of this organising strategy is that communication aids may be used infrequently (e.g. Light *et al.* 1985; Von Tetzchner and Martinsen 1996). Analysis of VOCA use in children's peer talk has highlighted the potential benefits of question–answer–response sequences, and prompt – VOCA turn – response sequences, for both natural speakers in understanding VOCA-mediated contributions, and for non-speaking children in being understood (Clarke and Wilkinson 2007, 2008). It is possible also that a further issue motivating the positioning of these VOCA-mediated turns is related to the inherent delays in speaker transfer where VOCAs are used. Non-speaking children's VOCA-oriented activities brought about following first pair parts of adjacency pairs, such as questions and meta-interactional prompts that make VOCA use relevant next, can be seen *as* pre-beginnings of forthcoming turns. Natural speakers' first turns prefigure a delay in speaker transfer, and anticipate an adjustment in the typical expectations for progressivity at speaker transition that may be approached by non-speaking children's use of non-vocal responses. Where VOCA-mediated turns are initiated outside such sequential contexts (Extracts 13.6 and 13.7) the speaking partner may produce talk co-occurring with possible pre-beginnings in a bid to clarify explicitly the status of the VOCA-user's actions as possible pre-beginnings. By providing structurally defined locations for delay in speaker transition, and seeking to determine explicitly where delay is relevant, these children are seen to actively negotiate locations in talk that may reflect what Robillard, a communication aid user himself, describes as the 'alternative time order' (Robillard 1994; see also Higginbotham and Wilkins 1999) that is inherent in the organisation of such talk. Notably, the significance and robustness of participants' orientation to delayed progressivity is changeable. Naturally speaking children's talk co-occurring with pre-beginnings has been seen to display their attention to enhancing the potential for progressivity in such locations. Despite having been granted the conversational floor, delay in the onset of the initiated next turn may lead to the participants, and the speaking participant primarily, orienting to such delay as potentially troublesome. For example, in Extract 13.7 Lucy is observed to bring about a negotiated departure from the explicitly identified condition of the talk, and thus a re-shaping of the direction of the subsequent talk, and expectations for progressivity in that talk.

The orderly accomplishment of speaker transition is an integral aspect of conversational organisation (e.g. Sacks *et al.* 1974; Schegloff 1996). For both children in these conversations, VOCA use challenges conventional practices in the organisation of transition space. The analysis has shown that these children are occupied with the organisation of speaker transfer, and some ways in which it is handled. Transitions between speakers where VOCAs are used can display distinctive sequential properties. Detailed sequential analysis can reveal how interplay between children's physical disabilities, the demands of VOCA use, and normative practices in (children's) conversation brings about distinct and novel forms of conversational organisation.

References

Atkinson, J.M. and Drew, P. (1979) *Order in court: The organisation of verbal interaction in judicial settings.* London: Macmillan.

Beukelman, D. and Mirenda, P. (1992) *Augmentative and alternative communication: Management of severe communication disorders in children and adults.* London: Jessica Kingsley Publishers.

Clarke, M.T. (2005) *Conversational interaction between children using communication aids and their peers.* Unpublished PhD thesis, University College, London.

Clarke, M.T. and Kirton, A. (2003) Patterns of interaction between children with physical disabilities using augmentative and alternative communication and their peers. *Child Language Teaching and Therapy,* **19**, 135–151.

Clarke, M.T. and Wilkinson, R. (2006) *Turn construction using voice output communication aids in interaction between children with cerebral palsy and their peers.* International Conference on Conversation Analysis, Helsinki, May.

Clarke, M.T. and Wilkinson, R. (2007) Interaction between children with cerebral palsy and their peers 1: Organising and understanding VOCA use. *Augmentative and Alternative Communication,* **23**, 336–348.

Clarke, M.T. and Wilkinson, R. (2008) Interaction between children with cerebral palsy and their peers 2: Understanding initiated VOCA mediated turns. *Augmentative and Alternative Communication,* **24**, 3–15.

Clarke, M.T., Price, K. and Jolleff, N. (2001) Augmentative and alternative communication: Principles in assessment. In M. Kersner and J.A. Wright (eds), *Speech and language therapy: The decision making process when working with children* (pp. 268–282). London: Fulton.

Goodwin, C. (1980) Restarts, pauses, and the achievement of mutual gaze at turn beginning. *Sociological Inquiry*, 50, 272–302.

Goodwin, C. (1981) *Conversational organisation: Interaction between speakers and hearers.* New York: Academic Press.

Goodwin, C. (1995) Conversations with an aphasic man. *Research in Language and Social Interaction*, 28, 233–260.

Higginbotham, D.J. and Wilkins, D.P. (1999) Slipping through the timestream: Social issues of time and timing in augmented interactions. In D. Korvasky, J. Duchan and M. Maxwell (eds), *Constructing (in)competence: Disabling evaluations in clinical and social interaction* (pp. 49–82). Mahwah, NJ: Lawrence Erlbaum Associates.

Higginbotham, D.J., Mathy-Laikko, P. and Yoder, D.E. (1988) Studying conversations of augmentative communication system users. In L.E. Berstein (ed.), *The vocally impaired: Clinical practice and research* (pp. 265–294). Philadelphia: Grune and Stratton.

Goffman, E. (1981) *Forms of talk.* Oxford: Basil Blackwell.

Harris, D. (1982) Communication interaction processes involving nonvocal physically handicapped children. *Topics in Language Disorders*, 2, 21–37.

Heritage, J. (1984b) *Garfinkel and ethnomethodology.* Cambridge: Polity Press.

Hjelmquist, E. and Sandberg Dalghren, A.D. (1996) Sounds of silence: Interaction in aided language use. In S. Tetzchner and M.H. Jehsen (eds), *Augmentative and alternative communication: European perspectives* (pp. 137–152). London: Whurr.

Hutchby, I. (2001) *Conversation and technology: From the telephone to the internet.* Cambridge: Polity Press.

Jefferson, G. (1986) Notes on latency in overlap. *Human Studies*, 9, 153–183.

Lerner, G. (1996) On the 'semi-permeable' character of grammatical units in conversation: Conditional entry into the turn space of another speaker. In E. Ochs, E.A. Schegloff and S.A. Thompson (eds), *Interaction and grammar* (pp. 238–276). Cambridge: Cambridge University Press.

Levinson, S.C. (1983) *Pragmatics.* Cambridge: Cambridge University Press.

Light, J., Collier, B. and Parnes, P. (1985a) Communicative interaction between young nonspeaking physically disabled children and their primary caregivers: Part I – Discourse patterns. *Augmentative and Alternative Communication*, 1, 74–83.

Light, J., Collier, B. and Parnes, P. (1985b) Communicative interaction between young nonspeaking physically disabled children and their primary caregivers: Part II – Communicative function. *Augmentative and Alternative Communication*, 2, 98–107.

Light, J., Collier, B. and Parnes, P. (1985c) Communicative interaction between young nonspeaking physically disabled children and their primary caregivers: Part III – Modes of communication. *Augmentative and Alternative Communication*, 3, 125–133. Communication Research Symposium in AAC Pennsylvania Toronto.

Mahon, M. (2003) Conversations with young deaf children in families where English is an additional language. In P. Gallaway and A. Young (eds), *Deafness and education in the UK* (pp. 35–52). London: Whurr.

Mehan, H. (1979). *Learning lessons: Social organisation in the classroom.* Cambridge, MA: Harvard University Press.

Pennington, L. and McConachie, H. (1999) Mother–child interaction revisited: Communication with non-speaking physically disabled children. *International Journal of Language and Communication Disorders*, **34**, 391–416.

Pennington, L. and McConachie, H. (2001a) Interaction between children with cerebral palsy and their mothers: The effects of speech and intelligibility. *International Journal of Language and Disorders of Communication*, **36**, 371–393.

Pennington, L. and McConachie, H. (2001b) Prediction patterns of interaction between children with cerebral palsy and their mothers. *Developmental Medicine and Child Neurology*, **43**, 83–90.

Robillard, A.B. (1994) Communication problems in the intensive care unit. *Qualitative Sociology*, **17**, 383–395.

Sacks, H. (1987) On the preferences for agreement and contiguity in sequences in conversation. In G. Button and J.R.E. Lee (eds), *Talk and social organisation* (pp. 54–69). Clevedon: Multilingual Matters.

Sacks, H., Schegloff, E.A. and Jefferson, G. (1974) A simplest systematics for the organisation of turn-taking for conversation, *Language*, **50**, 696–735.

Schegloff, E.A. (1979) The relevance of repair for syntax-for-conversation. In T. Givon (ed.), *Syntax and semantics*, vol. 12: *Discourse and syntax* (pp. 261–288). New York: Academic Press.

Schegloff, E.A. (2007) *Sequence organisation in interaction: A primer in conversation analysis*. Cambridge: Cambridge University Press.

Sweidel, G. (1991) Management strategies in the communication of speaking persons and persons with a speech disability. *Research on Language and Social Interaction*, **25**, 195–214.

Tarplee, C. (1996) Working on young children's utterances: Prosodic aspects of repetition during picture labelling. In E. Couper-Kuhlen and M. Selting (eds), *Prosody in conversation* (pp. 406–435). Cambridge: Cambridge University Press.

von Tetzchner, S. and Martinsen, H. (1996) Words and strategies: Conversations with young children who use aided language. In S. von Tetzchner and M.H. Jensen (eds), *Augmentative and alternative communication: European perspectives* (pp. 65–88). London: Whurr.

Wilkinson, R., Bloch, S. and Clarke, M.T. (in press) On the use of graphic resources by people with communication disorders. In C. Goodwin, C. LeBaron and J. Streek (eds), *Multimodality and human activity: Research on behaviour, action and communication*. Cambridge: Cambridge University Press.

Glossary of transcript symbols

This glossary is based on that of Gail Jefferson (2004). Any individual, additional symbols are annotated within the appropriate chapter by the author(s).

[*A left bracket* indicates the point of overlap onset at which a current speaker's talk is overlapped by the talk of another.

]   *A right bracket* indicates the point at which two speakers' overlapping speech end, if they end simultaneously, or at the point at which one of them ends in the course of the other. It is also used to parse out segments of overlapping utterances.

=   *An equals sign* indicates no break or gap. A pair of equals signs, one at the end of one line and one at the beginning of the next, indicate no break between two lines.

(0.1)   *Numbers in parentheses* indicate the time elapsed in tenths of a second.

(.)   *A full stop in parentheses* indicates a brief +/−0.1 second pause within or between utterances.

::   *Colons* indicate prolongation of the immediately prior sound. The longer the colon row, the longer the prolongation.

↑↓   *An upward or downward arrow* indicates a shift into, especially, a high or low pitch.

.   *A full stop* indicates the end of a fall in tone. It does not necessarily indicate the end of a sentence.

?   *A question mark* indicates a rising inflection. It does not necessarily indicate a question.

<u>Word</u>   *Underlining* indicates some form of stress, via pitch and/or amplitude.

WORD   *Upper case* indicates particularly loud sounds relative to the surrounding talk.

°word°   *Degree signs* bracketing an utterance or part of an utterance indicate a stretch of speech that is quieter than the surrounding talk.

–   *A dash* indicates a cut off.

><   *Right/left carats* bracketing an utterance or part of an utterance indicate that the bracketed material is spoken more quickly than the surrounding talk.

<>   *Left/right carats* bracketing an utterance or part of an utterance indicate that the bracketed material is spoken more slowly than the surrounding talk.

.hhh   *A dot-prefixed* row of h's indicates an in-breath. Without the dot, hhh indicates an out-breath.

fu(h)n   *An h in parentheses* marks a discernible aspiration or laughter within a word or in an utterance.

( )   *Empty parentheses* indicate that the transcriber was unable to hear or be certain of what was said.

(dog)   *Single parentheses containing either a word, phrase, or syllable count* mark where target item(s) is/are in doubt if an utterance was very unclear.

(( ))   *Double parentheses, or text in italic and a smaller font size*, indicate the transcriber's descriptions of the activity.

→   *A single arrow or series of arrows* before a line or lines indicates a place of key interest for the analysis.

Reference

Jefferson, G. (2004) Glossary of transcript symbols with an introduction. In Gene Lerner (ed.), *Conversation analysis: Studies from the first generation*. Amsterdam/Philadelphia: John Benjemans Publishers.

Index